The Nervous System

Books by Peter Nathan

The Psychology of Fascism (1943)

*Retreat From Reason: An Essay on the
Intellectual Life of Our Time* (1956)

The Nervous System

THIRD EDITION

Peter Nathan MD FRCP

*Honorary Consultant in Clinical Neurophysiology to the
National Hospital for Nervous Diseases, London*

*Honorary Consultant Neurologist to the
Royal National Orthopaedic Hospital, London*

*Honorary Consultant Neurologist to the
City Migraine Clinic, London*

Oxford   New York

OXFORD UNIVERSITY PRESS

1988

Oxford University Press, Walton Street, Oxford OX2 6DP

Oxford New York Toronto
Delhi Bombay Calcutta Madras Karachi
Petaling Jaya Singapore Hong Kong Tokyo
Nairobi Dar es Salaam Cape Town
Melbourne Auckland

and associated companies in
Berlin Ibadan

Oxford is a trademark of Oxford University Press

First edition © Peter Nathan 1969
Second edition © Peter Nathan Charitable Trust 1982
Third edition © Peter Nathan 1988

First published 1969 by Penguin Books Ltd.
Second edition published 1982 by Oxford University Press
First issued as Oxford University Press paperback, with corrections, 1983
Third edition published 1988

British Library Cataloguing in Publication Data

Nathan, Peter, 1914-
The nervous system.—3rd ed.
1. Vertebrates. Nervous system
I. Title
596'.0188
ISBN 0-19-282152-0

Library of Congress Cataloging in Publication Data

Nathan, Peter Wilfred.
The nervous system/Peter Nathan.—3rd ed.
p. cm.
Bibliography: p. Includes index.
1. Nervous system. I. Title.
612'.8—dc19 QP361.N37 1988
ISBN 0-19-282152-0 (pbk.)

Typeset by Colset Private Ltd.
Printed in Great Britain by
The Guernsey Press Co. Ltd.
Guernsey, Channel Islands

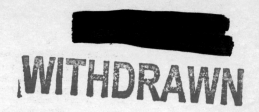

To Ursula, Nickie, Jennifer, and Brian

The quotations used at the beginning of many of the
sections of the book are from
Christopher Smart's poem, *My Cat Jeoffrey*.

Acknowledgements

I have much pleasure in thanking the following friends and colleagues for the photographs and drawings: Professor H. Hydén for Plate 1; the late Professor E. W Walls for Plate 2; Dr Alan Ridley for Plates 3 and 4; Dr Victoria Chan-Palay and Springer Verlag, Berlin for Plate 5; Dr David Landon for Plates 6 and 7; Dr Tony Pullen for Plates 8 and 9; Mr Leslie Frampton for Plates 10–14; the late Mr Sidney Woods for Figs. 3.1, 4.2, 6.1, 7.1, 8.1, 9.1, 10.1, 11.1, 15.1, 2, and 3, 17.1 and 2, 18,1,2,3, and 4, 21.1, 2, and 3, and 23.1; Mr Michael Woods, son of the late Sidney Woods, for Figs. 4.1, 5.1, 16.1; Mr Sidney and Mr Michael Woods for Fig. 5.2; Dr Antoinette Pirie and the late Professor Ida Mann for Fig. 3.3; Dr Juergen Tonnsdorf for Fig. 4.3; Professor Peter Matthews FRS for Fig. 8.2; the late Professor Norman Geschwind for Fig. 20.1; and Dr Gordon Shepherd and Oxford University Press, New York for Fig. 20.2.

I am grateful to the following scientific workers who have allowed me to quote from their work: Dr Macdonald Critchley; Dr Dalle Ore; Dr Michael Espir; Professor Robert G. Heath; the late Professor Wilder Penfield, OM, CMG, FRS; the late Dr Curt Richter; the late Professor W. Ritchie Russell; Dr W.B. Scoville; and Dr H. Terzian.

I should like to take this opportunity of thanking the following editors of scientific journals and publishers of encyclopaedias, journals and books: Dr Russell de Jong, editor of *Neurology*; Dr Bruce Lindsay, editor of the *Journal of the Acoustical Society of America*; Dr Robert Mayor, editor of the *Journal of the American Medical Association*; the late Professor W. Ritchie Russell, editor of the *Journal of Neurology, Neurosurgery and Psychiatry*; Dr Victor Soriano, editor of the *International Journal of Neurology*; Harper and Row for permission to quote from *The Role of Pleasure in Behaviour*, edited by Robert G. Heath; Major C.W. Hume for permission to quote from material by myself in *The Assessment of*

Pain in Man and Animals published by the University Federation for Animal Welfare; Professor Cyril Keele, editor, and Oxford University Press for permission to quote from *Applied Physiology* by Samson Wright; J. R. Newman, editor, and Thomas Nelson and Sons and Harper and Row for permission to quote from the *International Encyclopaedia of Science*; and Oxford University Press for permission to quote from *Traumatic Aphasia* by the late W. Ritchie Russell and Michael Espir.

I take this opportunity of thanking Sheridan Russell who criticized the book throughout its three editions from the point of view of the interested non-medical reader, and I am grateful to Dr Marion Smith and Martin Starkie and Dr Catherine Storr who read each chapter and criticized it in detail and whose advice in ways of improving the first edition was of great value.

Contents

List of plates   xi

Introduction   xiii

1   Functions and structure of the nervous system of verte-
    brates   1

2   Examining the world   5

3   Light receptors: looking   10

4   Sound receptors: listening   24

5   Olfactory receptors: smelling   46

6   Gustatory receptors: tasting   57

7   Cutaneous receptors: touching and feeling   60

8   Receptors for the inside world   70

9   Nerves and nerve fibres   83

10   Communication within the central nervous system   90

11   Standing and moving   104

12   Awake and exploring; relaxed and sleeping   127

13   Needs, desires, and emotions   140

14   Pain   152

15   The centre of the brain: the hypothalamus   164

16   Broadcasting information: hormones   189

17   General plan of the human brain   208

18   Exploring man's living brain   218

19   Sensation acquires a meaning   241

20   Speech and other symbols   267

21   Learning   299

22   Remembering   324

x **Contents**

23 **Personality and the brain** 348

Glossary 363

Index 373

List of plates

1 A living neuron dissected from the brain of a rabbit
2 Mid-line section though a man
3 A nerve fibre in the skin of a man's finger
4 Several nerve fibres ending in a sensory receptor in the skin of a man's finger
5 A neuron from the cerebellum. This type of neuron has several axons: the axons are thin; the dendrites are thick
6 Scanning electron microscope study showing a node on a myelinated nerve fibre
7 Scanning electron microscope study showing a neuron in tissue culture
8 Electron microscope study of a cat's motoneuron
9 Synapses between nerve-endings and a motoneuron in a cat
10 The brain of a fifty-year-old man from above
11 The same brain from the right side
12 The same brain from below
13 The same brain from the left side
14 An adult man's brain dissected to show the corpus callosum

Introduction

The nervous system is made up of the brain, the spinal cord and the nerves throughout the body. Neurology is the study of the nervous system. The disorders and diseases that bring patients to neurologists are paralyses, tremors, Parkinsonism, shingles and the pain that follows it, epilepsy and multiple sclerosis. Psychiatrists treat what are called mental diseases; these are neuroses and psychoses; and they also try to cope with personality disorders and anti-social behaviour.

The boundaries between neurology, psychiatry and psychology are fluid and indistinct. If someone starts behaving oddly, he may need the help of a psychiatrist, a neurologist or a neurosurgeon; it depends whether he is suffering from depression, from senile dementia, or a brain tumour. It is the neurologist who makes the diagnosis.

The word 'nervous' is used in ordinary language to mean anxious, apprehensive or frightened. This use of the word comes from a hundred years ago when a psychiatrist and a neurologist were one and the same person and it was generally thought that psychological and psychiatric troubles were due to something wrong with the nervous system. Even so, it is strange that people said there was something wrong with their nerves when they meant something wrong with their brains. Nice examples of various misuses of this word can be found in Conan Doyle, although he was a doctor. An opium smoker had 'every nerve in a twitter'; the hero of another story wrote 'My nerves which were steady enough on the field of battle, tingled as I thought of it'; the Hon. Philip Green had nerves like live wires, which indeed is what nerves are like. The prize goes to the poet Robert Browning who wrote to his fiancée, describing her as 'The recluse with nerves that have all been broken on the rack and now hang loosely'.

Books on psychoanalysis and psychotherapy can be understood by any one who has had no education in science: and that is one of the causes of their facile acceptance. But neurology, like the rest of medicine, requires some knowledge of physics, chemistry and anatomy.

As it is five years since the previous edition of this book, and as the subject grows so quickly, this third edition is published. More than a half of the book is new, and there are new Figures.

The first chapter of the book is introductory, starting with a concise explanation of what the nervous system does, followed by basic facts of its anatomy. The five senses are discussed in Chapters 1–7. Following the five senses, there is a chapter on the senses unnoticed by the Greek philosophers, the senses of the body itself, muscle sense, the sense of balance, the sensations of the visceral organs. Chapter 9 is on the physics of the nerve impulse; for this chapter some knowledge of physics and chemistry is an advantage. How neural messages are sent in the nervous system is the subject of Chapter 10. The result of receiving messages from the world around and from one's own body is almost always a movement of some kind. It may be shouting, it may be running away, it may be turning one's head to look. What we know about standing and moving is recounted in Chapter 11.

Philosophers and many psychologists used to believe that animals, including ourselves, did not react or behave until they were stimulated; they were just blanks waiting for stimuli, and they then reacted. That is exactly how it is not. Animals are inquisitive and go out to explore the world. They are seeking what is interesting to them. This exploration and seeking stimulation, and its opposite, lying resting at home and going to sleep, is discussed in Chapter 12. How animals are motivated is the theme of Chapter 13 and the anatomical bases of motivation is the theme of Chapter 15. Chapter 14 is devoted to pain. Chapter 16 is on endocrine glands and hormones, the general chemical messengers that affect the structure of the tissues and the animal's behaviour throughout its life.

With Chapter 17, we come to the higher levels of neural activity and the cerebral hemispheres of the brain. What has been learned about the brain by the electrical stimulation of parts of it during operations in conscious patients is reported in Chapter 18. Chapter 19 is about sensation and perception.

People tend to think of the function of the brain as organizing what are called the higher nervous activities: thinking, calculating, learning, remembering, reading, and writing. These functions are discussed in Chapters 20, 21 and 22. Chapter 23 concerns some aspects of the personality and the brain.

I would like to quote here an extract from the preface of a book by my colleagues Professors C. G. Phillips and R. Porter on 'Corticospinal Neurones': 'Because our subject is advancing rapidly, we know that parts of our book will have been overtaken by the time they appear in print, and we have simply had to give up worrying about this.'

Although the writer of any book imagines his ideal reader starting on page 1 and continuing absorbed to the hard-won words, 'The End', I have tried to write this book so that any single chapter may be read on its own or left out.

1 Functions and structure of the nervous system of vertebrates

The function of a nervous system is to keep its possessor informed about the world. All animals need to have a continuous supply of information about what is happening; and things are happening in two worlds, the world outside the body and the world of the body itself. The actual state of affairs around the animal is not reported; the nervous system provides a selected representation of the environment which is meaningful to that animal. Anything changing is noticed with vigilance, for it could be desirable or dangerous. Particular notice is always given to the behaviour of other animals, especially those of one's own group. Adaptation to one's environment, and this includes one's fellows, is a first law of life. It requires, among other attributes, memory and the continual filling of the memory store.

The function of the nervous system is to provide its possessor with the ability to move, both move around the world and move its own body. It arranges the movements of the visible parts of the body, the limbs and tongue, and the unseen parts, such as the stomach and other viscera, the bladder and the rectum.

Nervous systems of vertebrates consist of the brain and spinal cord, called the central nervous system, and the nerves running to and from the central nervous system, called the peripheral nervous system. There is another part of the nervous system, the autonomic nervous system. It consists of the sympathetic system, the parasympathetic system and the enteric nervous system which is the nervous system of the gut or alimentary canal.

In the earliest and simplest vertebrates the central nervous system was a tube, called the neural tube, which ran throughout the length of the body; it later became surrounded by bone. This bony case of the present spinal cord is called the spinal or vertebral column, and is made up of separate bones, the vertebrae. During evolution the front end of the neural tube enlarged into three swellings; they became the brain.

As the central nervous system is buried inside the body, it has to be kept in touch with the world and with everything that is happening inside the body as well. The peripheral nerves are the telegraph wires that do this. They are made up of cables of nerve fibres that bring messages to and from the central nervous system. The sense organs, such as the retina, the organs of the inner ear, and the sensory organs of the skin, are prolongations of the brain and spinal cord, pushed out onto the surface of the body so that the brain should be kept informed of what is going on. The nerves going to the brain and the spinal cord are named afferent nerves, as they carry messages to the central nervous system, and the nerves coming away from the central nervous system are efferent nerves, carrying messages to muscles, glands and viscera.

When these nerves develop in the embryo, they grow out from the central nervous system into the body. This would be like a telephone exchange sending out wires to push their way through the ground and come into your house. When the wire reaches your desk it starts to grow a telephone. Meanwhile the surrounding earth and your desk adapt themselves to the presence of this auditory sense organ. If one day someone were to cut your telephone wires, the telephone would start disintegrating before your eyes; and nothing could stop it until another wire grew out to reach the spot where the telephone ought to be.

Nerve fibres send their messages rapidly though not nearly as fast as telephones. It takes one-fiftieth of a second for the message of a flash of light exciting the retina to reach the visual part of the brain. The message conveyed by the nerve fibre is coded in pulses, like the morse code. These pulses are simply called nerve impulses. When the nerve impulse reaches the end of the nerve fibre, it puts out a chemical substance that acts on the structure to which the nerve is running.

The nervous system is made up of cells, like every other tissue of animals and plants. The principal cell is the nerve cell or neuron. There are two sorts, excitatory and inhibitory; the excitatory cell brings other cells into activity and inhibitory neurons cancel this out, tending to stop this activity. Neurons of the central nervous system are collected together in layers and in small groups; these groups of cells are called nuclei and one group is a nucleus. Both nuclei and layers of neurons are often called centres, particularly when their function is being thought of; and so one has visual centres, a vesical centre to work the bladder, and autonomic centres working the autonomic nervous system. To the naked eye, collections of neurons in nuclei or layers look grey and so they are called grey matter; nerve fibres are white and they constitute the white matter.

A photograph of a living neuron is shown in Plate 1. This neuron was dissected out of the brain of a rabbit by Hydén of Göteborg University in Sweden. The neuron has been magnified 1,800 times. The main mass of this cell is the cell body; the arm-like structures streaming out of it are the dendrites, branching prolongations of the cell. One of the cord-like prolongations of the cell body is the axon; this might be the tentacle in the bottom on the left. The axon is the long thin telegraph wire of the neuron, conveying the message to the muscles, glands or other neurons. The pale circular spot in the middle is the nucleus of the cell, and in the middle of the nucleus is the black nucleolus. The little black spots on the surface of the cell body and the dendrites are the nerve-endings of other neurons, passing excitatory or inhibitory messages to this neuron. Between these nerve-endings and this neuron is a minute gap, called the synapse (Greek for grasp).

The brain is an enormously enlarged part of the spinal cord. Where this enlargement starts is a part of the brain that is obviously an enlarged spinal cord; this is called the medulla oblongata, having no name in English. It is shown in Plates 11, 12, and 13. This basic part of the brain organizes basic functions—the heartbeat, the blood pressure, breathing, swallowing.

The position of the central nervous system in the body of man is shown in Plate 2. The lowest part of the brain, the medulla oblongata, is seen to lie behind the hard palate and the upper part of the cavity of the mouth. The cerebral hemispheres, of which the left one is seen here from the midline, are by far the largest part of the brain and they fill most of the cavity of the skull. The hypothalamus is in the centre of the front part of the brain. Running forward from it, the stalk of the pituitary gland can be seen. The various structures shown in this photograph will often be referred to in the subsequent chapters of the book; and reference to it will show why we speak of the parts as being in front, behind, above, and below.

2 Examining the world

All living organisms since the beginnings of life on earth have passed their lives under the influence of certain permanent physical features of the world. Such are night and day, the increasing duration of daylight as spring follows winter in the northern and southern hemispheres, various kinds of movement of the environment, winds, currents, waves, tides in the sea; there are sounds, usually made by other animals; there is the ambient temperature and barometric pressure; and, less obvious, there is gravity and the earth's magnetic field.

In some organisms these forces are felt by all the tissues of the body, in others they are felt by special cells, these cells and the tissues in which they are encased are called receptors. The receptors are either specialized cells connected to nerve fibres or they are the nerve fibres themselves without specialized cells.

No animal is sensitive to all aspects of the physical world. One has to keep reminding oneself of the various kinds of sensation that one is missing. We see neither ultraviolet nor polarized light. Our hearing is limited, other animals hearing lower and higher notes. And when we go out for a walk with a dog, we realize the existence of the world of smell so interesting to him but not to us.

In principle, animals have no sensory apparatus able to respond to features of the world that they do not normally meet. Animals that live in caves are mostly pale and blind. There would be no point in going to all the trouble of being pigmented if there were no one there to see you. These troglodytes concentrate on smell, taste, and touch. The tick can neither see nor hear, but its sense of smell is attuned to the sour smell of the mammals on which it feeds. It is also sensitive to warmth so that it can tell when it has landed on a warm-blooded creature.

Of the many kinds of animals that are sensitive to the same sort of energy, each class of animal does not have the same sort of receptor, nor does it have the receptors in the same part of the body. Many fish, for instance, have taste receptors not only in their mouths, but also scattered over the surface of the body. These are not so much to enjoy food with as to detect it, to find the particles of it suspended in the water. Fish with barbels, such as the sturgeon or the red mullet, have taste receptors on the barbels. The barbels are like the antennae of insects, on which there are olfactory receptors, the sense organs for smelling. Mosquitoes also feel radiant heat with their antennae. The receptors of those spiders who build webs are on their legs; they feel the vibration which is set up by the insect caught in the web with their feet and legs. Many sorts of butterflies and most flies taste with their feet. Flies have their olfactory receptors for smelling on their antennae and palps. When a fly finds some food, it steps into it so as to taste it. It then makes use of other taste receptors on the hairs surrounding its mouth. If the food tastes good, it sucks it up. When it is replete, it vomits a little and then defecates. If we behaved in this way, we would find a restaurant by smell and not by sight. We would go in and stand in the food. We would give a preliminary opinion on the food, put our moustaches in it, and then give a definite opinion on it. If the food was good, we would suck it up until we felt full, vomit some back on the plate, defecate on the floor, and go. Clearly, it takes all sorts to make a world.

We all have our limits; man is able to sample only certain aspects of the world. Mammals on the whole are less limited in their sampling of the environment than insects. Simpler animals may be able to use only one kind of sensory information. Female crickets recognize the male of their own species only by the chirping sound it makes with its wing-covers. If male crickets are placed beneath a glass from which no sound escapes, the females take no notice of them, even though they can see them. Wasps recognize female wasps entirely by their sense of smell. Blinded wasps can easily find the females. But wasps in which the antennae have been removed do not recognize female wasps; for on the antennae are the chemoreceptors sensitive to the smell of the female abdominal gland secretion. So important is the sense of smell that after the female's scent glands have been dissected out, many male insects attempt to copulate with the glands and not with the female herself.

Bees and ants can see ultraviolet light, but they cannot see into the red part of the spectrum as far as we can. Red appears black to them. Many insects can see the direction of polarized light. Man is so intelligent that he makes use of the receptors and sensory systems of other animals. He trains pigs and truffle-hounds to smell out truffles beneath the ground; he uses blood hounds to smell out the trails of men he wants to track down and St Bernards to find men lost on the mountainside. As we have only recently learned about animals being sensitive to sounds of very high frequency and insects being sensitive to polarized light, we may well learn of further sensitivities of living organisms and through them come to appreciate other aspects of the world.

Animals do not wait around to be stimulated. The nervous system is not a passive receiver of information; it actively selects. Animals use their receptors to explore the world. Books usually say that the eye is for seeing. It is not, it is for looking; the ear is for listening, not hearing.

Receptors are usually classified as exteroceptive, those sampling the environment, interoceptive, those signalling what is going on within the body itself, and proprioceptive, used for controlling the position of the body and its parts. Exteroceptive receptors are for taste, smell, vision and hearing. The proprioceptive receptors or proprioceptors are receptors within the inner ear used to report the position of the body in space and those used for sampling the position and the movement of the head, the limbs, and parts of the limbs. The interoceptive receptors convey information about the bladder, the gut, and the pressure the blood exerts against the walls of the heart, the blood vessels, and within the brain itself; others report on the amount of oxygen, carbon dioxide, and glucose in the blood, some are sensitive to the osmotic pressure of the blood, and others to the temperature of the circulating blood. There are receptors sensitive to stimuli that cause pain throughout most structures of the body. There are no receptors sensitive to painful stimulation in the brain itself. Patients carry on conversations unconcerned while needles are passed through their brains.

Receptors are also classified according to the sorts of stimuli to which they are sensitive. In this classification we have the chemoreceptors, for instance receptors sensitive to carbon dioxide or glucose; thermoreceptors, sensitive to changes in temperature; nociceptors, sensitive to stimulations that threaten to or actually do damage the body; and mechanoreceptors which are excited by pressure on the skin, by pulling or stretching the skin or merely indenting it. Many mechanoreceptors are hairs of the skin or hairs on the cuticle of insects. Insects have mechano-sensitive hairs on the legs which tell them about vibration. One hardly knows whether to call these hairs tactile organs or hearing organs. For mammals use hairs in the skin to report low-pitched vibration and similar hairs in the inner ear to report high-pitched vibration; the first is called touch and the second is called hearing, yet the mechanism is similar in the two cases.

Another way of classifying receptors is in accordance to whether they report a constant state or a changing state. Constant state receptors continue to send in impulses to the central nervous system as long as a certain state, such as a temperature, remains constant. Changing state receptors signal a change in the stimulus. These are the commonest sort of receptors, for all animals need to know about new events. Whenever a stimulus first affects the body, that is something new and may be important; so this kind of receptor sends in a volley of nerve impulses. It is of equal or almost equal importance to know when the stimulus goes, so that is signalled with equal intensity. The continued presence of the stimulus may be less important, and so this is signalled with fewer and fewer impulses. In some cases there is a constant, slow discharge of impulses; in others, they cease altogether.

There are two features of all stimulation—intensity and localization. Intensity is reported to the central nervous system mainly by the number of impulses sent within a certain length of time. If the brain receives 500 nerve impulses a second, it concludes that stimulation is less intense than when it is receiving 2,000 impulses a second. Localization in space, regarding both where stimulation is on the body and where the stimulus is in the environment around the body, is not a great problem; for the body itself and the brain are spread out in space. A cloud in the sky is at the top of the visual field and a worm on the ground at the bottom; they excite different parts of the retinae and are reported by different nerve fibres to different parts of the cortex of the cerebral hemispheres. It is the same with a thorn in the foot or in the finger. A different region in the brain is excited by the different regions of the body that have been pricked. Localization outside the body depends on having a pair of receptors, one on each side of the body. Tastes and smells are not clearly located in space; to do this well, one should have two noses and two tongues, one on each side of the head.

With two ears separated by the whole width of the head, we can tell where a sound is coming from. Two ears give us discrimination between sounds, allowing us to separate one voice out of a buzz of conversation or to hear it in a howling wind. Two eyes give a larger field of vision than one eye and they also provide stereoscopic vision or vision in depth. When our ancestors moved around among the branches of trees, stereoscopic vision must have been a great advantage. For in the forest, you need to tell which of two branches is nearer or farther away from you. But having groups of receptors on the two sides of the head brings its own problems. We have to make a fusion of what we receive from each sensory organ. Two eyes do not tell us that there are two cats in the room; we interpret the information by concluding that there is one cat. Our two ears tell us someone is talking to us, not that the sounds of his voice are coming to one ear at one time and to the other ear a fraction of a second later. We have to learn to make this interpretation in babyhood. In seeing, we learn to keep the visual axes of the two eyes parallel. When the young child does not do this, he is said to squint. This should be corrected as early as possible, in the hope that he grows up to use both eyes together.

What the central nervous system receives from its various receptors has to be integrated so that one can get a picture of what is happening. For one has to be kept continuously informed in order to act and live in the world.

3 Light receptors: looking

For he keeps the Lord's watch in the night against the adversary.
For he counteracts the powers of darkness by his electrical skin and glaring eyes.

Those bandwidths of the electromagnetic radiation that we experience as light have effects on the protoplasm of even the simplest single-celled organisms—in some cases light attracts, in others it repels. As animals evolved, it must have been an advantage to collect all the receptor cells sensitive to light in one place. To enable these cells to absorb the light effectively, a light-sensitive pigment developed in them. In the higher kinds of animal, this region became the retina.

The general arrangement of the eye remains the same throughout the animal kingdom. That is surprising. It appears to be that no better kind of eye could be formed during evolution. The simplest kinds of eye are pits in the skin lined with cells of light-absorbing pigment. These cells called light detectors or photoreceptors react to light and dark. Light affects the molecules of pigment and this reaction sends off nerve impulses to the parts of the central nervous system developed to cope with reactions to light.

The eye is a ball, of which one can only see the front part. This part consists of a transparent conjunctiva, which gets inflamed in conjunctivitis, a transparent cornea, and behind that a transparent lens. Lining the eyeball is the retina. As has often been said, the eye is like a camera. In both eyes and cameras, there is a light-sensitive film, with black backing to absorb the light that has passed through the film. Both have an iris or diaphragm to adjust the amount of light, and both have a lens for focusing. The lens in the eye of the mammal is elastic; its curvature can be adjusted by muscles within the eye, and this changes its focal length. It is slightly yellow; this is like a yellow filter, and cuts out some of the violet light. As we become older, the lens becomes yellower and blue light is not seen so well. Colours appear more orange. It has been suggested that Turner's later pictures all have this orange tone and are lacking in blues on account of this change in his lens, of which he himself would have been unaware.

The human retina is amazingly sensitive to light; we can see a single candle at night five miles away. The range of light intensity to which the retina can respond is equally amazing, for between the slightest amount of light just visible in the dark and the brightest sunlight, there is a difference in intensity of about ten thousand million to one.

Both cameras and eyes work with an optimum amount of light, and modern automatic cameras and age-old eyes automatically adjust the size of the aperture to let in this correct amount. Both film and retina absorb light; and both react to a certain bandwidth out of all the possible frequencies of radiation. This selected bandwidth brings about a chemical reaction in both of them. In the retina, this bandwidth of radiation is absorbed by a pigment in the photoreceptors; in the film it is absorbed by the emulsion in the gelatin.

There are some obvious differences between cameras and eyes. The camera is kept dry, eyes are kept wet. The eye selects; it does not record everything in the indiscreet manner of the camera. The camera has to be kept quite still, the eye has to be kept moving. It carries out little invisible movements at a rate of thirty to ninety a second. If this were not done the image on the retina would fade out, for it has to be transferred to different photoreceptors. Cameras work whether they are always in use or not; but eyes and the whole visual system have to learn in order to see. Chimpanzees brought up in darkness for sixteen months from birth are blind when they are first brought out into the light. It then takes them a long time to acquire sight and to learn to identify objects. Our vision has gone through a long period of learning when we were too young to remember how we were doing it. But some of our vision is innate and does not require learning or practice. Turning the eyes and the head towards a light or a sound is a reflex and does not need the higher parts of the brain.

With photography, once the light has been taken in, it is fixed; and once it has been fixed, this chemical reaction is irreversible. This is not so for the eye. After receiving light, the retina is ready again almost immediately for the next picture. It is not quite immediate, as we learn if we go out of strong sunlight into a dark room. For the first second, we cannot see properly. During this time the photoreceptors are becoming re-adjusted by means of a chemical reaction so as to be ready to absorb light again. When you go into a dark room, again, you see nothing. Gradually dark adaptation occurs, the photoreceptors re-adjust and you can make out the outlines of the objects in the room.

Although the retina is as thin as a sheet of paper, it contains three layers of cells. There is the layer of photoreceptors, called rods and cones as that is what they look like down a microscope. The next layer is that of the bipolar cells. They are connected to the third layer, that of the ganglion cells. There are also interconnecting cells at two levels: horizontal cells connecting the photoreceptors together, and amacrine cells connecting the ganglion cells together, all shown in Figure 3.1.

In each eye there are about 123 million rods and 6 million cones. Cones are scattered throughout the retina and are also concentrated at one spot in the centre. This is called the fovea and is about the size of the head of a pin. Cones are sensitive to colour and they are also the receptors for fine discrimination. In any cone, there is one of three kinds of visual pigment. Each of these is sensitive to a different wavelength of light. We have cones particularly sensitive to red, to blue and to green. Rods are also scattered throughout the retina but are not present in the fovea. They are insensitive to colour but very sensitive to anything moving. With rods alone, we would see only shades of grey, like newspaper pictures. The horizontally running cells are thought to play a role in the spatial aspects of vision and in colour vision.

The photoreceptors work by containing pigments that are affected by light. Photons of light are absorbed by the molecules of rhodopsin or visual purple in both rods and cones. This is a protein containing a chemical substance called retinene, which is a form of Vitamin A. When the light energy is absorbed, the shape of the rhodopsin molecule is changed; and this change in shape allows ions to pass through membranes, eventually starting off a nerve impulse along the optic nerve fibre.

At night and at twilight only rods are useful, for there is not enough light to excite the cones. Many nocturnal animals have only or mainly rods. The Australian opossum avoids the light of day and stays in the attics of houses, protected by law; at twilight it saunters bravely out. The South American night ape or dourou-couli possesses only rods and is nocturnal. The fish of the deepest seas also have only rods; they have very large retinae to catch all the light that penetrates the ocean depths. The owl and the pussy-cat see better in poor light than man does.

If we see a nocturnal animal with small eyes, then we can presume that it does not rely so much on vision. The common

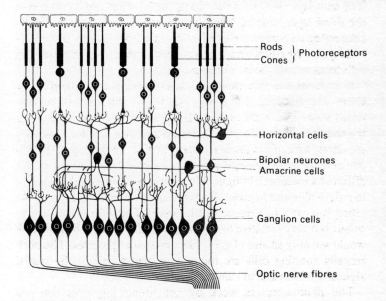

Fig. 3.1 Diagram of the retina. The light rays come from the bottom of this diagram and run through the retina to the photoreceptors at the top.

shrew has small eyes but it also has sensitive bristles on its snout; these are its feelers. It is also guided by smell and it sniffs the air continually. It hears, but it is not much interested in visual aspects of the world.

Although the photoreceptors all look the same under the microscope, they have different functions and different kinds of behaviour. Some of them are 'on' receptors, registering when a light is switched on, others are 'off' receptors, noting the light being turned off; and there are also 'on-off' receptors signalling when a light is switched on or off.

How the retina works is more easily investigated in animals with a less complicated visual system than man. A great step forward was made when the technique of recording from single nerve fibres was mastered. From then on, it was possible to listen to the messages passing along a nerve fibre and to send messages along it artificially and learn how it conveyed them. This technique was used for understanding what the eye sends in to the brain in the case of an ancient horeshore crab, left over from Silurian times, 400 million years ago. This crab has long optic nerves, so it is not too difficult to record the traffic passing along them by means of electrodes. In this animal, the eye consists of many visual units called ommatidia. An ommatidium consists of a lens with a transparent crystalline cone behind it, connected to photoreceptor cells. From each cell one nerve fibre goes to the brain. In the United States, where this crab lives, H.K. Hartline recorded the electrical events of these single nerve fibres when he shone a very narrow beam of light on each ommatidium. Each ommatidium sent off impulses in proportion to the intensity of illumination. Having got an ommatidium steadily discharging impulses in response to a constant amount of illumination, he found that its rate of firing could be decreased by illuminating the surrounding ommatidia. Although the central ommatidium was still receiving the same amount of light, it fired off far fewer impulses. When he stopped illuminating the surrounding ommatidia, its firing rate returned to the previous level. The brighter the light on the surrounding ommatidia, the fewer impulses were sent off by the central one. Every ommatidium has a surrounding ring of ommatidia that reduce its firing rate. This is a mechanism for enhancing contrast in what is seen.

The principle of an antagonism between the firing of central cells and that of the surrounding cells is a form of neural organization called centre-surround antagonism. It was first discovered in this crab's eye; then it appeared that it was a general form of organization used throughout nervous systems.

Seeing something and stimulating a receptor are not the same. It is calculated that a single photon can excite a single photoreceptor; but nothing would be seen. Seven photoreceptors have to be excited before we are aware that we have seen something.

The eye is used for looking; and what makes us look is catching sight of something moving. If you are a carnivore, then you are wanting to see something moving, for it may be something to eat. If you are a herbivore, you need to see something moving, for it may be something intending to eat you. Preying animals behave as if they know that the slightest movement betrays them. They move slowly so that their movements do not excite the movement-detecting receptors of the retina of their prey.

We look, we see, and we perceive. We look in the direction of the horizon, we see a little red form with a pointed top against a green lower and sky-blue upper background; and we perceive a gnome in the far distance. This simple example shows us that what we perceive is much influenced by our experience of life, by what we have been taught and by what we expect to see. On the other hand, the basic elements of looking are innate and reflex: these are the changes in size of the pupil in relation to light, a startle reaction to a sudden increase in light, and turning of the eyes and head towards the light source.

The fovea of the retina is the part used for putting things into sharp focus. The rest of the retina is mainly concerned with noticing movement. If photoreceptors are excited, a series of reflex movements occur so that first the eyes and then the head are turned to focus rays from the moving object on to the fovea.

Keeping a variable constant or within limits is a situation that occurs both in biology and in engineering; and biologists, including neurologists, have adopted the terms and concepts of the engineers. Naturally occurring self-regulating mechanisms are called control circuits. In these circuits the variable to be controlled has to be measured, and this is sampled by a sensor. A transducer encodes the information from the sensor. In the present example, keeping the rays of light on the fovea is the controlled variable. The photoreceptors are the sensor, and they encode the information as physico-chemical impulses in nerve fibres.

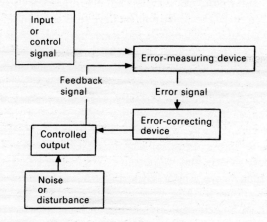

Fig. 3.2

A closed loop circuit is shown schematically in Fig. 3.2. In order to keep the variable constant or within controlled limits, the difference between the actual variable at any time and the reference signal is picked up by a sensor, is measured and corrected. When the feedback signal differs from the reference signal, this measured error causes the controller to initiate correcting measures. Such a system is working by negative feedback; the effect of the feedback signal is to decrease the error. Positive feedback is when the feedback signal increases the error.

In the case we are considering, the error that has continuously to be measured and corrected is a deviation of the eyes that would change the angle at which the rays of light reach the fovea. The error-correcting device is provided by the muscles of the eyes, the head and the neck.

Focusing the rays of light depends on changing the focal point of the lens. The curvature of the lens is controlled by a muscle within the eye. For near vision, the lens has to be made more spherical and for far vision, it is flatter. If the rays of light from an object do not focus clearly at the fovea of both eyes, we see double.

For looking at near or far objects, the size of the pupil has also to be adjusted by the muscles of the iris. If you hand someone something and say 'Look at this!', you can see his eyes roll inwards and downwards and you will see his pupils contract. The accompanying change in the lens cannot be seen. The size of the pupil is altered to deal with the extremes of illumination. Where the light is poor, the pupil is dilated to let more into the eye. If the light is very bright, the pupils are brought down to pinpoint size. This may seem to be as quick as a flash, but it is not. That is why photos taken by synchronized flash show pupils of normal size. The picture is taken before the light stimulating the retina sends nerve impulses to the centre of the brain and other impulses run along other nerve fibres to make the iris contract. But if you shine a light into the eyes of a friend, human, canine or feline, you will have time to see the pupils constricting. Start with someone young as the young have larger pupils than the elderly.

In the servo-mechanism of the pupil, the output that has to be continuously controlled is the amount of light reaching the retina. The error is the difference between the right amount and the actual amount of light. The error-measuring device is the retina itself. The servo-mechanism is made up of a part of the brain, the nerves to and from the eye, and the muscles of the pupil.

The conception of the nervous system and its various parts as examples of automatic control was the contribution of Professor Wiener of Boston. He got together communication engineers, biologists, neurophysiologists and anatomists and showed them that they were all dealing with the same problems, those of the communication of information and of servo-control. He called this subject cybernetics.

The total field of the environment that is seen is called the field of vision or visual field. A diagram of it is shown in Fig. 3.3 for man, bird and fish. Not all fish have this visual field: the flounder lying on the bottom of the sea has a panoramic visual field, taking in about 180° around his head. Dragon-flies have the same large visual fields, one for each eye. Most carnivores and birds of prey have their eyes in the fronts of their faces; they need to judge distance with accuracy once they have sighted their prey. Herbivores have very large fields of vision. They need to see both sides, in front, and behind, for they serve as food for other animals. Man has the eyes of a predator: set in the front of his face, with good distance judgement and a moderately wide field of vision. Eyes in the front of the face permit stereoscopic vision. As the eyes are a certain distance apart, each eye sees the world from a slightly different angle. The resulting vision in depth was probably developed by man's forebears as they lived in trees. Moving among the branches of trees demands accurate judging of the relative distance of intertwining branches. Stereoscopic vision depends on retinal image disparity, a difference in the images in the two eyes. It ceases when objects are more than seven metres away, for then the images in the two eyes become identical.

The image each eye receives is two-dimensional. The three-dimensional picture of the world to which we are accustomed is an interpretation, based on hours of learning throughout babyhood and childhood. This picture of the world has become so ingrained that when we lose the sight of one eye, we still see the world in three dimensions. Only when we have to do something needing the careful judgement of distance, such as pouring tea out of a narrow spout into a cup at arm's length, do we find that we have lost our ability to judge distance. If we need to rely on monocular vision, we can still do very well. We have all the clues given by perspective, learned during childhood. We judge the relative distance of two objects by seeing which appears to be the larger, by seeing the relative nearness of two objects to the horizon, by noting whether one object partially overlaps another. All such features of perspective were discovered by European painters. The best comment on them is a marvellous painting by Hogarth where all features of perspective are painted absolutely wrong. There are also variations in lightness so that a black and white photograph gives even one eye almost as good depth perception as a colour photograph. But not quite: for colour television gives us better depth perception than black and white. If we move our heads, we

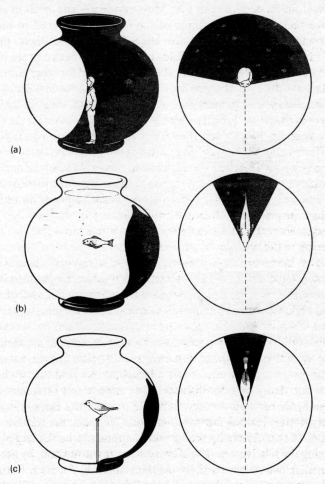

(a)

(b)

(c)

Fig. 3.3 If a man, a fish and a bird were placed in the middle of a goldfish bowl, each one could see everything white and nothing black. The white part is the visual field.

can make use of parallax. When objects are moving, we observe that those seeming to move faster must be nearer than those seeming to move more slowly.

The colour of objects comes from the reflection of certain bandwidths of radiation; the other parts of the spectrum are absorbed by the object. When we see something as red, the red light is being reflected and the rest of the light is being absorbed. We see it as red because we have cones and other cells able to react to red light. The redness, like beauty, is in the eye of the beholder.

We are very sensitive to minute differences in colour, and we can appreciate them even in poor light. Most mammals do not see colours. Cats can see green and blue. Reptiles, most fish, butterflies, and bees see colour. Bees cannot tell red from black but they see a colour in the ultraviolet that is hidden from us. Von Frisch points out that scarlet flowers are very rare among the indigenous flowers of Europe, because the insects that pollinate flowers cannot see red. But in Africa and America scarlet flowers are common; this is because flowers there are pollinated by birds which see red very well. In America this is done by humming birds and in Africa by the sunbirds. Interestingly enough, the strelitzia is pollinated by the sunbird's feet, as it lands on the horizontal petals. Red European flowers, such as dianthus and daphne, are pollinated by butterflies, which are the only insects able to see the colour red. Poppies, which are bright red to us, reflect ultraviolet light, and so bees can see them. Thus flowers and insects form good examples of symbiosis in evolution, the two developing together, each making use of the other.

On the whole, animals which are themselves brightly coloured can see colour, for colour is usually there for other members of the species to see. There would be no point in having colours to display if no one else could see them. Peacocks display for peahens, butterflies for butterflies. But certain animals are coloured especially for other species. Probably the wasp is indifferent to its own colours; they are there to warn birds to keep off.

Colour-blindness occurs in 8 per cent of men and 0.5 of women, a distribution indicating that it is sex-linked. Some colour-blind people see only black and white and yellow and blue; they cannot see red and green. Of course, colour-blind people see the mixtures of the colours they can appreciate. There is a very rare kind of colour-blindness in which men cannot see yellow and blue, but do see white, red and green. Equally rare are cases of total colour-blindness; they see only white and grey. Colour-blind people manage very well by making use of brightness clues.

Birds have very good sight, for their lives depend on it. Their eyes make up a large proportion of their skulls. Some can keep objects in focus hundreds of metres away and also within a few centimetres of their eyes. Probably the winner is the great condor, which from a height of 5,000 metres can see small rodents moving on the ground.

There are many aspects of the world around that we are very good at seeing. Our eyes are most sensitive to dark and light, and to angles and the orientation of lines forming angles. We are good at seeing if something is a little off straight and if one angle is slightly bigger than another. To represent the world to us the brain needs information about bright and dark edges, and contrasts in lumination. The retina has to take in these attributes of the environment and convert them to the code used by nerves. Then this has to be stored so that subsequent impressions, undergoing the same processing, can be compared. Otherwise, objects we see would not have continuity. All of this is the same for all sensory systems that are at all complicated.

All vertebrates are good at seeing movement. Around the edges of the retina there are only rods and only movement is seen. If you move your hand up and down on the very edge of the visual field, which is seen only by the edge of the retina, you will see the movement but you will not see your hand; you would not be able to identify the thing that was moving unless you looked. Looking means focusing the rays from the moving object onto the fovea. But one can also see movement when there isn't any. For instance, if one is put in a darkened room and there is only a single spot of light to see, soon one will have the illusion that the spot is moving. This is because in order to localize the spot, one needs a visual framework; without this framework, localization fails and the spot appears to move. This is a good example of how seeing something as complicated as something moving requires the functioning of the higher levels of the brain and demonstrates that it is not a matter of simply recording from the retina.

There are neurons of the retina that are sensitive to the direction of movement in depth, in fact there are four different kinds of cell with different sensitivities to the parts of this movement, just as there are three sorts of cones sensitive to different wavelengths giving rise to colour. Of course, this is important as all animals must look out for objects coming towards them that could damage their faces. This is a different sense from the usual perception of movement, of things moving from side to side. That clearly has different biological significance and it is subserved by different neurons of the retina and the visual system.

Eyes are not only for seeing and looking; the light they absorb has other effects on the body and on behaviour. In some animals, the effect of prolonged daylight is to suppress the activity of the pineal gland (*pineale*, Latin for a pine-cone). In fish, reptiles, and amphibians, the cells of this gland are photoreceptors. In mammals, the cells themselves are not sensitive to light but they have connections with the retinae, receiving an input of light from the eyes. As the pineal suppresses the pituitary, the increasing length of daylight has the effect of making the pituitary active. If you are able to detect the increasing length of day, you are getting information about the changing seasons. If you need to moult as summer is approaching or change the colour of your coat, if you have to raise a family and to find and protect a territory, you need this information. All of these activities need hormones secreted by the pituitary gland. This subject is discussed in detail in Chapter 17.

If the duration of daylight is artificially altered, the whole rhythm of the reproductive cycle in birds can be altered. Professor Thorpe slowly decreased the amount of light of the environment of greenfinches and chaffinches; he found that not only did they stop singing but that their testes had regressed to an inactive state. Then he gradually increased their daily ration of light until they were receiving sixteen hours of light per day in the middle of September. These birds were in full song in the middle of November.

There are some animals that have a third eye, on the top of the head. It is quite obvious in the reptile known by its Maori name of tuatara; it is also present in some lizards, frogs, toads, and iguanas. The third eye is believed to record the amount of sunlight. This information is necessary for the circadian rhythms of the body, which will be discussed in Chapter 15. During the millions of years of evolution, plant and animal life has related itself to the cycle of dark and light of night and day. Many rhythms of the body depend on this alternation. In those animals with a third eye, the rhythms seem to depend on this eye; for the rest of us, the two eyes in the face supply the information.

In simpler kinds of animals, light is received but not through the eyes. Some have photocells scattered over their bodies. If a shadow is cast over them, they reflexly withdraw. Such a reflex is inexorable and cannot be modified or altered by learning. Earthworms have no eyes but they have a light-sensitive receptor on each side of their front ends. They arrange their position and their movements so that the same amount of light falls on both these receptors. They avoid daylight and burrow back into the earth when they are brought to the surface by gardeners. But at night, when it is dark everywhere, they come to the surface of the ground. This is the time when they meet for sexual intercourse. In their preference for the dark of the night for this activity, they resemble human beings.

4 Sound receptors: listening

For his ears are so acute that they sting again.

Why—one might ask—was hearing evolved? Living creatures have always been faced with all the physical aspects of the world and so they have evolved reactions to them. The world is full of noises, and those animals that could hear them could make use of them in their struggle to keep alive. They could hear the approach of animals hunting them, they could hear the flow of water in streams and rivers, and they could keep in touch with their friends and relations. But not all animals hear. Hearing is largely confined to insects and vertebrates.

In physics, all aspects of a tone are described by its wavelength, its frequency, and its magnitude. For man and other animals living on land, sound is nearly always conducted in a gas, air. This is not a very good way of transmitting sound, for it travels more than four times faster in water and ten times faster in solids.

We measure the intensity of sound in decibels (dB), a term borrowed from telephone engineers; it is a term describing energy flow in acoustic systems or sound pressure level. A whisper 1.5 metres from the ear is about 10 dB. A sound of 1,000 Hz reaches the pain threshhold at 120 dB above its just detectable intensity. Our ears are most sensitive over a frequency range of 250 to 6,000 Hz. This covers the frequencies used in speech which are between 500 and 2,500 Hz; for music we need to hear between 40 and 16,000 Hz.

Every kind of animal hears only a certain range of frequencies, the range suitable for its purposes. There are limits of frequency and limits of intensity. Horses, rats, mice, cats, and dogs all hear higher-pitched sounds than human beings. Below frequencies of eighteen cycles a second, man feels sounds, he does not hear them. The upper limit of hearing for the young is 20,000 cycles a second;

at the age of sixty in Western societies, the upper limit is only 8,000 cycles a second. Man calls sounds with a frequency above 20,000 cycles a second ultrasonic, as he cannot hear them.

Sounds are detected by vibration receptors; in mammals these are movable hairs or cilia, implanted in hair-cells. They follow the frequency of the waves of pressure and thus detect the note. Waves of pressure spread out from a source like ripples on a pond spreading out from the stone dropped into the pond. The hair is moved by waves of alternating pressure like a water-lily rocked by the ripples.

As the ear is developed out of the skin, it is interesting to examine the skin to find out if it has any similar properties; and it is quite easy to do this. Just get three tuning forks having frequencies of 128, 256, and 512 cycles a second. Then get a friend to set them vibrating and apply them separately to the hairs on your forearm or leg, taking care not to touch the skin itself. Keep your eyes shut and your ears blocked up, so that you do not see or hear the forks vibrating. You will find that you can tell if the fork is vibrating or merely touching the hairs without vibrating (the fork with a vibration of 512 cycles a second may cause more difficulty). You will find too that you can tell the pitch of the note from the vibration imparted to your hairs. That is to say, you will not hear a note, but you will be able to distinguish which fork it is that is vibrating; for the hairs of the skin are sensitive to the frequency of vibration of the three forks. This experiment also shows us how apt hairs are as receptors for the vibrations of sounds.

The mammalian ear is best thought of as consisting of three parts, the outer, middle, and inner ear. All three parts develop in the embryo out of the surface epithelium, the covering that later becomes the skin. And so it is not surprising to find that the receptors of the inner ear are a sort of receptor used in the skin; they are pressure and movement detectors, hairs embedded in a base.

The outer ear is the part of the ear you can see—in fact what people call the ear. It is separated by a drum from a little chamber, the middle ear, and this is separated by another drum from the inner ear, which is deep inside the bone of the skull. This is the part containing the sound receptors and nerve fibres. A drawing of the ear is shown in Fig. 4.1. The three little bones—malleus or hammer, incus or anvil, stapes or stirrup—are in the middle ear. On its left is the external ear and on its right the inner ear.

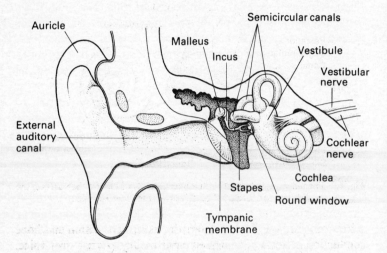

Fig. 4.1 Diagram of external, middle, and inner ear.

The pressure waves of sound pass down the funnel-shaped passage of the outer ear to affect the ear-drum. This drum, the tympanic membrane, is a flattish cone, like the cone of a loudspeaker. This membrane is connected to another membrane, the oval window, by the three little bones. The oval window seals the inner ear from the middle ear. The inner ear appeared so complicated to the early anatomists that they named it the labyrinth. It consists of the cochlear apparatus, the semicircular canals and the vestibular apparatus; it is the former that is used for hearing. Figure 4.2. shows the inner ear.

The middle ear is a chamber containing air, which is kept at atmospheric pressure by a tunnel connecting it to the throat. When the tunnel is blocked up, as occurs momentarily when we yawn or for some days when we get a cold, our hearing is impaired. It is not absolutely necessary for the pressure waves to pass through this air-filled chamber for hearing; vibration can be conducted directly to the inner ear, being conducted in the bone.

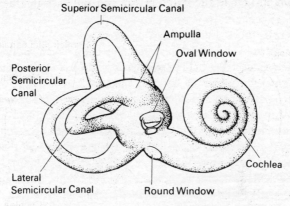

Superior Semicircular Canal

Ampulla

Oval Window

Posterior
Semicircular
Canal

Cochlea

Lateral
Semicircular Canal

Round Window

Fig. 4.2 The inner ear. The part on the right is for hearing and the parts on the left are for balancing and keeping the right way up.

You can examine the characteristics of air conduction and bone conduction of sound in yourself by listening to your own voice. Just read aloud from a book, and in the middle of reading, block up both your ears with your fingers. You will find that when your ears are blocked up and you are hearing by bone conduction, your voice sounds deeper; conversely it sounds higher when the sound is conducted through the air to your ears. Bone conduction damps the sound of higher frequency and so the low frequencies predominate. Now continue your reading, but whisper what you read; and again, block and unblock your ears. You will find that you can hardly hear your whispered voice when your ears are blocked. The reason is the same. Whispering makes use of the higher frequencies; there are so few low frequencies used that there is almost nothing to conduct, so you hear almost nothing.

In the outer ear, the waves of sound are conducted in air; in the middle ear, they are conducted in solids; and in the inner ear, in fluid. That the transmissions of sound-waves from air to fluid does not readily occur can be observed by anyone bathing on a noisy beach or in a swimming pool. The noise around you when your head is above water goes if you put your head under the water. The air-water interface forms an effective sound-barrier, most of the sound being reflected from the surface of the water.

When the sound-waves have to pass from air to fluid (and this has to happen in all animals who live in the air), a great loss of energy occurs. The middle ear contains the mechanism for compensating for this loss. This mechanism consists of the tympanic membrane, the three little bones hinged together to form a system of levers, and the oval window which seals off the fluid of the inner ear. The compensation is achieved by the great area of the tympanic membrane compared to the small area of the flat footplate of the stapes up against the oval window, and by the lever action of the three bones.

In man, the tympanic membrane is about twenty times the area of the footplate of the stapes. But as the membrane is firmly fixed all round its circumference, this whole area is not available for movement. The effective difference in areas of the membrane and the stapes footplate is about 14:1. The lever system of the three bones collects the pressure from the tympanic membrane and concentrates it down to the footplate of the stapes; it increases the energy arriving at the oval window of the inner ear by about 1.3:1. The total effect of the tympanic membrane and the little bones, with their relative sizes and elasticities, is that sound arriving at the inner ear is increased by 10–20 dB: this means that the loudness of the sound is doubled. This great increase particularly affects the sound of the middle frequencies heard by man.

There is an ear disease called otosclerosis in which the stapes gets fixed onto the oval window. Hearing is much impaired. If the person loses more than 30 dB, quiet speech is not heard. These people can be helped by surgical removal of the stapes and having a hearing aid.

The sound-waves pass from the middle ear, through the oval window into the inner ear. Here they pass along one narrow passage, called the scala vestibuli, round a very small corner into another passage, called the scala tympani, on to the round window, where the pressure is dispersed into the middle ear.

In the scala vestibuli there is a membrane, the basilar

membrane, which in man is 30–35 millimetres long. This membrane supports hair-cells of two kinds, globular ones along the inner part and slender tubular ones along its outer part. The cilia of the hair-cells touch the membrane above them, some of them penetrating it. This membrane is called the tectorial or covering membrane.

When the sound-waves are transmitted to the fluids of the inner ear, they send a ripple along the basilar membrane. This wave can be imagined if one thinks of the basilar membrane as a long, narrow sheet, fixed at both ends and also along both sides; but fixed loosely, so that a shake given it at one end sends a wave of movement along its whole length. This wave is complicated, for the membrane is of different thickness and consistency in its different parts and it is also coiled round the snail-like cochlea. The kind of wave pattern it probably makes in this membrane is shown in a spread out membrane in Fig. 4.3. When the membrane is raised into folds and ripples like this, the hair-cells in it are rocked about. As the basilar and tectorial membranes have different mechanical properties, being different in stiffness, tautness, thickness, and elasticity, the wave of pressure causes a different form of ripple in the two membranes. This difference in the movement of the two membranes displaces and twists the hairs of the hair-cells, causing a shearing movement between them and the tectorial membrane in which their tips are embedded. As the hairs are minute levers, their movements affect the hair-cells themselves. The hair-cells convert mechanical energy into nerve impulses, which are pulses of electric current.

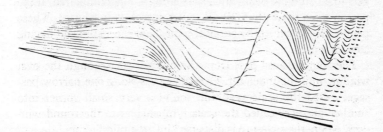

Fig. 4.3 A wave pattern in the basilar membrane of the inner ear.

The nerve impulses are conveyed to the brain by the auditory nerves. In mammals each auditory nerve consists of 25,000 afferent nerve fibres. These fibres are continually sending in impulses to the brain whether we are listening to something or not.

Every nerve fibre of the auditory nerve is activated by a single inner hair-cell or else by a very few hair-cells. As these hair-cells are each activated by tones of particular frequencies, so are the nerve fibres that are fired off by them. How these mechanisms enable us to hear a difference between two notes having a frequency difference of only three cycles a second, we do not know. For it is inconceivable that such a minute difference in frequency could produce different shapes of ripple in the membrane.

A further mechanism that we do not altogether understand is a kind of contrast enhancement acting at the level of the hair-cells. When one records, in the guinea-pig, the response of a single hair-cell to a tone to which it responds best, one notes the surprising effect of adding a tone of slightly higher or lower frequencies. This is to reduce the response of the hair-cell that is responding at its characteristic frequency.

Another problem is this. If each nerve fibre fires off with a tone of a certain frequency, what happens when that tone is much louder? We know that when this occurs, neighbouring nerve fibres are also firing off; but we do not hear the note indistinctly, mixed up with semitones above and below. Clearly, there must be some other mechanisms for hearing, perhaps some sort of filtering and correction within the central nervous system.

In reality, sounds hardly ever consist of pure tones. Naturally, the first investigations into hearing were made with the simplest material—clicks and pure tones. When later the effect on the basilar membrane of more complex tones was examined, it was found that the kind of ripple in the membrane was quite different from that brought about by pure tones. Even the fundamental of a note did not necessarily produce the same wave form as the fundamental played with its overtones. This example of hearing demonstrates how sensory mechanisms are complicated and remain difficult to understand.

The question has been asked: at what age does the new-born baby hear? The answer is that it can already hear when it is in its mother's womb. When sounds are made near the mother's abdomen, from the seventh month onwards the foetus shows changes in its heart rate. So that the sound could penetrate the mother's abdominal wall, low notes having long wavelengths were used. The bassoon part of Prokofiev's *Peter and the Wolf* was chosen, and played to babies in the womb. From the resulting changes in heart rate, it was clear that the babies heard it and responded to it. Some weeks after birth, the same music was played to the babies when they were crying. They would immediately calm down. Other music did not have this result.

This experiment shows us not only that the foetus could hear within its mother's womb but also that it remembered what it had heard a month or two before its birth. These observations lead us to ask what other intra-uterine events are experienced and remembered. And it makes the theories of psychopathology of Otto Rank and others, about birth trauma and its possible role in legends, less improbable.

The receptors of the basilar membrane can be damaged by a lot of noise going on for years. The noise made by everyone speaking at a cocktail party reaches 80 to 85 dB, 'not quite enough', as the two Canadian research workers who looked into the matter wrote, 'to cause permanent impairment of hearing'. But there is no doubt that the noise of civilized countries damages the receptors. In 1961, an expedition went out to a remote tribe living in Sudan near the western borders of Ethiopia. The purpose of the expedition was to examine the hearing of these tribal people, who live in the quiet of a stone-age culture. They were found to have far less deafness with old age than is usual in America and Europe, and infinitely less than those who work in noisy factories. The music made by rock-and-roll musicians is so loud that it damages the auditory receptors of those in the band. The noise level up among the musicians reaches 105 to 120 dB; this is the same as the noisiest industry, a boiler shop.

Animals note both the direction from which a sound is coming and the distance of the source of the sound. We learn to do this in childhood just as we learn to estimate the position and distance of what we see.

Animals which are around at night either have large eyes or they live by using their ears or, like the owl, they use both. The owl has its ears set far apart on its head; it is unique in that the structure of its two ears is different. These two anatomical features are used for localizing the little sound made by the scuttering mouse. The mouse does not hear the owl, which has special feathers to render its flight silent. Fish-eating owls do not fly so silently for the sound of flight is not carried into the water.

The curious shape of the external ear must contribute to our hearing. This is known to be so for the bat, which relies on hearing for its livelihood. Little research work seems to have been done on man's external ears. No one examined Van Gogh's hearing after he cut off one of his ears; and so this unique opportunity of comparing the hearing on the two sides was missed.

Our ability to localize sound is based on appreciating the slight difference in the arrival time and the intensity of the sound at the two ears. Most mammals turn their heads to increase the differences between the two ears when they want to localize a sound. And many can move their external ears so as to point the incoming sound-waves towards the passage of the external ear. Dogs are better than man at localizing sound, pricking up their ears and using them as direction indicators; man has to turn his head to help himself localize the source of a sound. Deaf people tend to turn their ears to the mouth of the speaker so as to get the sound into the funnel of the ear; they need to hear the higher frequencies of the overtones to hear speech distinctly. The old-fashioned ear-trumpet was good in this respect and it may well have been better than electric amplifiers which magnify all wavelengths. The best position of the head for sound-localizing is to have the sound source coming straight towards one ear, the sound-waves of greater length meeting the nose-neck axis of the head like a wave against a cliff. When this happens, the further ear will be in the worst position for hearing the sound. And so, when we are receiving a sound so that we get maximal stimulation of one ear and minimal stimulation of the other, we know from past experience that the source of the sound is at right angles to the antero-posterior axis of the head. These are not the only mechanisms for sound-localization by only one ear. The quality of a sound changes as things move off or come near. As a sound gets nearer, the bass notes get relatively louder than the treble.

The differences in time and intensity at the two ears do not tell one whether the sound is in front, behind, or above the head. The external ear supplies this information. If two identical sounds are delivered by earphones simultaneously to the two ears, the subject hears one sound and he locates it in the midline, inside or perhaps just above the head. From experiments in which these two variables can be changed, one has learned that the time of arrival is far more important than the relative intensity for localizing sounds.

For sound localization, the input from the two ears has to be brought to a common group of neurons. There is such a group in the medulla, just near the region where the auditory nerve arrives. From this group, the combined input is sent on to higher levels of the brain, such as the midbrain, the thalamus and the cortex. In the medulla, one kind of neuron has all nerve fibres coming from the left ear ending on a dendrite on the left and all those from the right ear on a dendrite on the right. This neuron can appreciate differences in the input from the two ears coming in at an interval of a ten-thousandth of a second. But this is not the only way in which accurate timing and hence localization of sound is done. Some neurons of this nucleus are excited only when inputs from the two ears arrive simultaneously; and others are inhibited by inputs from one ear and excited by inputs from the other.

The auditory area of the cerebral hemispheres reacts differently to sounds one is making oneself and to sounds produced by others. Some of the neurons respond to both kinds of sound but others do not respond to one's own voice. This means that many of the neurons can respond to sounds of the outside world, while one is screaming or speaking.

Compared with many other animals, man is not particularly good at hearing. Birds are far better at distinguishing a lot of notes packed into a short period of time. The lives of most varieties of birds are much shorter than ours, and everything about them takes place more rapidly. All animals are good at hearing the kinds of sounds important for them.

Chicks of penguins on their islands in Antarctica can recognize their parents from the sounds they make, and so can the guillemots on our coasts. In neither case can the human ear detect any differences in the sounds made by the parent birds. Large ranges of sounds cannot be heard by animals for which they have no meaning. There is an advantage in having only a restricted hearing for sounds of importance. These sounds alone will be heard, unsullied by the surrounding din. One might have expected that all animals would be happy to hear the noises made by the animals they eat. But the noise made by cicadas upsets the birds that eat them. Humans also dislike this sound when it is loud enough.

When the first amphibia left the Silurian seas two or three hundred million years ago, with their heads resting on the ground, they relied entirely on bone conduction of vibration for hearing. The vibrations in the earth were transmitted from the bones of their lower jaws to the bone surrounding the inner ear. In order to hear, they probably kept their lower jaws touching the ground. As animals evolved, they first raised their heads in the air and then their whole bodies. As long as these first terrestrial animals, the reptiles, kept their lower jaws to the ground, they heard by bone conduction. Once they raised their heads from the ground, other mechanisms for hearing were evolved; for hearing now meant sensing the vibrations in the air. But bone conduction did not disappear. Birds hear both with their heads and with their feet. And so they may become agitated before earthquakes begin, at a time when we hear nothing.

The first hearing organ of amphibia and reptiles was the saccule. As animals listened to the vibrations in the air, the saccule gained more receptors, with more nerve fibres connecting them to the brain. Then a tubular outgrowth developed from it; this was the beginning of the cochlea. With the evolution of the cochlea, there was an increased sensitivity to vibrations of higher wavelengths; these are the sounds propagated in the air.

When we follow the development of hearing among the vertebrates, we see that an improvement in hearing ocurred when the change from cold-blooded to warm-blooded species took place. The constant higher temperature allowed all neural events to be speeded up, and speed is an advantage in the struggle for living. It gets you away from a predator, it gets you more quickly on to your prey, it allows you to beat your adversary whoever he may be. At higher temperatures nerve fibres conduct impulses more quickly and muscles contract and relax more quickly. Each nerve fibre also recovers more quickly after the passage of a nerve impulse, and so it is ready to conduct another impulse sooner. This fact permitted the range of hearing to increase upwards: more rapid vibrations could be conducted by nerve fibres able to conduct faster. In fish, the auditory nerve fibres can follow the vibrating receptors only at very low rates of vibrations; in frogs the nerve fibres can follow up to rates of 500 vibrations a second, in turtles up to 1,000 vibrations a second, in mammals up to 4,000 to 5,000 a second.

It seems to be that the earlier, more primitive inner ear detected the pitch of a sound according to the principle of resonators. The individual receptors were tuned to vibrate at certain frequencies. They vibrated at the rate of the frequency of the sound, and the nerve fibres from these receptors conducted impulses at this rate. When the cochlea developed, the pitch of a sound was signalled by the movements of the membranes in which the receptors were embedded. In mammals both mechanisms are used. For low frequency sounds, volleys of nerve impulses pass to the brain in time with the pressure waves of the vibration. There is also a displacement of the basilar membrane as the sound wave passes along it. For high frequency sounds, signalling to the brain is only by the mechanism of displacement of the basilar membrane.

Whether snakes hear only by keeping their jaws touching the ground or whether they can also hear when their heads are in the air has not been agreed upon by zoologists. It seems certain that they do not hear the music played to them by snake-charmers. The real purpose of this music is to charm money out of the pockets of tourists. What elephants hear of the soothing songs from the lips of the mahouts who tend them, we do not yet know. Interestingly enough, African elephants can hear the same songs, for the negroes of the Congo learned them from Indian mahouts brought over for training by the Belgians before the First World War. The elephant does not use his big external ears only for hearing. He uses them to communicate, to warn us that he is threatening and will charge if we do not go away. They are also used as vanes from which to lose heat. The skin is relatively thin and it contains dilatable blood-vessels from which heat can be dissipated into the surrounding air.

Bees are able to hear by feeling the vibration in solids. Their buzzing, which to us is so characteristic of bees, is something they do not hear; they feel it. When they are standing on something solid, the vibration of the buzz is transmitted through the solid to other bees, and they feel it with their legs. As well as with their legs, they hear with their antennae, on which there are receptors specialized for certain vibrations. When a bee arrives back in the hive, other bees come up to it and touch its thorax with their antennae; in this way the foraging bee can tell the others where food is to be found. This way of communicating a message allows the bees to speak to a few individuals in a crowd alive with buzzing, where another additional buzz would be lost among the noise. In addition to this, bees have a way of screaming out the urgent news. If a bee discovers a rich source of nectar when the whole hive is short of food, it opens a scent gland in its abdomen and, flying off to the flowers, it leaves a scent trail behind it for all workers to follow. The queen bee has her own royal speech; its fundamental note is about 300 to 380 cycles a second, and its harmonics go up to 1,500 cycles a second. The other way in which bees communicate is by dancing the message, the language discovered and interpreted by von Frisch in Munich.

Most fish communicate by sound. They serenade each other, like crickets and man. Their different calls of alarm and of aggression can now be recognized, since research work has been done on underwater recording of their repertoire of sounds. Shrimps make a great deal of noise for their size. Fish cannot hear the high-pitched sounds made by the porpoises and whales that feed on them. In this respect, they resemble the fly whose composite eyes cannot detect the silk of the spider's web, but they are unlike the moths which hear the shrill cries of the bats that are searching for them.

To find out the source of a sound, fish have developed a way of feeling the movement of water particles. For sound in fluid is transmitted by similar waves of pressure as in air and it also displaces fluid particles. Fish can feel the movement of these particles by means of a row of receptors, concentrated in a line running along their sides, from head to tail. The receptors of this lateral line are just like the hair-cells of the rest of the vestibular system. In many sorts of fish these receptors are within a canal, sunk beneath the skin. As the fish has two rows of these receptors, one on each side of its body, it is able to tell the direction of disturbances in the water.

Echo-location

How bats are able to fly in the dark and avoid all obstacles was first examined in a series of experiments by the great naturalist Lazzaro Spallanzani in Italy. One night in 1793, in company with his brother and a cousin, he hung a lot of threads provided with little bells from the ceiling of his room. 'There was no moon and the shutters of the windows were closed so as to exclude even the faintest beam of light.' The bat flew around the room without touching the threads or the walls. It was able to fly around the room in complete darkness, as Spallanzani reported, 'with the same abilities in complete darkness as with the light of a candle'. To try and find out how bats could fly and avoid obstacles in the dark, Spallanzani next covered bats' heads with opaque hoods. This did prevent them from flying efficiently; they bumped against the walls and fell to the floor. He then took the hoods off their heads and covered their eyes with discs. He was amazed to find that these bats flew about quite happily. He then removed the eyeballs of a bat; this bat flew perfectly.

When these observations were communicated to the Natural History Society of Geneva, a surgeon, ornithologist and botanist, Dr Charles Jurine, confirmed their truth. He thought of plugging the ears of bats with wax. He then saw that these bats were unwilling to fly and when they did fly, they bumped into things and were unable to navigate. He concluded that bats are able to use their ears for navigation in the dark.

When Spallanzani heard about these experiments, he repeated them and confirmed the fact that bats 'collide and fall down if they have their ears plugged. Moreover, they behave in this way not only when blinded but even when they have their eyes.' He came to the conclusion that hearing 'replaces vision in these winged quadrupeds'. He let blinded bats fly around the campanile of the cathedral of Pavia and found that they could catch insects. He finally deduced that bats use echo-ranging or echo-location. 'Thus I think that the organ of hearing of bats is delicate to such a degree that they hear the noise of their wings and body when they are flying, and that they judge the distances from the quality of the sound, like Sanderson [a famous blind man of the time] who determined the size of a room on the basis of sounds reflected from the walls. In this way the sound of the wings reflected from the walls may cause them to know the distances and therefore to avoid them.' Like modern investigators of echo-location, he also thought of trying to jam their radar by making a noise. He beat a drum and got a lot of people to shout and clap in a room where bats were flying. To his disappointment it had no effect.

This early research work that answered the question correctly was forgotten. It was rediscovered by D. Dijkgraaf who went to Pavia to look into the eighteenth-century scientist's notebooks. There he also found Spallanzani's discoveries about swallows and eels.

The rest of the story was guessed correctly by Professor Hartridge in England in 1920. He proposed that 'bats during flight emit a short wavelength note' and this sound is reflected from objects in the vicinity. Twenty-one years later, the navigation of bats by echo-location was rediscovered in the United States by Griffin and Galambos.

Nowadays we are all familiar with sounds reflected from large objects. We hear it when we drive in a car past a row of trees or parked cars with gaps between them. The car we are sitting in produces the sound and it is reflected back from the objects along the side of the road. As trees and cars are separated by gaps that do not reflect sound, we hear a changing pattern of sound, a kind of rushing sound when there is reflection of the sound and a quieter sound when the sound is not being reflected. Auditory clues like these can be useful to blind people; with practice they can gather a lots of information about gaps in walls or doorways. They listen to the sound made by their own footsteps or to the taps they make with a walking-stick and they can hear when the sound is no longer reflected off the walls. A well-trained blind man can walk down a passage and avoid screens thrown half-way across the passage by listening to the sound of his own footsteps reflected by the screens.

The bat's ear has been changed from the usual mammalian pattern to make use of echo-location. The little bones of the middle ear are smaller, lighter, and more tightly bound together so that there is less movement between them; this probably reduces transmission losses. Another development is the increase in size of the muscles working this system of bones. The cochlea is relatively large in relation to the small size of the animal's head. Also it is acoustically isolated from the other bones of the skull; this reduces bone conduction of the noises generated in the animal's own body. The auditory parts of the brain are much larger than in other animals.

Objects as small as wires or insects will cause only extremely faint echoes, yet these are what the bat hears. They are very good at hearing the differences in frequencies and intensities of these faint sounds. The problem for the bat is how to hear a faint echo of high frequency very soon after hearing its own emitted orientation cry, and how to tell the one from the other. The bat copes with the problem by making its orientation cry very short so that it will not overlap its own echo. It also uses the muscles that work the bones of the middle ear to damp down the emission sound as it makes it but it does not use them to damp down the echo.

This is an example of a general problem—how to distinguish the sensory input coming back from one's own activities from the sensory input arising from the external world. Another example is that the visual world appears stable to us while we walk along, bobbing up and down.

The various species of bats make use of a large variety of sounds.

All are very high-pitched with short wavelengths. To bounce sound waves off objects, the wavelengths must be short. If the wavelength were much longer than the object it meets, it would not be bounced back; a wave of one-metre length would not be interrupted by a wire stretched in its way. This high-frequency sound must be given out in a narrow beam, like the light from a pencil-torch, so that it can be focused accurately enough to be reflected off an insect of 1 to 3 mm. long. They achieve this so well that they can tell if an insect of this size is flying towards them or away from them.

Bats are extremely sensitive to interaural differences, noting the difference both in intensity and in time when sounds reach the ears, essential information for the location of sound. In their brains, one lot of neurons reacts to the difference in the time of arrival of the sound, another lot to difference in intensity. If there are no differences noted between the two ears, the sound is coming from straight ahead; and that is what the bat wants to hear.

The common European horseshoe bat makes use of the Doppler effect. When either the source of a sound or the hearer of the sound, or both, are moving, the number of vibrations a second changes. If a whistling train comes nearer when you are standing on a platform, the number of vibrations a second increases, and it decreases as the train goes off. The result of this is that the whistle sounds higher as the train comes towards you and lower as it goes away. The horseshoe bat uses fairly long bursts of a few pure tones, and guides itself by this effect. It hears the note becoming higher as it approaches an object and lower as the object recedes. It is obvious that for echo-locating, the actual pitch of a note is unimportant; whether it is rising or falling is what the animal needs to know. Those bats that make use of the Doppler effect increase this effect by moving their ears. If one stops them moving them, they are lost; but within three weeks they learn to move their heads backwards and forwards instead, and are then almost as good at echo-location as they had been before.

The horseshoe bat emits the sound by humming through its

nose instead of shouting through its mouth. The strange-looking horseshoe nose is modified for the emission of its radar. It is made up of folded skin around the nose which acts as a sort of trumpet, narrowing the sound down to a beam. To locate the echoed sound well, bats make much use of movements of the ears and head, and one can interfere with a bat's ability to carry out echo-location if one prevents these movements.

Bats have a sense of smell. They use this for finding their mates and not for finding food. Many bats have eyes well adapted for seeing at twilight, but even these bats do not use sight for finding their way about or for catching insects. Most bats live in caves into which no light penetrates and so sight is impossible.

How successful this manner of hunting by echo-location is, is made clear to us when we find that bats can catch mosquitos at a rate of two per second. The final proof that bats do find their way about by this system of radar was obtained by Griffin and Grinnell. They jammed the bats' echo-location by high frequency noise. The result was that the bats preferred to stay at home and did not venture out. Some bats hover and they hunt for non-flying insects such as spiders. These bats have very large ears.

The prey of the bats have developed their own defences against their enemies. In the constant agony of nature, those eaten and those searchers for living food wage an equal battle. Whenever this was unequal in the past, either the one or the other species passed away. Moths' furry bodies and wings form a protection against echo-location. For unlike shiny bodies and wings, hair absorbs the sound of the bat's radar. Some insects have developed ultrasonic hearing organs that detect the echo-locating cries of the bat. Certain kinds of moth can jam the bat's radar by making their own ultrasound. Roeder and Treat of Tufts University in the United States have studied the battle between nocturnal moths and the bat. The moth's ears consist of two tympanic membranes; they are connected to two tympanic organs, each of which has only two neurons, an acoustic and a non-acoustic neuron. This animal's whole world of hearing, which is ultrasonic, is brought to its central nervous system by four nerve fibres. As Roeder and Treat realized: 'The small number of receptor cells in the tympanic organ makes it possible to define with some precision the total amount of impulse-coded information available to the moth.' They showed that with this simple apparatus the moth can distinguish the loudness of sounds, their duration, and the direction from which they are coming. The bat is first heard when it is 35–40 metres away. At this distance, the moth hears a warning sound of low intensity. This sound makes the moth fly away from the source of the sound. At this time, the moth tends to win, for the bat's echo-locating system does not work at this distance. When the moth hears a sound of great intensity, it either folds its wings and falls or else it spirals down to the ground. The bat may then be able to find it by echo-location, but it may or may not be able to pick it up from the ground. The design of this moth has evolved to aid its escape from its enemy. Its ears are in the middle of its body, just behind the attachment of the second pair of wings; and the auditory nerves are closely connected to the neurons that work the flight-muscles. The distance between these nerve-cells is very short and so the impulses from the ears reach the flight-muscles very quickly.

Not all bats live on insects. Some live on fruit. In the rainforests of South America, there are bats that catch fish by echo-location. And in South America are the vampire bats that live on the blood of men and horses. Fruit-eating bats rely on vision to find their way about and not on echo-location; they are around during the daytime. One sort of fruit-eating bat flies both by day and night. It uses its eyes when there is enough daylight; and when the sun goes down, it listens to the echoes of the clicking noises it makes with its tongue.

Instead of saying 'as blind as a bat', it would be better to say 'as careless as a bat'. Bats, it has been found, often pay no attention to their echo-location systems. If a new obstacle is put into a tower in which bats live, many of the bats fly into it and hurt themselves. Their echo-location systems are working perfectly; they do not bother to listen in once they have got used to the location of the objects in their accustomed environments.

Bats have existed for more than fifty million years. As complete skeletons of that age have been found which are the same as bats' skeletons today, we may safely assume that they were using echo-location fifty million years ago. This is confirmed by the fact that the shape of their skulls indicates that the part of the brain used in hearing was very well developed. At this time, the horse was the size of a present-day wire-haired terrier.

Some other small mammals, such as certain kinds of mice and shrews, also use echo-location; for some of them are active both by night and day.

Vertebrates which live in the ground specialize in hearing the lower frequencies of sound, for higher frequencies do not penetrate the ground. They probably make more use of conduction via the bones of their skulls. Dr Douglas Webster of New York University has studied the gerbil of Central Asia, the jerboa of North-Africa and the kangaroo rat of the southern United States, and he found out that these little mammals of the desert from quite different parts of the world deal with their acoustic problems in the same way. The range of hearing of the kangaroo rat is from 1,000 to 3,000 cycles a second, and in accordance with this selective sensitivity, its basilar membrane is most developed in the apical part of the cochlea. Dr Webster has shown that the sounds made by rattle-snakes that prey on kangaroo rats, sliding heavily over the ground, come within this frequency range.

Baron von Humboldt in his wonderful book *Voyage aux Régions Équinoxiales du Nouveau Continent* published early in the nineteenth century tells us about the nocturnal birds of Peru. These birds live in complete darkness in caverns, coming out only at night to feed on fruit. The bird, called by the Peruvians the guacharo, is about as big as a hen and has blue eyes. Von Humboldt relates how the local Peruvians are afraid to go into the caves where these blue-black birds are living, and they speak of dying as 'going to join the guacharos'. Unfortunately they are not frightened enough, for once a year during the summer they enter the largest cave with long poles and destroy the birds' nests. These birds are very fat; they have probably evolved the fat as a protection against cold, for it is cool in the caves where they live. The Indians killed the birds to obtain their abdominal fat, which they used for cooking.

Professor Griffin, literally following in von Humboldt's footsteps, proved that these birds fly in darkness, though not in silence. He reported: 'Our ears were bombarded almost constantly by a variety of squawks, screeches, clucks, clicks and shrieks.' For echo-location these birds use very short clicking sounds, averaging about 7,000 cycles per second, within the range of human hearing. Outside the caves, the birds use their eyes.

However, these Stygian birds are not the only ones that fly by night. The little swifts of the Southern Hemispheres, whose nests are stolen for the Chinese to eat, live in similar caves. Although they catch insects by day, they return at night to nest in the caves. They make clicking sounds for echo-location, which not being ultrasonic are heard by man. There is some satisfaction in noting that the men who kill the guacharos and who take the swifts' nests sometimes fall a hundred feet or more to the ground and either kill themselves or linger on with broken backs and limbs.

Echo-location in the sea is used by whales, seals, dolphins, porpoises, and sea-lions. Blind sea-lions get along quite satisfactorily. The sounds they make for echo-location are not the barking we hear at the zoo; they make a kind of ringing sound. The echolocation system of this group of animals that has been most investigated is that of the dolphin. This animal has no sense of smell, it has good sight, a sense of taste, and above all a marvellous sense of hearing. The dolphin, like the bat, lives by echo-location. Its sensitivity in using echo-location is amazing to us. It can distinguish between an aluminium and a copper plate in the water. Apparently it bases this discrimination on differences in reverberation qualities—something we would hardly have thought of. Dolphin can detect fish in muddy water so turbid that using sight is impossible; it does this with its eyes covered, distinguishing red mullet from other fish and being able to tell fish six inches and twelve inches long. The dolphin emits a beep-beep sound at a rate of about five per second when it is not particularly interested in its environment. When it realizes that there is something interesting around, it speeds up its exploratory sound to a rate of several hundred beeps a second, the rate becoming faster as it gets nearer the object. The part of the sound made by the dolphin that man is able to hear sounds, according to Professor Kellogg, like a canary. And if you whistle to it, it whistles back.

How whales communicate has been investigated during this century. In the neighbourhood of Bermuda, you may be lucky enough to hear the song of the humpbacked whale. It lasts up to half an hour. The first description of the sounds made by whales is that by Mr Fisher, who mentions it in his *Journal of a Voyage for the Discovery of the North West Passage* published in 1821. He describes the sound made by the white whale as 'a shrill ringing sound, not unlike that of musical glasses badly played'. Mr Fisher and his fellow explorers heard it by keeping their ears under water. Toothed whales and dolphins use low-frequency sounds for social communication; they make a great variety of sounds with presumably the same variety of meanings. The humpbacked whale sings a song of which the verse, repeated over and over again, lasts eight to twelve minutes. For echo-location these animals issue very high-frequency clicks, putting out about 700 clicks a second. The echoes cannot be repeated at this rate and so presumably they come back as a continuous sound.

These mammals that have returned to the water do not have the problems of air/fluid interface barriers which mammals living in air have. Arriving back in the sea after millions of years' evolution on land, they started off with the land-living ways of amplifying sound. Most mammalian systems amplify the sound twenty times before it is transmitted to the inner ear. Starting off with this advantage, one can see that they were in a good position to develop communication by echo-location.

5 Olfactory receptors: smelling

Our world is so visual that even our way of expressing ourselves is visual. When we understand something, we say 'Yes, I see', not 'Yes, I smell'.

Chemoreceptors have a very long history, for these receptors are probably the oldest of all. They are of most use to animals living in the sea where everything of interest is dissolved in sea water. This means not only everything of positive interest, such as food to be found and swallowed; it means also food to be avoided. For the reactions of vomiting and expelling food are laid down in the same basal parts of the brain as those of sucking and swallowing.

For the predator, scent is the most important of the senses; but for its prey, hearing and eyesight are equally necessary. When we watch the behaviour of animals with keen noses, we can see how all sense organs are used. A wind laden with odours passes by. The dog or the deer turns and faces the wind, pauses and sniffs. They are getting more of the odours into contact with their olfactory receptors so as to examine them in detail, to classify them, so as to know how to behave towards all that the odour implies.

Ancestral fish of the ancient seas had already developed a good sense of smell, though in the case of fish one cannot separate smelling from tasting. The fish shows the basic pattern of vertebrates. The organs for sampling the environment are in the front. The front end of the fish houses the nasal sac for tasting and smelling, for detecting particles or molecules in the water. There may be barbels for feeling the ground or the weeds streaming in the current. The result of receiving this news about the environment is some sort of behaviour. That is carried out by the rest of the fish. For most of the fish consists of the power pack, muscles encased in a streamlined, lubricated envelope; they bring the fish nearer the interesting object or whisk it away from danger. Some fish hunt entirely by smell. These include the dogfish, familiar to all biology students, and those fish that hunt by night when there is no light to see by. One of the schemes tried to keep sharks off bathing beaches is to put unpleasant smells in the sea; apparently the smell of man is not unpleasant enough.

Some fish have such a keen sense of smell that they can detect a substance when there are only a few molecules of it in the water. Although water spreads the molecules around just as air does, some mammals who have returned to the sea from the land, such as the porpoises and the dolphins, have no sense of smell. This sense, which their ancestors used on land, has lapsed to such an extent that these marine mammals no longer have olfactory bulbs; they have lost the very nerve tracts concerned with smelling.

Snakes have a good sense of smell. After they have bitten and injected venom into their prey, they do not always swallow it straight away. The poor frightened animal goes off and hides while it dies within an hour. The snake has to go and find it and it does so by smelling it out.

The sense of smell is so important to the mouse that the female, if she is deprived of it by an operation, no longer shows maternal behaviour and will eat her litter of young. Sheep, goats, and rats recognize their young by smell. To kittens each maternal nipple has a different smell, and so there is no squabbling to suckle; each kitten goes to the nipple whose smell it has rapidly learned. At this time, the kitten is blind and deaf but its sense of smell is acute.

Human babies can smell the female breast, distinguishing it from other parts of the body. If a breast is put under a sleeping baby's nose, it makes sucking movements in its sleep. By six weeks, the baby can distinguish the smell of the breast of its own mother from that of other women.

The world of insects is a world of smells. It is surprising to find that wasps and bees like the same flowers as we do. The smell of flowers developed just with the purpose of attracting insect pollinators and not to please us, though our noses may do a little pollinating as well. Insects have their olfactory organs on their antennae. In ourselves this would be equivalent to us having a long, mobile nose, a little like an elephant's trunk; we could then push this nose right up against the source of the smell. Von Frisch and his colleagues have discovered that some flowers have different smells in their different parts. Our crude noses note only one general smell. But insects with their little olfactory organs on their antennae can push these sense organs up against the various parts of a flower and thus locate the different parts according to their different smells. Von Frisch has found out that in a narcissus the yellow ring is not only a different colour from the white corolla but has also a different smell. Having found that bees could easily distinguish these two parts by their smell, he then found that if the yellow and the white parts of the flower were separated, humans could also distinguish two different smells. The bee can follow the scent of the flower according to the strength of the smell; and so the flower has arranged matters so that when the bee is smelling the strongest smell, it is most likely to pollinate the flower.

Those animals that make more use of smell than of vision have more olfactory receptor cells than photoreceptors. In vertebrates, the olfactory receptors are in a special region of the nasal mucous membrane right at the top of the nose. It is shown in the human nose in Fig. 5.1.

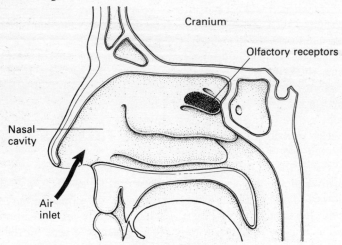

Fig. 5.1 Location of olfactory epithelium within the nasal cavity.

Really one has two noses: a left and a right nasal cavity separated by the nasal septum. The cavities join together at the top of the nose. If they had been kept separate on the two sides of the head, like the ears, we would have been able to locate the source of a smell by noting the difference in its arrival time at the right and left nasal cavity. But such matters are arranged by evolution, and the nasal cavities developed out of the primitive mouth. The advantages of having two noses must have been small, considering, too, that smells diffuse all round.

Odours reach the nasal cavities by two routes: they come in with the air we breathe, and they pass up the back of the nose from the throat. The smells of the outer world arrive mainly through the nostrils. The smells of our food and drink pass up the back of the nose.

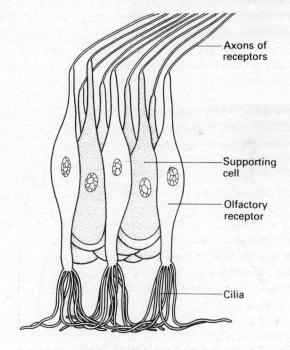

Axons of receptors

Supporting cell

Olfactory receptor

Cilia

Fig. 5.2 The olfactory receptors.

There are some people with congenital anosmia, people who cannot smell, like people born blind or deaf. The only abnormal feature of their olfactory systems is an absence of cilia, described below. There are also people who cannot smell certain fatty acids but can smell everything else. A drawing of the olfactory receptors in the nose is shown as Fig. 5.2.

The olfactory mucous membrane consists of the olfactory receptors and supporting cells; though their name of supporting cells need not imply that they have no olfactory function. The essential part of the olfactory receptor is the long mat of cilia or fine, hair-like structures. They are drawn in Fig. 5.2 as separated from each other, in order to demonstrate them; but in fact the cilia would be overlapping, forming a mat through which the incoming air has to pass. The olfactory mucous membrane is for smell what the retina is for vision. There are fifty million of these receptors in each of our nostrils.

Smell is the least understood of our senses. In vertebrates living on land, those substances that can be smelled have to be transferred from air into the mucus covering the olfactory membrane and from there to the surface of the cilia. This means that anything that we can smell has to be volatile, so as to get into the air, and soluble in water, so as to get in the mucus. The cilia are made of proteins and these proteins unite with the molecules of the odoriferous substance. Whether the substance will be smelled or not depends on the shape, size, and crystalline form of its molecule. Many molecules come in two crystalline forms, one being the mirror image of the other. This is like a key and a lock. The lock will accept only the key with the correct outline facing the left; the outline facing the right is no good. The protein molecules of the receptor membrane are built like the lock. They will accept only the molecules shaped in the right way. A substance consisting of molecules that fit the membrane will be smelled, and one with molecules formed in a mirror image will not be.

The olfactory membrane is different from the retina in that light excites the whole retina, odours affect particular parts of the membrane. This spatial organization does not mean that there is just one region of the membrane for one kind of smell, for any odour can affect different areas of the membrane.

From the olfactory receptors nerves pass up to the brain through small holes in the base of the skull. These are the smallest nerves outside the central nervous system. They connect to an outgrowth of the brain called the olfactory bulb, which can be seen in Plates 11 and 12.

The input from the olfactory cells not only excites the next lot of neurons, as one might have expected. It excites some and inhibits others, and the different odours have different effects. In addition, there are nerve fibres coming down from the brain which decrease the inhibition. How all of this works, we do not yet know.

Our ability to smell can be ruined by severe head injuries. There are two causes for this. The fine nerve fibres of the olfactory nerves can be torn as the brain is displaced within the skull by the force of the blow. Also this displacement may bruise the front ends of the temporal lobes of the brain and parts of the frontal lobes: these injuries may cause an inability to differentiate various smells.

External communication by chemical substances: pheromones

Pheromones (derived from the Greek words for 'carry' and 'excite') are substances that excite the sense of smell. An animal sensitive to a certain pheromone performs a particular act on receiving the smell signal. Pheromones tell others that a territory is occupied, they are used to signal dominance in a social group, some are used to spread alarm, others to induce sexual behaviour, to lay a trail, or as a warning that an animal is likely to attack.

One of the advantages of pheromones is that the signal itself, the scent, is left to transmit the information while the animal that gave the signal goes off to do something else.

One pheromone is well-known to all Americans and to others by repute: the stink made by the skunk. The skunk first threatens by turning its back, raising its hind-quarters and its tail. Its anal glands are aimed at its foe. If the foe does not beat a retreat, a strong solution of butylmercaptan is squirted at it. Any animal receiving this once would avoid a second encounter.

Zoologists first became interested in pheromones when they realized that there were alarm substances put out by a damaged member of a group in order to warn the others. Bees make a substance in their salivary glands that keeps other bees away. If this substance, of which the chemical composition has been worked out, is spread around, bees flee from the spot. When the skin of many varieties of fish is damaged, alarm substances spread in the water; fish flee from the area, except for predators who are attracted by the substance. When the alarm substance of the skin of the toad is dropped into water, it alarms toads, tadpoles and any fish that smell it. The dilution of the substance that is effective is infinitesimally small; a few molecules suffice. Alarm substances do not travel as far as sex attractants and they do not linger. This is nice to know. It would be a sadder world if the call to sex were brief and passing and the warning of danger were long-lasting and present everywhere.

Sex pheromones are probably the commonest kind of pheromone. They are used by insects, fish, snakes and other reptiles, amphibia, and mammals. They linger in the air or water and spread over long distances. There are two sorts of sex pheromone, one used by the female to bring the male to her side and one used by the male to encourage the female to copulate. Pheromones in moths and butterflies are contained in scent-scales or scent-plumes. Many varieties of insect and of mammal have special glands to make these chemical substances. Fabre, the nineteenth-century naturalist of Provence, one day found his house full of peacock emperor moths. He had put some females of this species under wire netting in his house. He then spent months trying to answer the question how these females had signalled to the males. Although he finally came to the right conclusion, that the sense of smell was involved, he concluded that this could not be the ordinary sense of smell, as he himself could smell nothing. It did not occur to him that there could be a smell that the male moths could smell and that he could not. This was an unfortunate moth to catch, for had he captured many other moths, he himself would have smelled something, for we can smell some of them; some smell like caramels, some like raspberries and some smell of vanilla.

The queen bee produces a pheromone that has two effects. It

makes the eggs develop into non-developing females, the worker bees. And it also acts as a sex attractant to the males during swarming.

The male moth is able to tell the direction from which a smell is coming. It does this by having two antennae and by estimating which of the two is receiving most stimulus. This is a similar mechanism to that by which one can tell the direction from which a sound is coming by having two ears.

There is a moth that was brought to New England from Europe and which has become a pest, denuding trees. The sexual attractant pheromone has been synthesized and is now used to trap the males; thus the lure of sex, not for the first time, leads eager males to their deaths.

The silkworm, being domesticated and available, has been studied more than other species with regard to sex pheromones. The male can smell the female up to 2,000 metres away. When he receives this exciting odour, he flutters his wings, waves the antennae which receive the odour, and flies off to try and find the female. The antennae of the male have 34,000 sensory organs, called sensilla, and these have 50,000 olfactory receptors, sensitive only to bombykol. This is the name of the pheromone, the Latin for a silkworm being *bombyx mori*. Bombykol is absorbed by these receptors, which then fire off nerve impulses to the brain. It has been calculated that 200 to 300 molecules of bombykol acting for four-fifths of a second suffice to bring out the typical pattern of behaviour of the male moth. The female silkworm can smell a lot of odours but she cannot smell bombykol; the male, on the other hand, responds only to this and related substances.

For monkeys, the attraction of the female for the male depends entirely on smell. The pheromone concerned is in the vagina. If a male rhesus monkey is deprived of the sense of smell he is no longer interested in the female. The literature of monkeys, if it existed, would be a literature of smell. But it is not only the female that attracts the male by means of a pheromone; the male emits an odour attractive to the female. There is a pheromone in the urine of the male mouse that brings the female into heat. The pheromone emitted by the female rat is attractive to the adult male rat but pre-pubertal and castrated rats pay no attention to it. The smell she emits depends on her sexual state, and so she makes use of a pheromone to broadcast her readiness to receive the male. The pheromone given out by the male pig, together with some other stimuli, induce an immoblization reflex in the sow so that she stands still during copulation.

The male hormone, testosterone, can be smelled by women far more easily than by men. Its smell is musky, similar to that produced by musk deer and the civet cat. But women who have had their ovaries removed become rather insensitive to this smell. When these women were given the female hormone, oestrogen, they could smell the substance again. Women can smell the most diluted solutions of musky substances about ten days before the period; at this time, the secretion of oestrogen is maximal. After the menopause when little or no oestrogen is secreted, women can no longer smell testosterone.

It has been suggested that the earlier age at which menstruation starts nowadays compared to fifty and a hundred years ago is due to the fact that boys and girls mix far more now than they used to. The odour of the opposite sex causes the secretion of hormones that induces puberty.

Sexual pheromones bring couples together. There are also aggregation substances that bring all the animals of a kind together. Then there are dispersal pheromones, used for instance by millipedes to chase animals of the same kind away. It is surprising to note that insects use insect repellants. These substances have not yet been chemically isolated and manufactured.

Mosquitoes detect human beings by their smell; they prefer the smell of some people to that of others. Women become more attractive targets to mosquitoes at certain periods of their menstrual cycles; but not only to mosquitoes: also to dogs, stags, goats, monkeys, and bulls. It may be that women misunderstand the intentions of bulls approaching them in lonely fields.

Right at the beginning of life, there is an essential communication between mother and offspring by smell. If the olfactory bulbs are cut out, rat pups and kittens do not suck the nipple. After the birth, the mother rat and cat—and no doubt other mammals—

lick their nipples. Their saliva on the nipples is smelled by the young and this constitutes a pheromone instructing it to suck. Clearly, this knowledge is inborn. If the animal's nipples are washed and her saliva is replaced by the saliva from a virgin rat or cat, this is no good; the young do not suck. In the rat, there is a particular region of the olfactory bulbs that is tuned to this smell.

Many mammals mark out their territories and home ranges by passing urine. The first thing a mouse does when it is put in a new cage is to mark the whole place with urine. The bear marks its territory with faeces smeared on trees. Similar pheromones are produced in deer near the eyes and on the breast. The males mark things in the environment with the secretion of these glands. If two males try to spread these secretions on each other, that is a prelude to a fight.

There are pheromones which when left in the home range of an animal act as warnings to others to keep off or they may act as trails left for others to follow. The male bumble-bee leaves trails in the air as he flies and he deposits the same substance on the plants he visits. Trail-laying has been studied in many different kinds of ants. Each substance is specific to the kind of ant producing it. Bees release a pheromone when they find a good source of nectar. They also take the smell of the flower back to the hive so that the other workers can search for that particular smell. Von Frisch found that this substance is sucked up with the nectar of the flower and that it also clings to the body of the bee. When the other workers in the hive learn about the source of food by observing the dance, they learn about the amount of pollen and nectar, about its distance from the hive and the direction in which to fly; from the smell brought in by the foraging bee, they learn which is the actual flower they have to seek.

Bees, ants, and termites recognize the members of their own colonies by their smell. If any other insect gets into a beehive long enough to acquire the right smell, it will not be evicted or killed but will be tolerated even if it spends its time raiding the eggs and honey. This recognition of one's own colony or family by smell is very common. No doubt, when the mother of many of the mammals we know best licks her young after birth, she covers it with a smell which she then recognizes as her own.

Ants live in a world of smells and produce several pheromones. Their alarm pheromone diffuses for about three to five centimetres, and fades out in about half a minute. Ants leave trails for others to follow, using this way of signalling a good food supply. This pheromone in the fire ant fades in about two minutes. It has meaning only for ants of the same species. E. O. Wilson, who has studied the communication systems of ants, considers that ants convey as much information in their chemical trail-laying as bees do with their communication by dancing. Ants respond to the alarm pheromone put out by aphids, trans-β-farnescene. They are called to the scene by this chemical substance, and then attack any insect preying on their aphids.

6 Gustatory receptors: tasting

The working of the alimentary canal is largely controlled by receptors scattered along its lining. They contribute to the production of enzymes needed for the digestion of the various sorts of food we take in. Most of the receptors in the viscera work without evidence of their activity reaching our conscious awareness; but when the tension receptors are strongly stimulated, their messages protrude into consciousness and we suffer the pain of abdominal colic. In addition to the tension receptors, there are chemoreceptors of all kinds; and receptors for sampling the pH or acid-alkaline balance of the alimentary contents.

The chemoreceptors in the oral end of the alimentary canal, the end that takes in food, send messages to parts of the brain to cause sensation; this is necessary to adjust behaviour according to the message received. Among our early ancestors, the fish in the sea, these chemoreceptors were in the mouth; for the world flowed into the mouth as seawater. When vertebrates left the sea, some chemoreceptors remained in the mouth and their messages were interpreted as taste; others moved to the top of the nose and their messages were smells. Our taste or gustatory receptors are on the top and edges of the tongue, on the epiglottis, the soft palate, and scattered around the throat. They are arranged in little goblets, called taste-buds. The actual chemoreceptors of taste are narrow cells ending in a fringe. These receptors wear away after about ten days and they are then replaced by epithelial cells, which metamorphose into taste receptor cells. Every taste bud has about fifty of these cells. Man has about 10,000 in all. They are drawn in Fig. 6.1. The function of the supporting cells is unknown; it may be that they serve to keep the environment right for the receptor cells.

The substance to be tasted has to be absorbed onto the fringes of the taste cells. To enter the cells, the substance must be water-soluble. It also has to be lipid-soluble and the molecules not too large in order to pass through the membrane.

Man has an even less developed sense of taste than sense of smell, for a larger number of molecules of a substance have to be dissolved in fluid for it to be tasted than for it to be smelt.

Cats are indifferent to sweetness and have no receptors for sweet tastes. One of my cats likes chocolate, so presumably it is not the sweet taste that it prefers. Most animals do taste and like sweetness; this is so for flies, butterflies, rats, mice, dogs, bears, and horses.

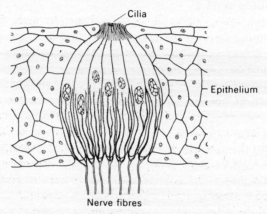

Fig. 6.1 The taste receptors within a taste-bud.

Animals, including man, are very sensitive to bitter substances. This has probably evolved as many poisonous substances in plants taste bitter; and equally the plants have evolved bitter tastes in order to preserve themselves from being eaten. The toad has a bitter skin. Although one toad may be eaten, others will not be, and so the race of toads is preserved.

The taste of sourness is related to the pH of the substance, though not all acids taste sour or acid. All the salts of chemistry taste salty if they are soluble in saliva and if they dissociate at least to some extent into ions; both the cation and the anion contribute to the taste of the salt. For instance, sodium bromide tastes different from sodium chloride, and sodium chloride tastes different from potassium and from ammonium chloride. But there are some exceptions to the rule that salts taste salty. Lead acetates, for instance, taste sweetish. Some metallic salts must be described as tasting metallic rather than salty. And Epsom Salts, which is sodium sulphate, tastes bitter rather than salty.

It is thought that man has four primary tastes, sweet, bitter, sour, and salt. Rats respond very quickly to any of these tastes, isolated and given purely. Their reactions are spitting or swallowing, licking or sucking. It is thought that these primary tastes are a sort of indication, telling the animal to go ahead and try more of the stuff or avoid it.

Most gustatory nerve fibres are activated by more than one of the primary tastes. It is reckoned that a combination of primary tastes gives us another taste, just as we see orange and not a combination of red and yellow.

The contribution of smell to our ability to taste is made clear to us when we have a cold. At a certain stage the mucous membrane of the nose is swollen with fluid or covered with mucus or pus; then the molecules of odoriferous substances cannot get at the receptors to excite them, and so we cannot taste our food properly.

As we get older we probably lose some of the sensitivity of all our receptors. This is so for hearing and smell, and it is very marked for tasting; many of our taste-buds disappear. The acuteness of the sense of taste in children may be one of the causes of their hatred of nasty-tasting medicines.

7 Cutaneous receptors: touching and feeling

For eighthly he rubs himself against a post.

The skin is not only the covering of the body; it is also a large area of receptors, constantly examining the world and sending information to the central nervous system. Its information is used for the automatic adjustment of the body which takes place without causing any sensation. It is used to control the temperature; some is used to aid in the control of the muscles; and some goes to alert the brain, telling it that more information is about to come in and to get ready to receive it.

What we feel and what afferent nerves bring to the central nervous system are two different things. The general principles of cutaneous or skin sensation were first studied early in the nineteenth century before anything was known about receptors and the central nervous system. Weber concluded from experiments on man that the senses are organized to take notice of differences between two stimuli rather than the absolute intensity of a stimulus; they are tuned to comparison and contrasts. Weber concluded from his experiments that a just discernible difference in the intensity of stimulation divided by the intensity was a constant, expressed as $\Delta I/I = $ constant. Later, Fechner concluded that the intensity of a sensation increased proportionally with the logarithm of stimulus intensity, expressed as $S = K \log I$. These relationships are true except beyond the usual ranges of stimulus intensity; they are now known as the Weber-Fechner law.

The sensory apparatus of the skin has to report three sorts of information. It reports the nature of the stimulus, saying: 'you have been touched', or 'you are being tickled', or 'you are being burnt'. It reports the intensity of the stimulation, saying' 'this stimulus is slightly warm; this one is very cold'. And it reports the position of the stimulus, saying: 'you have been stimulated on the tip of the left little toe'.

Some receptors of the body are the nerve fibres themselves; others are nerve fibres joined to a non-neural cell, which is needed to start off the message. Both kinds are in the skin. The non-neural structures or cells have various shapes and many names. A simple nerve fibre receptor is shown in Plate 3. The dark-staining cells are the layers of the skin. The nerve fibre is the dark wire entering this layer from the deeper regions of the skin. This photograph was made from a small piece of skin punched out of the fingertip of a man. The specimen has been killed and stained especially to show up nerve fibres. Although this photograph shows a twig of a nerve fibre running through the superficial layers of the skin, it fails to show the dense network of nerve fibres that there is throughout the skin. It is reckoned that under any spot of the skin, there are forty nerve fibres; and so any natural stimulus to the skin always excites a large number of receptors and nerve fibres.

A receptor that is sensitive to any deformation of the skin is illustrated in Plate 4. In this case the receptor is a non-neural cell, derived from the end of the afferent nerve fibre. This receptor belongs to the class of mechanoreceptors.

There are also receptors throughout the alimentary canal reporting events in both the mucous membrane and the muscular wall of the viscus.

In the last twenty years knowledge has been acquired by putting electrodes into the peripheral nerves of man, recording what is passing along the nerves when the skin and the muscles are stimulated, and finding out what the person feels.

The nerve fibres from the skin clearly fall into two categories, large and small. The large ones are the mechanoreceptors; they are excited by bending of the hairs, stretching or deforming the skin, by anything touching or moving along the skin. The small fibres are thermoreceptors and nociceptors; they report warmth and cold and any dangerous or noxious stimulation that causes pain.

Mechanoreceptors are like the pickups of record-players. They convert the energy from a mechanical movement to an electrical signal in a nerve fibre. In the fingertips, which are very sensitive to mechanical stimulation, one single impulse in a single nerve fibre can cause a perceptible sensation. In the palm, many more impulses are needed. In real life, there is never just one impulse and one nerve fibre is never excited alone. This is because the density of nerve-endings in any region of the skin is so great that no object would excite just one nerve fibre.

Warm thermoreceptors fire off impulses when the skin is warmed and stop firing when it is cooled; cold receptors do the opposite, firing on cooling and stopping firing when the skin is warmed. The terms warm and cold are rather vague for at a skin temperature of 33°C, which is comfortably warm, many cold receptors are firing. Warm and cold fibres are among the steady-state receptors, firing off constantly with different skin temperatures. Warm fibres fire between 33° and 45° and cold fibres from about 34° down to 18°. Within these ranges various fibres fire off constantly at different temperatures. Feeling cold in the hands depends more on the activity of these steady-state cold fibres than on the cold fibres that fire only when the temperature is dropped. This information about the temperature of the surface of the body is provided not only for conscious awareness; a lot of it is used for the automatic and unconscious control of body temperature.

Cats sample the temperature of the air with their noses; one can see them deciding on this evidence whether to go out or not. Hibernating hamsters have cold receptors in their noses that fire off when the temperature goes down to minus 5°.

Although we use the term tactile fibres and warm and cold fibres, we do not speak of pain fibres, but of nociceptors, receptors that report damaging or noxious stimuli. The reason is that these fibres do not necessarily cause pain and that one can have pain without exciting these fibres.

Pain depends on many impulses arriving within a short time and also on the amount of tissue damaged. Small fibres reporting damage to the skin are called polymodal nociceptors, as they are fired off by many kinds of stimuli. Chemical substances, both those caused by damage to tissues and those introduced into the skin by stinging nettles and poison ivy, stimulate the smallest polymodal nociceptors. The sensation we experience does not depend only on which kind of receptor or fibre is firing off. Although the firing of a nociceptor almost always causes pain, firing of other receptors can cause pain, if they fire rapidly and often enough. This effect of the summation of impulses probably underlies something we all must have noticed. You may be leaning against the sharp edge of a desk. At first all you feel is the pressure against your thigh. But suddenly the region which is pressed upon becomes painful, and you have to move. The effect of impulses arriving repeatedly from mechanoreceptors has been to cause pain.

The incoming nerve fibres form synapses with neurons of the posterior horns of the spinal cord. Each one of these neurons receives impulses from many incoming nerve fibres. The area of the skin from which a posterior horn neuron can be excited is called its receptive field. The relations between these nerve fibres from the peripheral nerves and the posterior horn neurons are not fixed, like architecture; they are changing all the time. These changes result from the many events that affect the input to the spinal cord. The messages of the incoming nerve fibres are not just relayed to the brain. At these synapses there are various forms of excitation and inhibition (to be discussed in Chapter 13), which change the messages into a form of the kind that the central nervous system copes with.

The layers of neurons of the posterior horns are largely organized according to the kinds of receptors they receive. There is one layer mainly devoted to mechanoreceptors; impulses from stroking or pressing or touching the skin go to the neurons of this layer. There are two layers most concerned with noxious events, which finally cause us to experience pain. Neurons in one of these layers receive impulses from the skin, from muscles and from the viscera. These neurons are those that underlie the phenomenon of referred pain. Referred pain is pain felt in the skin or the body-wall though it comes from a viscus; it is thus referred from the viscus to the wall of the body. The reason for the reference is that impulses from viscera, muscles, and skin end on the same lot of neurons. As the brain more often receives impulses from parts of the body of which we are aware, such as the skin, the chest wall, or the arm, maybe it interprets the arriving impulses as coming from these parts of the body and not from the viscera.

Intensity of stimulation, as was said in Chapter 2, is signalled to the central nervous system by the rate of sending of impulses: the stronger the stimulus, the larger the number of impulses that are sent within a certain time; and also the larger the number of nerve fibres used to send in the impulses to the central nervous system.

There may be a change in the quality of sensation when more impulses per second arrive and when the sensation becomes more intense. This is the case for sensation from the viscera. The very same nerve fibres from the bladder signal all the sensations we can get from that organ. When these nerve fibres are sending a few impulses per second, we have the feeling that we need to pass urine. When more impulses come in, we get an urgent need to do so. When a great many impulses come in, we get pain in the bladder.

How we can tell whereabouts in the skin we have been touched or pricked depends finally on the representation of the skin of the body in the cerebral hemisphere. Touches on the left big toe are felt in one part of the cortex, and touches on the back of the neck in another part. Different parts of the cerebral hemisphere are related to different parts of the body. And so when nerve impulses come to one part, we know that they originated in the big toe and when they come to another part, they must have come from the little finger. The sensation that the little finger has been touched is only a part of the information received. Many parts of the central nervous system have received the same information, parts having nothing to do with our consciousness, with sensation.

Any point in the skin is supplied by very many nerve fibres. When a point on the skin is stimulated, the nerve fibres beneath this point are stimulated unequally. For no two points on the skin come equally within the territory of all the same nerve fibres. This can best be shown in a diagram. In Fig. 7.1 each nerve fibre A, B, and C, supplies a little area of skin measuring a few square milli-metres; and these areas partially overlap. If the skin is touched at point X, it is in the receptive areas of the nerve fibres A, B, and C. No other point in the whole body is exactly in that position in the fields of these three nerve fibres. The number of branches of these three nerve fibres it might excite might be 10 per cent of A, 20 per cent of B, and 15 per cent of C. In reality, it is much more complicated than this; for any point on the skin is supplied by a great many nerve fibres. For instance the small region of pulp of a human front tooth contains 500 to 600 nerve fibres. The amount of overlap of the terminals of nerve fibres differs in different tissues and in one tissue it varies according to position. There are, for instance, more nerve fibres in any area of skin of the hands and feet than in the upper parts of the limb.

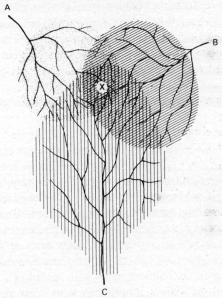

Fig. 7.1 Diagram to illustrate how any point in the skin has a unique relation to a minimum of three nerve fibres and no other point in the body has that same relation.

Our ability to localize a stimulus is organized further by the neurons in the posterior horns. The three nerve fibres drawn in Fig. 7.1 connect, let us say, to three different neurons of the posterior horn and each of these three neurons receives impulses from a large number of incoming nerve fibres from neighbouring areas of the skin. The receptive fields of these neurons also overlap similarly to the nerve fibres shown in this Figure. Any point in the skin lies within the receptive field of several neurons; here again, it would be in the centre of the field of one neuron, in the lateral part of the field of another, and the medial part of another. These receptive fields are often changing, in accordance with the excitability of the neurons and with all the events that affect them.

The mechanism of surround inhibition is used to localize a point stimulated in the skin. When one small group of nerve fibres coming from one point in the skin is excited, the neighbouring neurons are inhibited. This interaction takes place at the first synapse, where the arriving nerve fibres enter the spinal cord. The same mechanism occurs at many higher synapses as the input is taken up through the central nervous system. The effect of this surround inhibition is to make the most active group of neurons stand out clearly against a background of relative silence, and this enhances the contrast between the point of the skin stimulated and the surrounding skin.

How we localize the point of stimulation does not depend only on the nerves of the skin itself. For most touches or pricks, pinches or shoves excite the nerves deep to the skin as well. If some of the nerves of the skin have been cut through by accident, say by a knife or jagged glass, touch or pressure can still be localized fairly accurately, even though the skin itself is insensitive to very light touch, warmth, cold, or burning. This is because the nerves of structures deep to the skin, of muscles, tendons, and bones, may be uncut; and their information is adequate to tell us whereabouts we have been stimulated.

The sensation of pins and needles comes from depriving a nerve of its blood circulation. If a nerve is pressed on so that a length of it cannot get enough blood, the area of skin supplied by the nerve 'goes to sleep' and feels numb. When the pressure is removed the nerve fibres fire off impulses spontaneously. The sensation of pins and needles is due to these spontaneous showers of impulses in the nerve fibres from the skin.

When a peripheral nerve is cut through either by accident or by disease, the effects appear in the muscles and skin. All the muscles supplied by that nerve are paralysed and they atrophy. There is no feeling in the denervated area. Owing to the division of the sympathetic nerves which accompany the peripheral nerves, the skin becomes dry; for it can no longer sweat. The little muscles that erect the hairs of the skin are paralysed and so, even when the skin is cold, these muscles cannot be contracted to make the skin hairs stand up and conserve a layer of warm air. Also the blood-vessels are paralysed. At first they are dilated and the denervated area of skin is pinker than the surrounding region. Later, blood-vessels deprived of their controlling nerve fibres constrict, and the area becomes pale and cold. Eventually the skin becomes smooth and inelastic and the nails have white stripes and become ridged.

Thermoreception

Throughout the animal kingdom, one sees how a general pattern of structure or of function can become specialized in certain directions. In one species, a certain structure is particularly well developed; in another, a certain kind of behaviour is developed, and this necessitates the development of certain kinds of receptors. In vipers and rattlesnakes of America and in Australian pythons and boas, receptors for warmth have become specialized detectors. In the New World snakes, they are collected together in a pit between the eye and the nostril and in the Australian snakes they are in scales along the upper and lower jaws. Being sensitive to radiant energy, they detect the prey by the heat it gives out. The warmth given out by a rat is easily detected. As the snake has two pits, it gets a stereoscopic perception of the warm object; this allows it to estimate the distance of its prey with accuracy. A blindfolded viper will strike at a lighted electric bulb and not at a cold one; but if the facial pits are covered, it does not strike at all. The warmth of a human hand in front of the facial pit will excite the receptors in it, but if the hand strokes or touches the skin of the pit-organ, nothing happens. The pit viper has as many thermal receptors in an area of about half a square centimetre as we have in 200 square centimetres of skin. These receptors are spontaneously active all the time and always sending off nerve impulses. When there is a change in the radiant energy reaching them, all that has to happen is for this spontaneous discharge to be changed in amount and rhythm.

Electroreception

Among the various senses that man has not got is electroreception. Anyone who has had an electric shock will feel like denying this; but, in company with other land animals, we do not have special organs and receptor areas of our brains evolved to sense the electric field around us. That some fish can detect and make sure of feeble electric fields in the water was suggested by Lissman in 1958. This sense of electroreception occurred very early in evolution and disappeared in most recently-evolved fish.

Two groups of fish, mormyriforms of Africa and gymnotiforms of South America, put out an electrical field from electrical generator organs. This field is distorted by objects in the environment and that is perceived by the fishes' electroreceptors. Fish also use electricity to communicate with their fellows; and in this case they change the frequency of the emitted pulse.

Electroreception is related to the lateral line. There are three related afferent nerves, one from the lateral line bringing information about flowing particles of water, one from the electroreceptors, and one from the inner ear, concerned with hearing, vibration, and balance.

The largest electric potentials in living things are those of the electric eel of the Amazon river; it can discharge 600 V.

Magnetic field detection

The earth is a great magnet, the magnetic field originating in its core. There are changes in this field due to magnetic storms. They come from charged particles leaving the sun after giant solar flares. Any organism that can feel the earth's magnetic field can use this information for orientating itself in the world and for finding its way about. And animals that can sample the total intensity of the magnetic field at any place have information about the earth's latitude, the location north to south; but this information is upset by magnetic storms.

Bacteria and algae are very sensitive to the earth's magnetic field. Bees and termites in their constructed homes are sensitive both to the magnetic field and to gravity; termites have no other links with the outside world. Pigeons and other birds certainly use the magnetic field to know their latitude. They prefer to use the sun but they rely on magnetic information when the sky is very overcast. Making use of the excursion of the sun, they also have an accurate sense of time. Fish can orientate themselves by sampling the magnetic field. In addition, sharks, skates, rays, and catfish detect their prey by noting changes in the local magnetic field. Catfish can predict earthquakes; that was discovered in Japan in the nineteen-thirties. The fish probably detect electric potentials and it is likely that they increase before earthquakes. In certain earthquake areas, the local electric potentials always increase before earthquakes, and so one ought to keep catfish in those places.

Many animals, such as bees, monarch butterflies, and pigeons, have cells containing magnetite in their bodies. This is the iron oxide of the lodestone; and that was the stone that the Chinese discovered could be used as a compass.

Dr Robin Baker of the University of Manchester discovered that man too has a magnetic sense of direction. He blindfolded students and took them on journeys in trucks or buses. Then he took the bandage off their eyes and told them to point towards their homes. They were surprisingly accurate, pointing in the right direction. They were better at getting the direction right when they had been blindfolded; if they had had the usual visual clues or tried to work it out intellectually, they did not do so well. Even those who went to sleep on the outward journey did almost as well as those who kept awake. Man does not think much of his geomagnetic sense, preferring to trust himself to the features of the environment of which he is consciously aware. Curiously enough, this is the same also with birds that can feel the earth's magnetic field.

8 Receptors for the inside world

The receptors we have so far been reviewing keep the animal in touch with the outside world. There are also receptors to keep the central nervous system informed about what is happening in the inside world of the animal's own body.

All receptors are sensitive to those forces they are likely to meet and to no others. The receptors of the eye react only to light and those of the cochlea only to sound. It is the same with the receptors evolved to control the body. The receptors within the bladder do not respond to temperature, but they do respond to contraction and stretching of the muscle of the bladder wall. The receptors of the intestines are insensitive to temperature and to gentle touches; intestines can be torn or cut through in conscious patients without them feeling anything. But they are sensitive to stretching, to contraction, and to certain chemical susbstances.

Equilibrium receptors: keeping the right way up

For he can set up with gravity which is patience upon approbation.

That we stand upright with our heads above our necks and our necks straight above the trunk seems so obvious that we do not realize that this position has to be automatically maintained. Gravity is constantly acting to pull us down and so we have mechanisms designed to counteract it. It is due to gravity that Australians and New Zealanders do not feel that they are walking about upside down, though they are.

The inner ear is not only for hearing. It is also the organ of equilibrium. In it are receptors sensitive to movement, to acceleration and deceleration, to rotation and gravity. The part of the labyrinth concerned with posture and balance is called the vestibule. It consists of three structures, the utricle, the saccule, and the semicircular canals, of which there are three on each side, in the three planes of space. They are shown in Figs. 4.1 and 4.2. The three semicircular canals can be seen, but the saccule and the utricle are on the far side and so are not seen in this view. In all vertebrates, one of these canals is in the horizontal plane; its angle varies with the usual head position of the animal. In fish, the head is in the same plane as the body and both are horizontal; in the giraffe, the head is usually tilted forward and downwards, and so the position of the horizontal canal is arranged accordingly.

Being properly orientated in space needs more than that. It requires a visual as well as a vestibular input and it relies also on an input from the skin and the deeper tissues of the limbs and trunk. These inputs together form a self-stabilizing control system. As the evolutionary scale of animals is ascended, the vestibular system becomes less and vision becomes more important for the maintenance of balance. In fact we pay so much more attention to what we are seeing that when we are sitting in a stationary train and see the train alongside moving off, we have the strong impression that we are moving in the opposite direction. If we relied only on the accelerometers of our vestibular system, we would not get this illusory sensation.

Every movement one makes alters the centre of gravity and tends to upset one's equilibrium. The utricle, saccule, and semicircular canals contain the receptors that report the disturbance that occurs when we move. As movements tend to upset one's balance, compensatory action has to be taken. Certain muscles have to be contracted and others relaxed; the main purpose is to keep one's head straight up and the rest of the body in line with the head and neck. The computing mechanism that determines the muscular readjustment consists of the large masses of neurons within the cerebral hemisphere, called the basal ganglia.

The utricle and saccule are position-registering organs and are sensitive to linear acceleration, including gravity. The semicircular canals are sensitive to angular or rotational acceleration; they act like three spirit levels, set at right angles to each other. Unlike man-made spirit levels they are curved, not straight, and the fluid they contain is not spirits but endolymph, made from body fluids. (Incidentally, some aquatic insects do use an air-bubble, just like a spirit level; around the bubble are hair-cell detectors, which are displayed by movements of the bubble). Every movement of the head stimulates at least one canal on each side. When an acceleration becomes a constant speed, nothing more is reported than when the animal is still. If we keep our eyes shut when we are in a lift or an aeroplane, we do not feel that we are moving once the speed has become constant.

The balancing organs have one kind of receptor, the statocyst. In this fluid-filled cyst, the receptors are hair-cells. These hairs or cilia are embedded in various kinds of jelly. In the semi-circular canals, they are embedded in firm jelly that almost fills the canal. The receptor cells with their hairs embedded in the jelly are illustrated in Fig. 8.1.

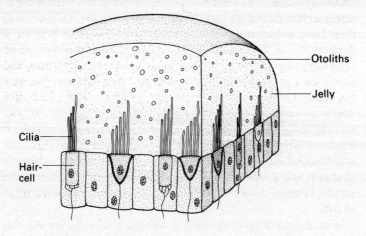

Fig. 8.1 The receptors used throughout the vestibular system.

The jelly of the utricle and saccule contains crystals of calcite; these are called otoliths. This jelly has the consistency of toothpaste. There are two kinds of cilia, a longer one called a kinocilium and many shorter ones called stereocilia. The tips of the cilia are embedded in the jelly and surrounded by the otoliths. The shearing movement between the cilia and this jelly is the stimulus that excites the receptor cells. When this movement goes towards the longest cilium, the kinocilium, the nerve fibres increase their basic rate of discharge of impulses, and when it is in the opposite direction, the discharge rate is reduced. Thus the brain is informed in which direction the cilia are being dragged.

In 1893 a physiologist in Vienna, called Kreidl, put prawns in an aquarium in which the ground consisted of nickel filings. During moulting, prawns replace their otoliths with grains of sand from the bed where they are living. Kreidl's prawns put nickel filings in. Then Kreidl replaced gravity with an electromagnet. He concluded from these experiments that, normally, gravity excites the hair-cells by pulling these otoliths down onto them.

Similar tricks can be played on fish to find out how the nervous system copes with two different inputs. Nearly all fish have a dorsal light reflex. This means that they automatically place themselves so that their dark backs are above, getting the full light, and their light bellies are below. The reason is clear. If you are a predator below the fish, there is a chance that you will not see its light belly as you look up at the sky and the general lightness, and if you are a predator from above, coming out of the sky, you may not see its back against the dark greyness of the water. Fish, like nearly all animals and plants, are sensitive to gravity. If you arrange things in an aquarium so that the light does not come from above but from one side, you give the fish a new problem. The usual relationship—light from above, gravity from below—is changed, and so the fish is faced with a disparity between two inputs. In man, this is a cause of sea-sickness, but it may not be so in fish.

With regard to gravity, when in fish the head is horizontal and in man vertical, the saccular and utricular receptors of each side of the head will be stimulated equally. When the head is tilted to one side, different groups of receptors on the two sides of the head will be stimulated. These receptors go on signalling as an animal is turned through 360°. They are position detectors. Other receptors of the saccule and utricle respond only at the beginning and the end of the tilting of the head. They are movement detectors. The effect of the input from the two utricles is to adjust the position of the head with regard to gravity and to the movements of the animal. The head then pulls the neck; afferent nerve fibres from the joints of the neck cause contractions of the muscles of the trunk, and so the posture of the whole body is suitably arranged to follow the new position of the head.

In the semicircular canals, the sensory organ is placed at the end of each canal. The canals are filled by two kinds of fluid, a rather viscous endolymph below and a covering jelly above. When the head is moved in any direction, this jelly remains relatively stationary, having more inertia than the endolymph. The difference in flow between these two substances bends the hairs and this movement excites the hair-cell receptors. The nerve fibres from these receptors are discharging nerve impulses all the time, whether the receptors are being excited or not. When the head is moved in one direction, the rate of discharge of nerve impulses is increased, and when moved in the opposite direction it is decreased.

The function of the semicircular canals and utricles is tested in patients by syringeing the ears with hot and cold water and by means of a rotating chair. Hot water causes currents in the endolymph of the lateral semicircular canal towards the ear being syringed, and cold water causes currents away from the ear. The effects of normal acceleration and deceleration are imitated by the rotating chair. These ways of stimulating the vestibule cause a movement of the eyes call nystagmus. This is a slow drift of the eyes away from the point on which the patient is trying to fix his gaze, which is followed by a fast correcting movement. When nystagmus is in an up and down direction and when it is marked, there is a movement of the eyelids at the same time. When the left ear is syringed with hot water, the stimulation of the lateral semicircular canal causes the eyes to move slowly away from the left; the patient compensates for this and moves the eyes rapidly back to the left. Stimulation of the left ear with cold water produces the opposite movement of the eyes. If the semicircular canal or the nerves connnecting it to the brain are not working properly, this nystagmus will not be normal.

You can see nystagmus any day by looking at the person opposite in the underground, when the train slows down as it arrives in the station; this is called train nystagmus. As he looks at something on the wall of the station and the train goes by, his eyes keep flicking sideways, while the train takes him past what he is gazing at.

Provided equal and opposite inputs from the vestibule of each side come to the brain, we maintain balance and stability without being aware that any of this system is working. But if there is any sudden disturbance of the balance of the two inputs, we get vertigo and nausea and we may walk as if we were drunk. In seasickness, there is a conflict between inputs from the eyes, the vestibular system and other proprioceptors; and above all, between the stimulation of these receptors by being moved passively and by moving actively. Deaf-mutes, who have not got connections from the vestibular apparatus to the central nervous system, lack the main component of conflict; and so they do not get seasick. In Cinerama, one may get seasickness. Here one is sitting still and one's vestibular apparatus is not being stimulated. But if you watch an aeroplane flying up and down or from side to side, you may get nausea and a headache. Your eyes tell you that you are moving up and down and from side to side and your vestibular apparatus tells you that you are sitting motionless. But you can also get travel sickness without an apparent conflict. Riding on a camel makes many people sick at first; in this case there is repeated stimulation of the utricle and saccule from the up and down movements of the camel's way of walking.

Your eyes alone cannot inform you if you are moving or the environment is moving past you. You have to deduce this by taking note of other inputs and drawing a conclusion. As you sit in a train and the train just outside the window starts moving off slowly, you cannot tell from your eyes whether you are moving or the other train is moving. You find out by taking note of the input from your vestibular apparatus. If either you or the other train is moving slowly, the cues may be inadequate; but if either speeds up, it becomes easier to tell. The accelerometers of your inner ears tell you whether you are being accelerated or not; and you fit this knowledge in with the input from your eyes. This examination of your position in the environment by comparing the inputs from different receptors is a particular example of a general principle:

our knowledge of the environment is worked out; it is a hypothesis, which we are continually testing.

At least half the astronauts get motion-sickness in space. There is no stimulation of the otolith receptors because gravity, their usual stimulator, has been removed. But the semicircular canals are reporting acceleration. There is thus a conflict between the lack of otolithic information and the information reaching the brain from the canals. This strange combination of inputs has never been experienced before and it conflicts with the stored physiological memories of consistent inputs from the whole vestibular apparatus. This situation can cause nausea, sickness, headaches, and cold sweating.

One of the American astronauts was a physician, Dr Joseph Kerwin. He reported his experience as follows: 'I would say that there was no vestibular sense of the upright whatsoever. I certainly had no idea of where the Earth was at any time unless I happened to be looking at it. I had no idea of the relationship between one compartment of the spacecraft or another in terms of a feeling of "up or down".'

In astronauts who had been away in space for seven or eight weeks, postural mechanisms were upset. This upset was perhaps the result of the nervous system soon adapting to a lack of vestibular contribution and then, on return to earth, having suddenly to incorporate vestibular inputs.

Man manages surprisingly well when he is deprived of the vestibular receptors. There is a disorder of the labyrinths called Menière's disease. If all other treatment has failed, the vestibular nerves are cut, and no more impulses from the disordered organ reach the brain. Most of the patients who have had these nerves cut are able to compensate for the loss of this input. One of the difficulties they have comes from an incoordination of the input from their eyes and the movements of their heads. Normally, as we walk and our heads go up and down, what we see keeps jumping up and down; but we are unaware of this. But these patients find that what they look at when they are walking goes up and down, and they have to stop in order to see things clearly in the distance. We would probably never have realized that there is a problem here if these patients with their vestibular nerves cut had not found it. When these patients shut their eyes, they have some difficulty with balance, and this is made far worse if they have to walk on an uneven surface. With their eyes shut, the patients are relying on the receptors of joints, muscles, and ligaments. They then find it difficult to walk downhill or downstairs. Once they start falling, they find it very difficult to correct.

Proprioceptors of muscles, tendons, and joints

Posture and movement depend on proprioceptors of the muscles, tendons and joints, on the vestibular apparatus and on the eyes. Every movement has to be correct for force, speed, and position. These aspects of movement are continously reported to the central nervous system; and the receptors that do this are the muscle spindles and tendon organs.

The tendon organs report the contraction of the muscle fibres. When the muscle is relaxed, they are quiet. When there is any pull on the muscle, either because it is being stretched or because it is contracting and pulling on its attachments on both ends, they send off impulses to the spinal cord.

Muscle spindles are named after the spindle used in spinning. They are in parallel with the main muscle fibres, being fixed to them at each end. Within the spindle there are two kinds of receptor, named primary and secondary; they are drawn in Fig. 8.2. The primary receptor consists of a thick nerve fibre coiled around a thin muscle fibre and the secondary is similar, the nerve fibre not being so thick. There are about ten of these modified muscle fibres in a spindle. They are thinner than ordinary muscle fibres. The nerve fibre from the primary receptor to the central nervous system is the fastest conducting nerve fibre in the body. Each one divides into more than a thousand little branches when it enters the grey matter of the spinal cord. The two receptors of the spindle send different messages to the spinal cord. Both send in volleys of impulses when the main muscle is stretched and also when the stretch has been removed.

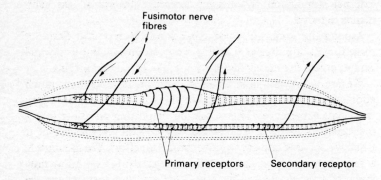

Fig. 8.2 Diagram of a muscle spindle. Two muscle fibres are drawn, surrounded by a capsule of connective tissue. The primary receptors are in the middle of the thin muscle fibres of the spindle and the secondary receptors at the ends. For the sake of simplicity, the secondary receptor is shown only at one end, on the right; all afferent fibres from the spindle are shown on the right and efferent fibres to the muscle fibres of the spindle are shown on the left.

The primary receptor is more sensitive to the rate of the stretch and it fires only slightly when the stretch has reached a constant level. It therefore acts as a reporter of the start and end of a movement. The secondary receptor reports a steady state of stretch; it fires off impulses steadily as long as the muscle is being pulled. When the muscle contracts, the pull is taken off the spindle and so both its receptors stop sending in messages. But the tendon organ is still being pulled on, and so it reports this information.

The sensitivity of the receptors depends on the tautness of the whole spindle and the receptors are kept taut by the small muscle fibres on each side of the receptors. The nerve fibres from the spinal cord going to these muscles are called fusimotor nerve fibres (the Latin for spindle is *fusus*). When the muscles are ordered to contract, orders are sent at the same time to the fusimotor neurons to make the spindle muscles contract; that tightens up the spindles, so that they can still act as measuring and reporting devices.

The spindle sends off impulses both when the muscle is being stretched and when one is actively contracting it. One imagines that the parts of the brain concerned with afferent information from parts of the body can distinguish between inputs from external stimulation and inputs derived from one's own commands to move.

Around the joints there are three kinds of receptor. Some of these fire off impulses as the joint is moved throughout its normal extent; others fire only when the joint is in extreme positions.

We are aware, at some level of consciousness, of how much effort we put into a movement. We know how much is necessary from past experience. This sensation of putting an effort into a movement is called muscle sense. We become very aware of it when we are tired and every movement is an effort. We use muscle sense when we weigh an object in our hands; for we know how much effort is needed to hold the hand out unsupported and we expect a certain additional effort when a weight is added. It is obvious that in such a case the effort we expect to put into it depends on our previous knowledge of just that weight. On first meeting a piece of aluminium we are amazed how the hand moves up to oppose the weight, for we are expecting to put out the correct amount of effort to counteract the weight of iron or lead.

Some people who are psychologically tense keep their muscles contracted most of the time. This gives them aches and pains and they may feel tired and exhausted. Further, they feel their own physical tension and that makes them feel yet more tense and anxious. These people may be making their spindles contract too much and continually, or they may be activating their main muscles. This constant contraction can be in most or in only some particular muscles. If the muscles of the jaw are kept contracted, pain in the face results or pain in or around the jaw-joint, which is just in front of the ear. Many headaches are due to constant contraction of the scalp muscles or the muscles of the neck. This muscular overactivity may be relieved by making the person aware of the fact that he is contracting his muscles and then training him not to do it. It can also be stopped by injecting local anaesthetic or just saline into the tender muscle, or by acupuncture.

When a doctor examines your knee-jerk, he is suddenly stretching the quadriceps muscle. This simple test is examining the primary receptors of this muscle, the afferent nerves to the spinal cord, the integrity and excitement of the local region of the spinal cord, the fusimotor neurons and the motoneurons of the quadriceps, the ability of the quadriceps to contract and relax, and the spread of excitability within the spinal cord which causes relaxation of the hamstring group of muscles, those that antagonize the action of the quadriceps.

If all the afferent nerves from the limb are cut, the person does not use the limb. The limb lies inert, just as if it is paralysed. Yet the efferent nerves are intact and so the limb could be moved. The continuous information coming in from the muscles, tendons, and joints is so important that the spinal cord and the brain do not move the limb unless this input frequently comes in. Eventually, the patient may learn to use the limb again. Not only are our purposive movements disrupted by cutting the afferent nerves but all the more automatic parts of posture and movement are equally disturbed. This cutting of afferent nerves not only may occur with accidents and with gun-shot wounds, it can also occur with certain neurological disorders. The most typical example of this is the third stage of syphilis. In this disorder, afferent nerves from the skin are cut through by the disease process, and the patient can burn himself and stick pins into his skin without feeling it.

Receptors for controlling the internal environment

Other variables of the body have to be kept within certain limits; they are monitored by receptors connected to the central nervous system by nerve fibres. These are the blood pressure, the temperature, breathing, the turgidity of the cells of the body, the chemical constitution of the blood and of the alimentary canal, the amount of glucose and amount of hormones in the blood.

The first and main way of controlling the body's temperature is the way used by all cold-blooded animals: the seeking of an environment that is comfortable so that the body neither gains nor loses heat. We are always doing this, whether we notice it or not; our newspapers are full of advertisements suggesting to us ways of keeping warm or cool.

The second way of controlling temperature is by having thermoreceptors in the skin, some of which send off impulses with constant temperature and others with changing temperature.

These receptors cause reflex alterations in the local blood supply and adjust the hairs of the skin to conserve or to get rid of heat. They also cause distant similar effects via sympathetic nerves.

Breathing is a fundamental activity which is arranged automatically and which we can also influence when we pay attention to it. There are four main controls influencing automatic breathing. It is partly controlled by stretch receptors in the lungs and in the bronchial tree. It is controlled also by the feedback mechanisms and reflexes used for the control of all muscles. The depth and rate of breathing is under the influence of chemoreceptors in the medulla oblongata which are sensitive to the carbon dioxide and the pH of the blood; and they are influenced by baroreceptors, noting the pressure in the large blood vessels and heart.

Much of the control of the internal environment of the body depends on chemoreceptors, receptors sensitive to chemical substances. Chemoreceptors for sampling aspects of the environment, those used for smelling and tasting, have been described in Chapters 5 and 6. There are others in the gut. One kind is sensitive to acids and another kind to alkalis; they are used to control the digestive ferments or enzymes needed to digest food. More important are the pH-sensitive receptors in the brain and the great blood vessels, which are necessary to keep the acidity-alkalinity of the blood plasma between narrow limits. To keep this pH constant, there are three mechanisms. In the blood plasma there are buffers; these are salts which are partly ionized and partly non-ionized, the two forms of the salt being in equilibrium. If an acid or an alkali is added to such buffered solutions, the equilibrium is shifted; but the pH of the total solution remains unchanged, as the added acid or alkali is neutralized. The second method of controlling the pH of the blood is to excrete carbon dioxide in the breath. If carbon dioxide is retained, the pH will be lowered, as this gas goes into solution in water, forming a weak acid—carbonic acid. The third method is to excrete acid or alkaline salts in solution in the urine.

Chemoreceptors in the large blood-vessels are sensitive to the amount of oxygen and of carbon dioxide present in the passing blood. If the amount of oxygen is reduced or the amount of carbon dioxide is increased, these receptors discharge nerve impulses at a greater rate. The brain responds by increasing breathing to take more oxygen into the lungs and to get rid of more carbon dioxide; it also increases the heart rate and constricts the smaller blood-vessels.

In the hypothalamus there are chemoreceptors which monitor the amount of glucose in the blood; there are others sensitive to the amount of the various hormones that circulate in the bloodstream. These receptors are situated close to the neurons that control the secretion of each particular hormone. The receptors sample the amount of the hormone that reaches them; and the amount of hormone to be secreted and passed into the bloodstream is then adjusted accordingly.

9 Nerves and nerve fibres

General features

All nerve fibres have two functions. The surface membrane of the fibre acts as a wire, transmitting messages as electrical pulses. The inside of the fibre is a tube along which materials conveying information pass in both directions. If we were to copy these two functions in the communication systems made by man, we would be using the wall of the water-pipes to pass the electric current of a telephone or telegraph wire. Yet the nerve fibre is more efficient than that. For this pipe passes not one but many substances along, moreover passing some in one direction and some in the other, and at different rates.

The peripheral nerves consist of bundles of thousands of nerve fibres. Some convey impulses away from the spinal cord towards the muscles and others in the opposite direction. Some of the fibres leaving the spinal cord are sympathetic fibres going to blood vessels, sweat glands, and to the hairs of the skin; they make these hairs stand upright with fear or when the body is cold and needs a protective layer of warm air around it. The fibres conveying impulses to the central nervous system come from the muscles, tendons, and joints; most of them come from the skin, reporting everything that touches the body, burns it, cools it, or affects it in any way.

Transmitting the message along the surface of the nerve fibre: conduction

> For by stroaking of him I have found out electricity.

The nerve fibre is usually likened to a telegraph wire; and the analogy is excellent. Both nerve fibres and telegraph wires are electric conduction systems designed to conduct messages rapidly over long distances. In both of these systems, the message is sent as a code, formed of pulses of activity spaced in time; and in both systems the pulses are of constant size and are conducted along the wire at a constant speed. In both systems, the wires have to be insulated; if the insulation gets damaged, the carrying of the impulses breaks down. Here the analogy ends, for the nerve fibre is more complicated than the telegraph wire. It is not just a passive conductor of electrical events; it is both the accumulator and the wire. In telegraphy, the current is carried in a solid wire made of metal; in the living conducting system the nerve fibre itself generates the electrical signal; it is a self-generating system.

What actually happens when the nerve fibre is transmitting impulses is a problem that scientists have been examining for over a hundred years. Before the First World War, Nernst suggested that the nerve impulse consisted of an electric current carried by ions through the membrane of the axon. In 1936, Hodgkin and Huxley at Cambridge working on the giant nerve fibres of the squid proved that this was right.

One of the main constituents of our bodies is a solution of common salt, sodium chloride. This solution surrounds all cells of the body and so it is called extra-cellular fluid. The solution inside cells is different, for it contains far less sodium and far more potassium. These two different solutions are separated by the cell wall or cell membrane. This membrane is selectively permeable to ions: potassium ions pass through with ease, chloride ions less easily, and sodium ions only with difficulty. The balance of ions outside and inside the axoplasm is maintained by the continual ejection of sodium ions from within the axonic membrane and by the continual intake of potassium ions. Owing to the different concentration of ions on the two sides of the membrane, there is a difference in electrical potential across it, the inside being negative and the outside positive. This difference of potential is called the resting potential. When the fibre is excited, there is at the point of excitation a transient increase in the conductance of the membrane for sodium. Positively-charged sodium ions then pass inwards through the membrane. This alters the electrical circuit so that the membrane potential is reversed. This process is then stopped by an increased conductance for potassium ions; this reverses the potential bringing back the state as it was before. These two events constitute the action potential. The physics of these events has been worked out, and it is even known how much current is carried by a single ion. After many action potentials have passed along a nerve fibre, sodium is expelled from within the membrane and potassium is brought back.

In the sensory nerves the action potential is started off by events in the receptor. For the function of the receptor is to change the energy that it takes in to electrical energy. It does this by producing a difference in potential, which is called the generator or receptor potential. The size of the generator potential is proportional to the strength of the stimulation of the receptor. When the generator potential reaches the adjacent part of the nerve fibre of which it forms a part, it excites the membrane, causing the action potential. The changes of the action potential take place in one direction only—ahead of the region of the membrane where these events has just taken place. The reason for this is that the membrane cannot be depolarized until it has been repolarized; the electrochemical events cannot be repeated until they have finished taking place and the resting state has been re-established. And so the little patch of electrochemical activity finds membrane in front of it free to be affected and membrane behind it not free to be affected, as the events have not quite finished taking place there. This ensures that the spreading electrochemical activity will pass along the membrane only ahead of the change in electrical potential to the part of the nerve fibre that has not yet been affected by these events.

These electrical events are always of the same extent, producing the same amount of current whenever they occur in one and the same fibre. A strong stimulus does not set up a big nerve impulse and a small one a small impulse; in any nerve fibre the size or amount of the nerve impulse is always the same. This is due to the size and physical make-up of the nerve fibre. But what can be altered is the number of impulses sent along the nerve fibre per second. Events are transmitted in the nerve as a frequency code.

Once the electrochemical changes taking place at the membrane of the nerve fibre have started, they spread along the fibre to its endings; they are self-propagating. This fact—that the nerve impulse is conducted throughout the length of a nerve fibre without being altered on the way—is an example of the all or none principle. The all or none principle states that an event either takes place or it does not; it is the same on all occasions and it cannot be altered in amount. One consequence of the all or none principle of impulse conduction is that when an alteration has to be made to a message, it canot be made during its passage along the nerve fibre. Changes to messages have to be made at the places where the neurons meet, where the message is passed from one neuron to the next. A corollary of this is that when it is important to take a message from one place to another unchanged, one nerve fibre is used. When it is important to influence the message, to let messages interact, then chains of nerve fibres are used, so that at each junction or link in the chain, modifying influences can be introduced.

As we have seen, one of the characteristics of a nerve fibre is the number of impulses it can send in a certain time; another is the rate at which it transmits the nerve impulse. The manner of conducting nerve impulses we have described so far is slow; in mammalian nerve fibres the rates are less than two metres a second. This way of conducting nerve impulses is used when rapid messages are not needed; it is probably used when continual impulse transmission is needed, as for giving a background of excitation or its opposite, inhibition.

Faster nerve conduction was not achieved by making larger nerve fibres with larger diameters. A new step in evolution occurred: the covering of nerve fibres with a myelin sheath. (A diagram of a neuron with a myelinated fibre is shown in Fig. 9.1.) The neuron must be thought of as being in three dimensions and the nerve fibre must be imagined as being far longer than is shown here. The myelin sheath is not continuous; it stops at regular gaps called nodes. One of these is shown at immense magnification in Plate 6. The myelin sheath is an insulator, like the plastic covering of a wire. In a myelinated fibre the action potential occurs only at the nodes. Depolarization jumps from node to node; and so this is called saltatory conduction. A nerve fibre with longer internodal lengths will conduct impulses faster than one with short internodal lengths. In large nerve fibres with long lengths between

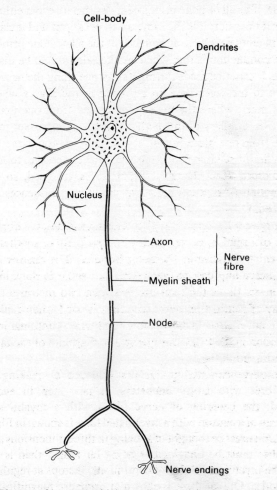

Fig. 9.1 Diagram of a neuron with its myelinated nerve fibre. Surrounding the axon is the myelin sheath, which is interrupted regularly at the nodes. The gap in the diagram is to indicate that the nerve fibre is longer than can be shown on the page.

nodes, the rate of impulse conduction goes up to 100 metres a second (225 miles per hour).

One might compare a nerve fibre with short internodal lengths and one with long lengths to a local train stopping at all stations and a fast train that stops at only a few main stations. It is obvious that the train stopping at many stations will be slower than the train covering large distances between only a few stations.

There are, then, two different kinds of nerve fibre throughout the nervous system, myelinated fibres that conduct impulses fast and unmyelinated fibres that conduct slowly. Myelinated fibres are used when information has to be sent quickly. The unmyelinated fibres are used for prolonged and continuing occurrences.

Nerve fibres used for conveying sensory information to the brain and spinal cord cover the whole range of conduction rates, with non-myelinated fibres conducting as slowly as half a metre a second and myelinated fibres conducting by saltatory conduction at 100 metres a second. The nerve fibres of the autonomic system and all nerve fibres to and from the viscera are small and slow conducting. When we blush, we do not do so as suddenly as we jump when we step on a sharp stone. It is unnecessary to signal with speed to our fellows our embarrassment or humiliation, but it is important to get our foot rapidly off the cutting edge of a stone. So fast-conducting nerve fibres are used for this and slow-conducting ones to dilate the blood vessels of our cheeks.

The amount of electricity used in nerve conduction is very small. Electricity is used in the body for signalling and not for power and work. The muscles provide the power. When they have received the small electrical signal, their molecules of protein contract and the whole body can be lifted by the muscles of one arm.

Local anaesthetics are solutions of various chemicals that prevent the passage of ions through membranes. In this way they block the conduction of nerve impulses and so the impulses that would eventually cause pain can no longer pass along the peripheral nerve fibres and so never reach the brain.

The electrochemical events that constitute the nerve impulse take a certain amount of time to take place; as one nerve impulse cannot follow another until these events have occurred, the number of impulses a nerve fibre can transmit is limited. This is one of the factors setting limits to the capabilities of nervous systems. Within such limits, the number of impulses transmitted within a certain time is very varied; one nerve fibre might transmit 500 impulses a second and another 10 impulses.

The disease of disseminated sclerosis or multiple sclerosis is a disorder in which there is damage to the myelin sheaths of nerve fibres within the central nervous system. Over a distance of a few centimetres the sheath of myelin is ruined. These nerve fibres are left like wires that have lost their coating of insulation. At first impulses can be conducted slowly through the short length of demyelinated fibre, but eventually conduction fails. The manifestations of multiple sclerosis depend on whereabouts the demyelintion has occurred. If it is in the optic pathway, then vision is upset; though complete blindness is rare. If it is in the spinal cord, there may be some paralysis or numbness or other kinds of disturbance of sensation.

10 Communication within the central nervous system

Neurons

The investigation of the nervous system by means of the microscope began about a hundred years ago. When the anatomists looked down their microscopes, what they saw was a thick, tangled mass of fibres. As they made thinner sections and teased nerve fibres out until only a few were there at a time, they came to realize that they were looking at two sorts of cells: there were neurons; and there were other cells, the function of which is to look after, feed, and repair the neurons. Once all workers had come to this conclusion, a controversy arose as to whether neurons were continuous throughout the central nervous system, forming a vast and complicated network, or whether every neuron was separated from every other one, with a gap between them where they met. This latter view is now recognized as being the correct one. It was the view of Cajal, the founder of the Spanish school of histologists. One of the ironies of history is that the contrary and erroneous view was supported by Golgi who invented the method of staining the nervous system for microscopical investigation, which Cajal used to establish the correct view, a view Golgi bitterly opposed. And in 1906, Cajal and Golgi shared the Nobel Prize for their respective contributions to knowledge of the nervous system.

An electron micrograph of a living neuron is shown in Plate 7. This neuron has been grown in tissue culture. A small piece of tissue is cut out from a living embryo and grown in physiological and germ-free conditions. Often the embryo used is the chicken in the egg as it is so easily available. The advantage of using tissue culture is that the neuron appears isolated and separated from a mass of nerve fibres and other surrounding matter. This neuron has to be thought of as being in three dimensions.

Neurons are classified as belonging to one of two classes: those with long axons and those with short. In man a long axon might be one metre long; in a whale or a giraffe it would be far longer. Neurons with short axons make a great many connections locally. One, first described by Golgi, is shown in Plate 5. This kind of neuron has several axons and each of them breaks up into many beaded branches. The cell body of a neuron with a long axon cut through and photographed is shown in Plate 8. When the cell body is cut through, some of the nerve-endings of other neurons on the membrane surrounding the cell body can be seen. This neuron is a motoneuron of a cat, stained, and shown by electron microscopy. In this photograph, one sees three circles: the central dark one is the nucleolus, the next one is the nucleus, and the largest and most exterior one is the membrane of the cell body. Outside the cell body, dark staining ovoids and circles are seen; they are small nerve fibres passing by the cell body. The nerve-endings, measuring about 1 μm across, are shown by the arrow.

One of the most beautiful neurons, called a Purkinyě cell, is drawn in Fig. 10.1. It is called after the Czech anatomist who

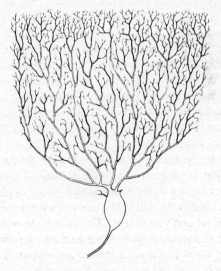

Fig. 10.1 A neuron from the cerebellum, named after its discoverer, Purkinyě

discovered it early in the nineteenth century. The branching dendrites, covered with spines, look like a flat fern. The drawing shows it in its widest extent; in the plane at right angles to this, the dendrites are slim, like a Lombardy poplar. On the dendrites of each Purkinyĕ cell, there are reckoned to be 120,000 spines. Continuing to think of resemblances between neurons and plants, we might see the dendrites with spines on them as the branches and the spiky leaves of a gorse bush. Each spine receives one nerve-ending. Passing through these dendrites are hundreds of thousands of nerve fibres, forming synapses as they pass. Other nerve fibres also connect to these cells; they spread around the branches before reaching the dendrites, like a vine. That is what the Purkinyĕ cell receives. A neuron that connects to Purkinyĕ cells sends its axons and branches to 300 to 450 Purkinyĕ cells.

One should think of the surface of the cell body, dendrites, and spines as looking like a mosaic. The little blocks of glass and stone of the mosaic would be the knobs of the nerve-endings on the surface of the neuron, and the cracks between the blocks would be narrow lines on the surface that are not covered by nerve-endings of connecting nerve fibres. The area of a cell body with its dendrites offering an anchorage to nerve-endings is very large. It has been worked out that on every motoneuron supplying muscles of the cat's hindlimb, there are 33,000 nerve-endings.

Neurons, being such long cells, are accompanied by supporting cells. In the central nervous system these cells are called the neuroglia; in the peripheral nervous system they are called Schwann cells, after the nineteenth-century anatomist who first described them. Nerve fibres are wrapped round and round by layers of these cells, and every nook and cranny between the neurons and nerve fibres in the central nervous system is filled with neuroglia. In the peripheral nervous system the Schwann cells make the myelin sheath; this sheath provides the insulating layers around myelinated nerve fibres.

Passing the message from neuron to neuron

In the central nervous system, every neuron sends out numbers of branches that end on other neurons. As was mentioned above, the place where a nerve-ending affects another neuron is the synapse. There, the message is passed on; and there it can be influenced, reduced, increased, or obliterated. The synapse is sometimes called a relay, for the message is relayed there to the next neurons. Between the nerve-ending and the cell body or dendrite, there is a gap. This gap is from 10 to 50 nm (100 to 500 Å) wide and is called the synaptic gap or synaptic cleft. Structures and events are named in relation to it: those before it are called pre-synaptic and those after it post-synaptic.

Neurons conduct impulses in one direction only. Afferent nerves take impulses to the central nervous system and efferent nerves take them out to the viscera, glands, and muscles. Within the central nervous system, impulses are sent away from the cell body along the nerve fibre to the nerve-endings on the next neuron. The nerve fibre breaks up into many branches and the branches finally end as twigs, connecting to one or to thousands of neurons.

There are two general patterns of connection between neurons: divergence where a neuron receives from a few neurons and makes connections with thousands of other neurons; convergence where a neuron receives nerve-endings from thousands of other neurons and sends its connecting axon to only a few neurons. The synapse is an arrangement for spreading messages far and wide or for channelling them down into a few or only one pathway. The more synapses there are on a pathway, the more modifications can be brought into the respon: es to stimulation and into behaviour. A similar situation would arise if there were only one road between Manchester and London with no possibility of turning off, or if there were a road with many crossings. If there is only one road the jourrney is quicker as there is no stopping at the crossroads; but it is also unmodifiable. Once on the road, you have to continue to the destination. If there are crossroads, the journey is slower; but all sorts of modifications and ways round can be made.

When the nerve impulse in an excitatory nerve fibre reaches the synapse, it delivers a standard amount of excitation. This is the excitatory post-synaptic potential. An inhibitory neuron does the same, delivering a standard amount of inhibition, which is the inhibitory post-synaptic potential.

In general the central nervous system is set at a high level of excitability and it is constantly restrained. When increased activity is needed, the brakes are released. The central nervous system has four general ways of acting: an increase or decrease of excitation and an increase or decrease of inhibition.

Single impulses are not the coinage of the nervous system: information is conveyed by volleys of impulses. Whether a volley of impulses fires the post-synaptic neuron or not depends on the kind of neuron it is and its state of excitability at the time. This is a changing state, depending ultimately on the chemical environment of the cell. Some neurons go through rhythmical phases of increasing and decreasing excitability; the neurons that work the respiratory muscles are an obvious example.

The impulses arriving at a neuron add up; the inhibitory impulses cancel out the excitatory ones. If a neuron is firing off impulses at a constant rate, the rate will be increased by excitatory impulses and decreased by inhibitory impulses arriving. The excitability of many neurons rapidly decreases if no excitatory impulses arrive. Both excitatory and inhibitory neurons tend to be fired off by excitatory nerve-endings and to be stopped by inhibitory endings. Inhibiting an inhibitory neuron is referred to as disinhibition.

The message a post-synaptic neuron sends on is not usually just the same message that it received. It may increase it by discharging impulses for a longer time than the duration of its input from the pre-synaptic neuron. In this action a post-synaptic neuron is more like an amplifier than a simple relay.

Some neurons seem to be firing most of the time; they do so to keep an adequate excitability at the synapses where their nerve fibres end. In such a case the neurons on which these nerve fibres end are ready to fire off and they can easily be triggered by the arrival of volleys of impulses. This is so with regard to the neurons of the spinal cord that organize movement. There is an ever present background of impulses coming in from the brain, keeping the system ready to respond to orders to move.

The excitation and inhibition described so far are called post-synaptic, as they take place on the neuron immediately after the synaptic gap. There is also another kind of inhibition, pre-synaptic inhibition. With pre-synaptic inhibition, the nerve fibre running to the post-synaptic neuron is inhibited before the synaptic gap, so that it cannot deliver its full quota of excitation. The inhibition takes place either at the very beginning of the axon as it leaves the cell body or near the end of the axon just before its termination. This kind of inhibition occurs on excitatory neurons; it is not yet certain whether it occurs on inhibitory neurons or not. Pre-synaptic inhibition can be so effective that it blocks all the impulses that would otherwise be delivered and completely obliterates the message. Most nerve fibres end up as many small branches, like the branches and twigs of a tree. Some of these twigs could be blocked by pre-synaptic inhibition, leaving the impulses to pass along other branches and twigs. This would be a mechanism for directing the excitation to one neuron and not another or to the dendrites of a neuron and not the cell body.

One might think of a synapse in the following way. Suppose someone is trying to lift a weight with his outstretched hand. The weight is the post-synaptic neuron and his hand is the exciting neuron. If you help him by adding your lifting power to his, together you might succeed in lifting the weight, whereas alone he could not have done it. In this case, you are an excitatory nerve-ending adding your quota of excitation to his. But suppose you push the weight down as he tries to lift it. Then you are an inhibitory nerve-ending. Whether the weight is lifted or not depends on the relative power of his lifting and your pushing it down. Now, say instead of pushing the weight down, you pushed his wrist down, so that he could not lift the weight up; this would be pre-synaptic inhibition.

The post-synaptic membrane is not equally excitable all over. The peripheral parts of the dendrites are relatively inexcitable. Excitation delivered far out on a dendrite may be insufficient to fire the neuron but it may just be enough to increase its excitability momentarily. In this way continually arriving impulses could keep the neuron sufficiently excited to be triggered off when volleys of impulses arrive nearer the cell body. Thus the nerve-endings on far-out dendrites provide a background excitability that is needed to make a neuron fire off. The spines on the dendrites are thought to be excitatory regions kept separate from the rest of the surface of a dendrite. This synaptic region has a privileged position, there being no interference from other arriving nerve-endings.

Some nerve fibres travel a long distance and then have just one or two nerve-endings; the nerve fibres supplying muscles are of this type. Others have nerve-endings throughout the course of the fibre. This is the common pattern of sympathetic nerve fibres. The railway analogy would be a train taking goods just from London to Glasgow for the first type, and a train dropping off goods at every halt and station along the line for the second. The actual number of endings along the line for a sympathetic fibre is 330,000 nerve-endings per cubic millimetre of fibre. This means that such a nerve fibre influences the structure it is supplying along the whole length of the nerve fibre. Thus a sympathetic fibre supplying the wall of an artery affects every muscle fibre it touches.

Chemical transmitters at synapses

As was said above, there was a controversy at the end of the nineteenth century and in the early years of this century about whether the nervous system of vertebrates consisted of a continuous network of neurons or of separate neurons. When it was eventually proved that the latter view was right, the question had to be answered how one neuron was connected to another.

The nerve-endings of any nerve fibre cover only a very small area of the post-synaptic membrane, for the nerve cell body is much bigger than a nerve-ending. This means that the amount of current a nerve-ending delivers is small. In synapses of crustaceans and fish, this current is enough to fire off or inhibit the next neuron. But in reptiles and mammals, a different mechanism has been evolved to increase the effectiveness of the nerve-ending.

Early in this century, physiologists had come to the conclusion that nerve fibres probably have effects on post-synaptic neurons by putting out chemical substances at their endings. They saw that the effects of injecting adrenalin on certain tissues was the same as stimulating the sympathetic nerves; and so it seemed likely that the sympathetic system worked by a similar local injection of these substances. Much research work has gone to prove that this is so. That the parasympathetic system works by secreting a chemical substance was shown by Loewi in 1921. The crucial experiment came to him in the middle of the night. He jotted it down, but in the morning he could not read his writing. Fortunately the idea returned during the following night. It was known at that time that stimulation of the parasympathetic nerve to the heart slowed down the heart beat and could finally stop it beating. Loewi stimulated the parasympathetic nerve to the heart of a frog, collected the fluid from the ventricle and passed it into the heart of another frog. When he stimulated the parasympathetic nerve, the rate of the heart slowed, as was expected; then the second frog's heart, receiving the fluid from the first heart, also slowed down. The conclusion was that stimulating the nerve to the first heart had produced some fluid that slowed the rate not only of the first heart but also of the second. This substance was later found to be acetylcholine. In other experiments Loewi showed that stimulation of the sympathetic nerves to the frog's heat produced a substance that increased the heart rate. It was not until 1948 that it was realized that this was noradrenalin.

In vertebrates impulses are passed from one neuron to another by means of vesicles of chemical substances. These substances are called neurotransmitters. They are stored in vesicles at the nerve-endings, and they are put into the synaptic cleft when a nerve impulse arrives. Some of them can be seen in immense magnification in Plate 9. One of them can be seen actually uniting with the pre-synaptic membrane, thus releasing its contents into the synaptic cleft. In the photograph, the synaptic cleft is so narrow that it is difficult to see. Of the four layers of membrane below the vesicles, the uppermost layer, which is nearest to the vesicles, is the membrane of the nerve-ending; this is pre-synaptic membrane. The other three layers of membrane are on the target cell; they are post-synaptic membrane. The synapse is between

..e uppermost layer and the next layer of membrane below it.

When the nerve impulse arrives at the nerve-ending, it triggers off a series of happenings. The first of these is an increased conductance through the membrane for calcium ions. Calcium ions flow from the extra-cellular fluid of the synaptic gap into the nerve-ending. This entry of calcium ions makes the synaptic vesicles unite with the membrane. The vesicles of transmitter are then released into the synaptic cleft. They pass across the infinitesimally small distance of the synaptic cleft and bind with the post-synaptic membrane. The place where this occurs is called the receptor or the target. Just by the receptor is a part of the membrane called an ionophore, as it carries the ions that take the current. When positively-charged sodium ions pass into the membrane of the post-synaptic neuron, excitation results; and when negatively-charged chloride ions pass in, inhibition results.

The arrival of impulses at the pre-synaptic nerve-ending with the emission of transmitter does not usually fire the next neuron; it alters its excitability making it more likely to fire when further excitatory impulses arrive. The mechanism of pre-synaptic inhibition is the same. Vesicles of inhibitory transmitter are put out by a nerve fibre onto the nerve-ending of another fibre. They prevent the second nerve fibre emitting all of its transmitter vesicles into the next synaptic gap.

Nearly all nerve-endings put out more than one kind of transmitter, many or perhaps most emitting three to five. Further, the membrane of the post-synaptic neuron, made up of thousands of kinds of protein, has various ways of reacting to the transmitters. Acetylcholine, for instance, can excite the membrane of one sort of neuron and inhibit that of another. It may have different effects on different parts of the neuron. A part of the membrane may react quickly and briefly and a nearby part slowly and for a longer time. Thus the kind of effects achieved even by one transmitter can be very varying. In spite of the leading role played by the receiving membrane of the post-synaptic neuron, some transmitters are always excitatory and others are always inhibitory. The most important inhibitory transmitter in the brain is gamma-aminobutyric acid, or GABA.

After the transmitter reaches the target membrane, it has to be changed so that it does not go on working. If it remained around, rapidly repeated effects on muscles or neurons could not be achieved. As a nerve-ending may deliver many hundred impulses a second, the membrane being affected must be able to respond to each impulse, and so the transmitter must be activated and inactivated at a rate of at least several hundred times a second. There are several mechanisms for doing this. When noradrenalin and acetylcholine affect the post-synaptic membrane, prostaglandin and adenosine triphosphate can be released; and they inhibit the further release of noradrenalin and acetylcholine. There are also enzymes at the synapse that can denature the transmitter. For instance, an enzyme breaks down acetylcholine into its components, acetic acid and choline; to all intents and purposes choline has no transmitter properties, being 1/1000th part as active as acetylcholine. In the case of adrenergic, noradrenergic and dopaminergic nerve-endings, most of the transmitter is brought back into the nerve-ending to be used again.

After the discovery of acetylcholine, adrenalin, and noradrenalin, it was concluded that the functions of the alimentary canal depended on nerves putting out these chemical substances onto the muscle cells forming the canal. However, in the nineteen-thirties, Gaddum and von Euler, working in the National Institute of Medical Research in London, demonstrated that the motility of the intestinal tract could still be increased when the action of acetylcholine was chemically blocked. It was soon discovered that the effects attributed to adrenalin and noradrenalin could also occur when these transmitters were blocked. Clearly, the original idea that the autonomic nervous system put out only acetylcholine, noradrenalin, and adrenalin was wrong. Further work showed that there was another transmitter used in the alimentary canal; it is thought to be adenosine triphosphate.

At that stage of knowledge, the transmission of impulses from one neuron to another was thought of like this. The neuron receives nerve impulses from another neuron or from a receptor. These impulses are received as quanta of transmitter substance. The amount of excitation the neuron receives depends on the amount of transmitter it receives within a certain time. It then transmits impulses along its length; this is done on the all-or-none principle. With each impulse, it emits a standard amount of transmitter to act on the post-synaptic receptors of the membrane of the next cell.

This conception needed some modification when it was realized that a great many non-myelinated nerve fibres, including those that put out adrenalin, noradrenalin, serotonin, dopamine, and acetylcholine, had nerve terminals of a sort along their course. For they do not terminate at one place but supply structures by emitting the transmitter during their course. These transmitters are put out by little bulges on the nerve fibres, called varicosities. This way of affecting the various structures is more diffuse, a solution of the transmitter spreading to a large number of cells in the vicinity. For example the outside coat of blood vessels is bathed in a solution of noradrenalin coming from the sympathetic nerves. In the alimentary canal this is the system of neural control that is used; and it is also used throughout the autonomic nervous system and in the brain. The varicosities are not fixed structures but change, like an orange being moved along a stocking.

In the last twenty years, this whole concept of transmission has had to be altered on account of the discovery of neuromodulators. Transmitters act by briefly changing the characteristic of the membrane of the target cell, increasing or decreasing its conductance of inorganic ions. They alone carry out the synaptic interactions between neurons. The modulators do not act by crossing the synaptic gap. They affect either the pre-synaptic or the post-synaptic membrane. They increase or decrease the release of the neurotransmitter or increase or decrease the sensitivity of the target membrane to the transmitter. They continue to act for a relatively long time. The transmitters work for a matter of milliseconds, the modulators for seconds or minutes. They can alter the size and duration of the action potential. Hormones acting on the nervous system reach their targets in the bloodstream, and they act for minutes or hours.

We now see that the amount of transmitter released by any pre-synaptic neuron may well not be a standard amount per nerve impulse and that every impulse does not have the same inevitable effect. In addition the standard amount of transmitter diffusing across the synaptic gap does not have the same effect on every occasion.

Although peptide neuromodulators are the most recently discovered elements in transmission of nerve impulses, they are probably at least 400 million years old. For man has the same peptides as fish and amphibia; and neuropeptides occur in plants that are older than any animal.

A few neurons just put out one peptide modulator, though most neurons put out many peptides together with non-peptide transmitters. For instance, the parasympathetic regulation of glands such as the salivary glands is done by putting out acetylcholine as the transmitter and vasoactive intestinal peptide, or VIP, as the modulator. VIP increases the amount of acetylcholine released and makes it more effective. VIP dilates blood-vessels and is likely to be the main factor causing erection of the penis and tumescence of the genital organs in both sexes. In some cases of impotence, the amount of VIP in the man's genital organs is below normal. VIP is also important in controlling blood pressure, for by dilating the blood-vessels it reduces blood pressure. There are other transmitters and modulators that dilate blood vessels, such as adenosine triphosphate. There are also peptide modulators that constrict blood vessels, such as neuropeptide tyrosin. Half of the nerves supplying the coronary arteries orarteries of the heart have tyrosin as the transmitter. This may be important in causing angina and coronary artery thrombosis or blocking of the arteries, with damage to the heart muscle. It may also cause the constriction of blood vessels that occurs in migraine, causing the disturbance of vision and other strange sensations occurring in one half of the body. What makes this likely is that this peptide delays the emptying time of the stomach; and that also occurs in migraine, causing the nausea and gastric upset.

When neurons are damaged or die, certain pathological states occur and we label these as diseases. As neurons produce their effects by putting out transmitters and modulators, we can in many cases supply these chemical substances to the patient and thus counteract the disease. The most successful replacement of this kind has been the treatment of Parkinsonism. In this disorder, many kinds of neurons degenerate. One of the main ones is the neuron that emits dopamine, an inhibitory transmitter belonging to the same series as adrenalin and noradrenalin. This transmitter is replaced by taking l-dopa. The patient finds that his stiffness is much better and his movements are improved.

In the brains of schizophrenics, the number of neurons having dopamine receptors in their membranes is abnormally increased. There is also a decrease in the peptide transmitters, cholecystokinin and somatostatin, in the temporal lobes of the cerebral hemispheres.

In the psychosis of depression, noradrenalin and adrenalin in the brain are decreased or else their functioning is disturbed in some way. This depression is treated by giving drugs that increase the amount of these transmitters in the brain. Most cases of depression are due to an inherited disturbance of these transmitters, though it is not yet known in what way they are disturbed or if they are secreted in insufficient amounts. Although there is this inherited tendency to become depressed or manic, it often needs events in the person's life to bring on each episode.

An indication that mental or psychiatric disorders might be caused by the absense or the wrong working of a neurotransmitter appeared when reserpine was used in the West for the treatment of high blood pressure. In India and Ceylon, a plant called in Europe *Rauwolfia* had been used for centuries by native practitioners of medicine. When this plant was investigated by pharmacologists, a substance named reserpine was isolated; it became the first effective drug for lowering the blood pressure. But an unwanted side-effect was depression. If quite normal people became depressed when they were taking this substance, then it became clear that the state of depression could be induced by a chemical substance, and it might be induced too by a chemical substance made in the body. People in general find it difficult to imagine that their moods and mental behaviour are due to chemistry. Further research on reserpine and related substances showed that it stopped the storage of mono-amine transmitters in the central nervous system. These discoveries opened up the era of the treatment of mental disease by drugs.

Transporting substances inside the nerve fibre: trophic activity

The nerve fibre is not only a telegraph wire; it is also like those vacuum tubes they used to have in shops which whizz bills in little capsules all around the place. But it is more cleverly designed than that, for it can send substances in both directions at the same time and at different speeds. This traffic inside the axon is called axonal or axoplasmic transport, or axoplasmic flow.

Under a strong microscope, particles can be seen streaming along nerve axons and dendrites in both directions. This is happening at rates between 50 and 400 mm a day; protein in solution is passed at the slower rate. Adrenalin, noradrenalin, serotonin, and some other transmitters are made in the cell body and then sent along the axon to the nerve-endings. Some transmitters are made also in the nerve-endings themselves. The enzymes made in the cell bodies that are needed for the synthesis and breakdown of the transmitters are made in the cell bodies and passed along the axoplasm.

The neuron differs from a man-made factory in that it not only makes a few products but it also keeps making itself. In the cell body it makes the materials of the nerve fibre for the surrounding neuroglia; it sends these substances along the nerve fibre continuously. Also material is taken along the axon to be passed on to the tissue supplied by the nerve fibre. If taste-buds do not receive this protein they disappear; and if muscles do not receive their protein, they turn into fibrous tissue.

There is also a passage of chemical substances from the tissue back along the nerve fibre to the cell body. This can pass beyond the cell body back across the synapse to the pre-synaptic neuron and even further back. A substance made in a muscle fibre could pass back into the brain or from the eye back to the occipital lobe of the cerebral hemisphere. This might constitute a chemical feedback system, the substance going back to the cell body informing it how much and what kind of substance it should send down the nerve fibre to the tissue.

11 Standing and moving

For God has blessed him in the variety of his movements.
For, tho he cannot fly, he is an excellent clamberer.
For his motions upon the face of the earth are more than any other
  quadrupede.
For he can tread to all measures upon the musick.
For he can swim for life.
For he can creep.

Plants are merely moved; animals move. Movements are brought
about by muscles, and muscles are made to contract by nerves
coming from the spinal cord and brain.

In general, small animals move more quickly than large. Small
birds move their wings far more rapidly than large birds, and the
largest birds prefer to glide and soar on currents of air. One of the
smaller humming-birds beats its wings eighty times a second. It is
very small, weighing only two grams. There is a very short distance between the wing muscles and the spinal cord, so that the
nerve impulses soon reach the muscles. In larger humming-birds
this distance is longer and so the rate of wing-beating can be
slower. One weighing twenty grams beats its wings eight to ten
times a second. The speed of flight achieved by some birds is
amazing. The fastest speed achieved by any animal is the 150 to
200 miles an hour of the large spine-tailed swift of Asia.

Each nerve impulse arriving at the muscle fibres makes them
contract once. This is so for all vertebrates and nearly all insects; but
wasps and bees, flies, mosquitoes, and some bugs, including the
aphids of our gardens, work their wing muscles on a different plan.
These muscles contract at a faster rate than their receipt of nerve
impulses. This system allows the honey-bee to beat its wings at a
rate of 200 to 250 beats a second, the mosquito at a rate of 580 beats a
second, and the midge that holds the record at 1,046 beats a second.

How fast can human beings carry out similar alternating movements? This question was examined by H. Hartridge, a physiologist, and James Ching, a pianist, who wanted to know about trills. They found that when they did up and down movements of the index and middle fingers alternately, they could do eighteen movements a second, nine up and nine down. The maximum rate for bending and straightening the elbow was eleven movements a second. The muscles themselves can work faster than this. The limiting factors were thus within the central nervous system and the time taken for messages to travel from the spinal cord to the muscles.

How the nerves work the muscles

Throughout biology one sees a few mechanisms and a few structures being used in many different ways; there is a general pattern with many variations on it. We have already seen how some of the characteristics of membranes surrounding cells are developed and used in different ways. The passage of ions through the membrane, some passing easily and others with difficulty, governs the mechanism of the nerve impulse: and at synapses this selective permeability to ions is used to excite and to inhibit the post-synaptic membrane. The warmth receptors of the skin which are used for controlling body temperature are used in certain vipers to detect the warmth emitted by their prey.

An example of this variation on a basic theme can be seen in the way nerve impulses are delivered at the neuro-muscular junction. For here, where the motor nerve reaches the muscles, there is a modified synapse. When the nerve impulse reaches the nerve-ending in the muscle, it puts out a small amount of acetylcholine, which substance unites with the membrane covering the muscle fibre. This is similar to a synapse in the central nervous system. The region where the nerve fibre joins a muscle fibre is called the motor end-plate. It is an enormously enlarged synapse, thrown into folds. The nerve-endings are similar to those in the central nervous system but they are far larger and are full of vesicles containing acetylcholine. When acetylcholine unites with the post-synaptic membrane, depolarization spreads along the membrane of the muscle fibre. From the membrane an electrical event passes to the muscle fibre and evokes a biochemical event. That makes the proteins of the muscle fibres contract. At this point, we take leave of the peripheral nervous system and enter the realm of protein molecules; that realm is outside the territory of this book.

The skeletal muscles, those you can see beneath the skin, are all cholinergic, being made to contract by the secretion of acetylcholine. There are many other sorts of muscle in the body; they make up the bladder, the uterus, the gut, the heart, and the bloodvessels. The muscle fibres that make up the viscera and the bloodvessels are called smooth or unstriated muscles, the skeletal muscles being known as striated muscles, owing to their appearance under the microscope. Every striated muscle fibre receives a single branch of a motor nerve. In the case of the visceral muscles, a bundle of muscle fibres is supplied by a single nerve fibre.

The muscle of the heart is controlled by both the sympathetic and the parasympathetic systems. The sympathetic speeds it up and the parasympathetic slows it down.

Reflexes for posture and movement

> For thirdly he works it upon stretch with fore-paws extended.

In biology and in engineering there are at least two classes of self-regulating systems--stabilizing and tracking systems. Both of them are used for maintaining posture and for moving. Two examples of stabilizing systems have been discussed so far—the balance of the body and the adjustment of the amount of light to the retina. A typical tracking system is following a moving stimulus with a rifle. Tracking implies that the target or reference input is continually changing; the output, usually including the eyes and head, has to follow these changes rapidly and accurately. In a stabilizing system, the output has to be maintained at the pre-set level. In both systems, the controlling elements have to be informed of what is happening. It would be useless to send out instructions without seeing that they were being followed. Feedback is an essential part of both systems. For moving, feedback is needed from the moving limb. The central nervous system has to be kept informed about the rate and amount of movement, about the position of the limb and its component parts, and about the force it is exerting. Feedback is not used throughout the extent of all movements, though it is used when one is learning a delicate movement, or when one is tracking. It seems to be the final stage of a movement that most needs control by feedback.

For certain movements, the skin is also an important source of feedback. When we feel something, we move the fingers and thumb and rub the surface of the object. These movements are partly controlled by the input coming from the receptors of the skin. There is also internal feedback, that is feedback from the groups of neurons organizing the movement, occurring before the movements have actually started and continuing throughout the movement.

Tracking includes aiming at an object not where it is but where it is going to be. You can observe this by going and playing with your cat. If you get the cat to follow a piece of string, it will follow it as you move it round the sofa. It quickly learns that the string is going to come round the other end of the sofa; and it then waits for it to appear and pounces on it when it comes into its visual field. This behaviour, based on anticipating the future position of the object, is quite different from following an object that remains in view. It is based on the knowledge or assumption that the moving object is going to continue in its course; and the co-ordination of the cat's movements is arranged to meet it at a time in the future, that is, future in relation to when it was seen disappearing round the back of the sofa. This remarkable achievement has been mastered by all hunting animals; obviously it was very useful during evolutionary development.

Posture is based on reflexes. The word 'reflex' was introduced in the last century by a neurologist from Nottingham called Marshall Hall to designate the response of a muscle or group of muscles to a stimulus that excited an afferent nerve. He explained that he chose this word as the muscle reflected the stimulus, just as a wall reflects a ball thrown against it. Since the introduction of the word a hundred and fifty years ago, the meaning has become enlarged and also more rigorous. It is now used to mean an inborn, immediate, stereotyped response of muscles or glands to a particular stimulus affecting the nervous system. The word is used only when the stimulus and response are simple; then, if the stimulus is known, the response is predictable.

Contrary to what people seem to think, reflex responses are not the same on every occasion. The response can diminish or increase, involving fewer or more muscle fibres, lasting a shorter or longer time. If one keeps on tapping the tendon below the knee-cap to induce the knee-jerk, the amount of response at first increases and then decreases. When it has become very small, it can be brought back to its original size by suddenly increasing the strength of the tap on the tendon or by stimulating the leg in any way.

All land vertebrates make use of the very force, gravity, that is pulling them down to the ground to keep upright. Pulling a muscle induces stretch reflexes. Stretch reflexes keep the head up and the limbs taut; they hold the abdominal wall and abdominal floor in, so that the viscera do not flop down and forwards. They adjust the amount of contraction and relaxation of muscles all over the body. A diagram of a spinal stretch reflex is shown in Fig. 11.1.

When a muscle is pulled on or stretched, the stretch stimulates the receptors within the muscle spindles. They discharge impulses to the spinal cord. The impulses end up on the motoneurons of the muscle, excite them, and they make the muscles contract. When the weight or the stretch is taken off the muscle, the spindle receptors cease to be stimulated, impulses from the muscle spindles no longer reach the motoneurons, they stop firing off impulses, and the muscle relaxes. Thus pulling the muscle makes it contract, and relaxing it causes it to relax. So that the spindles can be used as the receptors for stretch, they have to be kept taut; this is done by muscle fibres within the spindles. As was mentioned above, Figure 11.1 shows the main muscle fibre, above it the spindle receptor with the small muscle fibres at its two ends, the afferent fibre from the spindle receptor ending up on the main motoneuron. It also shows a small motoneuron; this is the one controlling the small muscle fibres of the muscle spindle.

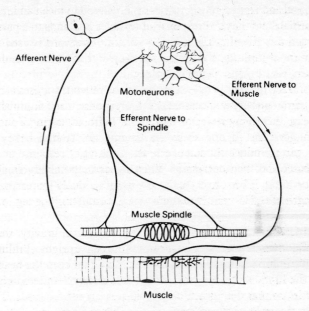

Fig. 11.1 Diagram of spinal stretch reflex.

This stretch reflex has only one synapse between the afferent nerve fibres and the motoneurons. Such monosynaptic reflexes are rare; for most reflexes have several synapses in the reflex arc. But this is the best-known of all reflexes, for it is the reflex examined when the doctor does your knee-jerks. In this case, the quadriceps muscle is slightly stretched by the tap on its tendon below the knee-cap. The stretching of the muscle fires off the motoneurons of the quadriceps and makes the muscle contract.

A new-born baby can walk if it is held up. Take a baby and hold him so that his feet are planted on a table. This firm contact causes a reflex contraction of the extensor muscles of the lower limbs; and it is so effective that the baby takes it own weight. Then lean your baby forwards and at the same time extend his head by pushing his chin up. He will then walk beautifully and enjoy it. This reflex walking lasts only about two months. It cannot be induced in all babies, so do not worry if your baby doesn't show it. Just change him for another.

There are other reflex games one can play with babies. For example, hold the baby just by a table; move him so that the front of his leg touches the edge of the table. Lo and behold, the baby reflexly lifts his leg and places the foot on the table. This reflex, occurring in many vertebrates, is called the tactile placing reaction. It too goes off in a few months as the nervous system matures.

Neurologists group the muscles of the trunk and limbs into flexors and extensors; in the limbs there are also adductors, abductors, and rotators. The movements of vertebrates are based on a pattern of contraction of one set of muscles with simultaneous relaxation of the antagonist muscles; this is called reciprocal innervation. This term means the contraction of a muscle or a group of muscles with simultaneous relaxation of muscles having the opposite function. Reciprocal innervation occurs in the eye-muscles when we turn our eyes to look at something. If we look to the right we contract the muscles that pull the eyes to the right and inhibit those pulling them to the left. One cannot turn one eye in any direction without at the same time turning the other eye in the same direction. Reciprocal innervation is organized at a low level of the central nervous system; and so this basic arrangement does not have to be worked out by the brain when it sends down a message saying 'Look right'.

Although reciprocal innervation forms the basis of movement, there is not always complete inhibition of the antagonist muscle. At the end of a movement, antagonists often work together with the main muscle, called the agonist, which is carrying out the movement; this is to achieve greater control so as to stop the movement at the right time and place. In fine movements such as those of the fingers performing accurate work, agonists and antagonists are used together throughout the movement. Also reciprocal innervation has to be set aside when one is standing, for it is necessary every now and then to contract all muscles together.

Following the vast amount of work that Sherrington did to elucidate the bases of movement, it was thought that every sort of movement was based on reflexes. But now it is apparent that this is not so. Forty years ago von Holst concluded that there was a network of neurons in the grey matter that generates an alternating or cyclic pattern of movement. He explained on this basis the rhythmically repeated movements of walking, running, galloping, hopping, swimming, flying, or creeping, the repetitive movements of breathing and purring, of feeding and chewing. He proposed that these movements were not reflexes as they did not need the input in the posterior roots. In experiments on fish, he demonstrated that properly co-ordinated swimming occurred after all the posterior roots had been cut. These are not simple movements as they need the correct timing of the fins, the tail, and the whole trunk. Further, they still occurred in a normal way after the spinal cord had been cut through and separated from the brain. Thus the mechanism for these movements must have resided in the spinal cord.

Mammals in which the spinal cord has been cut across cannot stand. But chickens which have had their heads cut off can run around the farmyard minus a head; their legs work perfectly, their wings flap in conjunction, and even their balance is adequate. The movements continue until all the blood is pumped out of the carotid arteries, and the loss of blood brings these reflex movements to an end. Snakes continue to perform their serpentine movements and move along the ground after their heads have been cut off. Beheaded eels are capable of all the movements of which eels are capable when possessed of heads. If a frog or toad is decapitated while it is copulating, its headless trunk continues to clasp the female, faithful beyond death.

These examples show us that the essential alternating movements of locomotion are organized within the spinal cord. This is so for all quadrupeds; whether it is the same in monkeys, we are not sure. The higher levels of the nervous system organize our walking. That is perhaps the reason that it takes us so long to learn to walk.

Accidents or disease can cut through the spinal cord, separating it from the brain. This leaves the patient with two separate central nervous systems. He has his brain and a certain length of spinal cord above, and the rest of the spinal cord below; and there may be no neural connexion between the two. If there is complete division of the spinal cord into two parts, the lower part produces no movements at all for months and eventually rather feeble reflex movements. But if there are any nerve fibres bridging the gap and connecting the lower part of the spinal cord with the upper part, reflex movements return and eventually become excessive. This form of paralysis is called spastic; the opposite form in which the limbs lie loose and floppy is flaccid. In spastic paralysis, many muscles contract simultaneously and so the limb may be held stiff. The reason is that motoneurons are generally very excitable. They fire off spontaneously and also in response to every sort of stimulation; and they continue firing for a far longer time than normal. As these motoneurons command the muscles of the limbs and the back and abdomen, the abdominal wall may contract and become as hard as a board, the back may be arched, the two legs held firmly pressed together, either extended straight out or bent up. In the normal undamaged nervous system, there are mechanisms that control this spread of excitation throughout the spinal cord. These mechanisms no longer work when the spinal cord is separated from the brain.

In the patients with the spinal cord divided, a condition known as paraplegia, the bladder and bowels work automatically, the patient being unable to control them. They carry on independently, as in a baby. When the central nervous system is intact, this control is organized by many parts of the brain. The front parts of the cerebral hemispheres are the region of most importance for voluntary control. When circumstances prevent us from emptying the bladder and we have to keep it full for an hour or so, it is this part of the brain that stops reflex emptying of the bladder. Like all skilful movements, this control has to be learned and practised. Using this region of the brain, we also make the bladder or rectum empty when we decide it is a convenient moment. Many other animals have acquired these kills. We may observe this in the dog. This animal uses urine to map his territory; as we all know he has difficulty in passing a tree or lamp-post without leaving his mark. The quantity of urine secreted is insufficient for this social use; and so we see the male dog cocking a leg and going through all the movements of emptying the bladder, even though there is no urine to pass.

Reflexes above the spinal cord

Although the basic patterns of walking and running are built into the spinal cord, there are many total movements organized above the spinal cord. For instance, there are reflex movements set off by sight and sounds. These reflexes occur at a place in the brain called the *colliculi* (the Latin word for hillocks). They are in the midbrain (see Fig. 17.1) and can be seen in Plate 13, just beneath the pineal gland. A sudden noise makes us turn our eyes and head in that direction. We do the same when a flash is seen to one side of us. This movement is arranged reflexly; we do not have to think about it. In the colliculi a single neuron responds both to the light and to the sound, and it responds very strongly when it is excited by both. But if a sound comes from one place and a flash from another, then the built-in reflex movement does not occur.

Whereabouts in the brain some of these reflex movements are organized has been learned from very deformed babies in whom all the higher parts of the brain have never developed. These babies can breathe, suck, swallow, and vomit. When the skin around the corner of the baby's mouth is touched, the head is turned round towards the stimulus, the mouth is opened; and if it is touched with a nipple, a finger, or a stick, this object will be sucked. A baby like this can yawn, cough, belch, and sneeze. It also can perform the reflexes built into the spinal cord. It empties its bladder and bowels, like a normal baby. It sleeps and can be woken up.

Many of the movements organized by the spinal cord and the lower part of the brain are working before the baby is born, as every mother knows. Some mothers-to-be have had a teacup kicked out of their hands, the kick coming from within.

Human embryos removed by operation can be kept alive for many minutes; and important researches on these specimens have been carried out in the United States. From these investigations, we now know that movements already occur in human foetuses aged 7½ weeks from conception. The first movement obtainable is a movement of the neck away from the stimulus when the mouth is touched. The 9½ weeks old fetus opens the mouth when stimulated around the mouth; at 10½ weeks, this stimulus produces swallowing movements as well. At this time it bends its toes and its fingers when the sole or the palm is stimulated. A little later, stimulation around the anus makes the foetus contract the sphincter muscle, closing this orifice.

Reflexes developed when the baby is still in the womb are all ready to be used after birth. The sucking reflex evoked by touch on the baby's lips and the complicated swallowing reflexes evoked when anything touches the back of the throat are ready for immediate use. There are reflex movements evoked by light. During the first few days of life, the baby turns its eyes and head towards a light; but if the light is too bright, it will shut its eyes. Within fifteen days, the baby will follow objects moved horizontally in its field of vision, first with its eyes, and then by turning its head. Within a few moments of birth, the baby turns its eyes, both together, in the direction of a noise made near one of its ears.

But the baby is not just a reflex organism. It arrives ready to explore. It explores the mother's body to find the nipple. Later it starts looking, listening, moving its arms out to touch and feel. It is active, not passive.

Reflexes are not just for standing and walking, for sucking, coughing, swallowing, and vomiting. For instance, there are flexion reflexes, having the purpose of removing the limb from something likely to damage it. If something very hot touches you, you find that your hand is pulled away so quickly that it has all happened before you know anything about it. By means of electrical recording it is possible to time the events in this reflex to an accuracy of a thousandth of a second. It can then be calculated that the hand is pulled away before any information reaches the cerebral cortex to tell you what has happened. If you tread on a thorn, it takes about a twentieth of a second for the nerve impulses to get to the spinal cord and back to the muscles pulling your foot away, but it takes a fifth of a second, four times as long, for the impulses to get up to the brain and return to the muscles of the limb. In a giraffe it takes even longer; it would take a third of a second for impulses running in the fastest-conducting fibres to reach the brain from one of its feet.

The organization of the total response to a painful stimulus follows the usual pattern employed among the higher mammals. At first, there is an emergency response, effective, possibly too crude. The event is then reported to the higher parts of the central nervous system, where it can be considered and fitted in with everything else that is going on at that moment. Further action is then taken. This takes longer, but it has the advantage that it fits in better with the total situation at the time. These higher level contributions are not reflex. They break through reflex responses and substitute something better suited to the whole situation.

Animals with fur or feathers have a scratch reflex, designed to remove insects and other irritants. The pathway of this reflex within the spinal cord is a long one, for something irritating the animal at the back of the head brings the hindlimb forward to scratch this bit of skin. The scratch reflex can easily be evoked in dogs by tickling the skin of the back or sides; you can often get it by tickling them just behind the shoulders. Then the dog stops whatever he is doing, distributes his weight on three legs, and scratches for as long as you go on tickling him.

Reflexes designed to take care of the body are organized not only for damage arriving from outside. There are reflexes to get rid of irritants already in the body: sneezing to get things out of the nose, coughing to get them out of the trachea, and vomiting to get them out of the stomach.

Changes in reflexes

Reflexes are not inevitable and fixed; but the very first part of a reflex may be difficult to change. They can be controlled, diminished, suppressed, amplified, and developed. This can be done by all those factors that we call mental, emotional, or psychological, including suggestion and hypnosis. The more neurons and synapses there are in a reflex pathway, the more modifications can be introduced into the reflex. We can do very little to change the knee-jerk and nothing to alter the pupil's reaction to light and dark. But we can train ourselves to suppress the gag reflex, the reflex that makes us retch when something touches the back of the throat.

The more complicated and delicate the movement, the more

learning is used, and the greater the part played by the higher levels of the brain. The highest levels of the brain can also control many simple reflex activities. The control of otherwise automatic reflex functions is a speciality of Indian fakirs and those adept in yoga. Reflexes can also be altered and controlled at spinal level. When the spinal cord is cut across in very young kittens or puppies, a great deal of compensation for this injury to the central nervous system can occur. With care and training these animals can be taught to walk and stand. The reflexes needed for these skills can be developed in these baby animals far more easily than in adult animals. Kozak and Westerman carried out some important investigations into the changes that can be induced in built-in reflexes of the spinal cord of the kitten. They showed that by rubbing the skin for ten minutes daily or putting a hindlimb in ice-cold or hot water daily, they could alter or suppress the built-in reflexes. This constituted one of the many examples of proof in the laboratory for what has been obvious to clinical observers for a long time: that patients with the spinal cord divided show similar changes in reflexes. Doctors and physiotherapists who treat these patients see many examples of how they can alter, suppress, and encourage various reflex postures and movements. They can train the bowels and the bladders of these patients to empty their contents reflexly in response to various forms of stimulation or to do so daily at a certain time.

Standing

Standing depends on balancing, particularly for two-legged creatures like ourselves; and moving requires even better balancing. We only have to move an arm or bend the head backwards, and we have altered the centre of gravity.

There are various servomechanisms that are acting to keep us in the upright position. What goes on beneath our conscious awareness can be brought to light if we fix electrodes over two or three muscles of the legs and record their activity by converting it to sound and playing it through a speaker. When the person is quietly standing, there is silence or almost silence. But if he is given a slight push or even raises an arm, suddenly a thunderstorm of activity occurs. Both the silence and the burst of muscular activity occur without us being aware of them. Like many other reflexes, these postural reflexes have to be practised and developed; the baby and the young child spend a lot of time doing this.

Standing is based on many reflexes. For one of these, the extensor thrust reflex, impulses coming from the foot go to the spinal cord and make all muscles of the leg contract together, so as to turn the limb into a rigid pillar. When the foot leaves the ground, the muscles of the foot are no longer stretched, the muscles relax and the limb becomes loose again.

When we stand, gravity is pulling on our bodies and limbs, tending to make us fall to the ground. But this pull on the muscles evokes their stretch reflexes; the muscles then contract and oppose the pull of gravity. Thus the very force that tends to make the animal fold up and fall is used to keep it standing upright.

When we are standing still, we are not actually still but are swaying slightly. This is controlled by vision although we are unaware that this is happening. For when one closes one's eyes, the swaying increases. When the sway reaches a certain degree, equilibrium is threatened; and then proprioceptors of the lower limbs notice it and they stabilize the ankles by contracting the muscles around the ankle joints and also the muscles of the thighs. These reflexes are not present in the new-born baby but start to occur during its first few months of life.

When we start walking, we lean forwards so that the centre of gravity comes to lie in front of the feet. This can be seen when one watches a mother teaching her baby to walk. She stands in front of it and pulls it slightly forwards by its arms. This displaces the baby's centre of gravity forwards, and it either has to take a step forwards or fall down. Both happen. Eventually the former happens more commonly than the latter. In walking, the foot that was left behind gives the propulsive force to move the body forwards. Then this foot leaves the ground and swings forwards. When it reaches the ground in front of the other foot the heel strikes the ground first. Then the weight of the body is put onto this limb. In normal walking both feet are on the ground together for about a quarter of each step; for the rest of the time we are balancing on one limb. The main difference between running and walking is that in running both feet are off the ground at the same time and both feet are never on the ground simultaneously.

The reflexes necessary for standing and stepping, including reciprocal innervation and holding the legs stiff as pillars, are organized by the spinal cord.

Once we have mastered the skill of standing, only very few muscles are used. The muscles are contracted just enough to correct the tendency to sway and to keep the centre of gravity in the central line of the body. This economy of the use of muscles is an example of the effect of practice and training. The more used to carrying out a posture or a movement one becomes, the more relaxed one is, the less muscles one uses, the less work is done, and the less tired one becomes.

There are some essential differences between a statue of a man made of metal or stone and a man of flesh and blood. The real man can balance, and if he is pushed off balance, he corrects the tendency to fall. All animals which walk on two legs, such as penguins, bears and men, must control the centre of gravity all the time, for it changes with every step and every movement of the trunk and upper limbs. One of the most impressive sights is that of an ostrich or a crane firmly planted on its stilt legs with its head bent right over and its beak touching the ground. But the less beautiful sight of a human being in the same position is really more astounding. For whereas nearly all the weight of the bird remains above its legs and feet and only a very small proportion is bent over in front, with human beings this is not so. If one bends forward with the upper limbs also hanging down, probably a half of one's total weight is hanging well forward of the legs and feet. Many receptors contribute to these postural reflexes. The final co-ordination is organized by the basal ganglia within the brain. When the body or any part of it is tilted, or when the ground is uneven, the basal ganglia arrange muscles to compensate for the changing conditions. The basal ganglia are always receiving impulses from the labyrinths. In man, when the labyrinths are destroyed or damaged, the eyes can compensate for the organ of balance. When the labyrinths are destroyed and the basal ganglia have been damaged by some disease, the patient needs his eyes even to keep his head upright; when he closes his eyes, his head falls forward. When the basal ganglia are damaged, the patient is liable to fall if he is pushed, as the compensating adjustments of the muscles are inadequate and late.

The contribution of the cerebellum

For he can jump over a stick which is patience upon proof positive.

It might be said that the cerebellum is an aesthetic organ—for the beauty and grace of movements, the astounding skills of the ballet dancer and of the daring young man on the flying trapeze are the contribution of the cerebellum.

The cerebellum looks like a miniature version of the cerebral hemispheres and so it was called the little brain or cerebellum. It is shown in Plates 11, 12 and 13. It originally developed to organize the information coming from the vestibular apparatus and the lateral line organ in primitive fish. In all animals it remains near the vestibular apparatus; and one of its functions is to co-ordinate movements with the changing centre of gravity and to keep the animal upright and in a correct posture. The cerebellum underwent much development with the evolution of birds from primitive reptiles: for birds' rapid movements in three dimensions of space demand perfect timing and balance.

Movements are controlled not only at the level of the muscles and the spinal cord; there is also monitoring within the central nervous system. One is aware of how much effort one is putting into a movement, without any input coming back from the limb being moved. It is thought that when a pattern of movements is intended or started by the cerebral hemispheres, a replica of the instructions is also sent off to certain parts of the brain. Certainly a part of the cerebellum is involved in this internal feedback. This copy of the instructions is called the efference copy. As the spinal cord is carrying out the instructions, it rapidly sends back information from the part being moved to the cerebellum and other relevant parts of the brain and this is compared with the pattern of movement of the efference copy. The two should agree. Visual, auditory, and vestibular inputs also go to the cerebellum. All of this information is worked on by the cerebellum and the result is sent back to the cerebral hemispheres.

The correct tension of the somatic muscles, called muscle tone, mainly depends on the cerebellum. For it has a great influence on the small motoneurons that work the muscle spindles.

Tracking movements based on vision are carried out by the cerebellum. The cerebellum makes an internal model of the movement which relates the components of the movement to where the target is just going to be. To keep the movement properly adjusted, it samples the error intermittently.

When the cerebellum is damaged or degenerates, the error between the movement being performed and the original programme of the movement is no longer continuously corrected. Further, the postural adjustment programme sent out from the cerebral hemispheres is no longer implemented. This is similar to when a person is drunk, for alcohol affects the cerebellum as well as the cerebral hemispheres. And so, with cerebellar disorders, the patient walks as if he is drunk. As he stands, he keeps his legs wide apart, giving himself a broad base on which to balance. When he moves, the movements are not performed harmoniously; the different muscles may not come in at the right time. The force and extent of the movement is abnormal; the movement goes too far or not far enough. The hand overshoots as he tries to reach for something. This is most marked at the end of a movement. The accurate arrival on target is replaced by an oscillation. His speech is affected in the same way; the flow of the sentence is broken up into short jerks, for breathing is poorly co-ordinated with the muscles of the larynx, throat, and mouth. If the middle part of the cerebellum is damaged, when the patient sits he tends gradually to fall over. He does not experience any difficulty in remaining upright, as the work, or the absence of work, of the cerebellum does not come into consciousness. He just slowly falls.

In degeneration or disorders of the cerebellum there is a tremor, rather like Parkinsonism, but even worse. There can be tremors of the head and upper trunk so that the afflicted patient cannot sit still. This is a prominent symptom of multiple sclerosis.

A patient with one half of the cerebellum severely damaged is aware of the defects in movement just mentioned. In addition, he is aware that his movements no longer occur unconsciously and automatically. He has to think about the movements and consciously guide them. Movements tend to run out and need restarting. It is like a car in which you keep having to restart the engine as it frequently stalls.

The contribution of the cerebral hemispheres

> For he can jump from an eminence into his master's bosom.
> For he can catch the cork and toss it again.

For nearly all kinds of movement, the cerebral hemispheres are in command. But in many mammals in which the matter has been investigated, the cerebral hemispheres are not necessary for walking, or perhaps one should say, the movements of walking. In Russia, Shik, Orlovsky, and Severin removed the forebrain of cats (shown diagrammatically in Figure 17.1). When they stimulated electrically two small regions between the midbrain and the pons, the animals carried out the movements of walking in a normal manner. As the intensity of the stimulation was increased, the walk changed to a trot and finally to a gallop. Normally, this region of the midbrain is subordinated to the parts of the brain that lie further forward. The higher levels command the lower regions to walk or run and they set the apparatus of the spinal cord off to produce the movements of walking, running, and galloping.

Innate movements, which are the same on every occasion, are organized at the lower levels of the central nervous system. They need no contribution from the cerebral hemispheres. Examples are the total movement patterns of crying, sneezing, coughing, swallowing, belching, and vomiting. Some other total conjunctions of movement are innate. A young child may throw itself down on its back, and yell with rage; it has never seen anyone else doing this.

If the organization of a movement is innate, that does not mean that it is present at birth. It means that it manifests itself without needing learning and imitation. In higher vertebrates, many kinds of movements are innate, though they become manifest only at certain times after birth. Walking, running, jumping are innate in man; normally they are learned with encouragement from others, but doubtless infants left to their own devices would acquire these movements on their own. Swimming, curiously enough, is not innate; for although all races develop it, human beings who have not learned it drown. Man's cousin, the chimpanzee, cannot swim and is frightened of water; he also dislikes rain. The orang-utan cannot swim either. It is not known for certain whether the gorilla swims or not; there are reports that they cross rivers. Presumably people in Thailand must know about the gibbon's ability to swim. Certainly a male and female gibbon I knew in Bangkok were not afraid of the rapidly flowing water of a river by which they lived, and they would spend a lot of time fishing floating debris out of the river.

Even complicated sequences of movements may be innate. Squirrels bury the nuts they do not want when they are replete, and press down the earth over their hidden treasure. Every part of this sequence of movements is innate.

Many simple movements that we take for granted have to be learned. We have to learn to move our two hands together and, perhaps more difficult, to do different things with the two hands. The baby has to learn to look at and listen to an object that is making a sound and reach for it with its hands, grasp it, and bring it to its mouth. After he has learned these skills, he begins to move objects around. It takes him weeks to know the feel of a cube or a ball; and this knowledge is not automatically transferred from one hand to the other. He then learns to manipulate the objects. Much of this is learned as the child plays. For children's play is not a mere diversion like the golf or tennis of adults. It is an important and essential part of neural learning. All higher mammals play and use this play to train both the sensory and motor parts of their nervous systems. One can see this occurring with otters, dogs, cats and foxes.

When we practise a series of movements, such as those needed for playing the piano, information about the movement, as it is being performed, is then compared with the pattern of impulses being sent out. Since all movements are improved by practice, it seems that the pattern of signals sent to the relevant parts of the nervous system must be stored. Otherwise we would be like children trying to do something for the first time whenever we tried to repeat a pattern of movements. There must be a kind of memory for movements. But we do not know how practice improves the efficiency of any skill. It is needed to acquire even those skills we learned so long ago that we have forgotten all about it, the skills of sitting, standing, walking. Practising must be done at the right time. Experiments done in the United States have shown that monkeys brought up with their limbs encased in cardboard cylinders never learn to use them properly, remain abnormally clumsy, and cannot acquire all the deft movements characteristic of their race. In such an experiment, repeated and necessary information has been withheld from many levels of the nervous system at a time when it was essential; if this information comes later, it comes too late.

We know from the various animals with which we are familiar that their young are born with every degree of prowess in movement. The new-born goat can stand at birth and in a few hours it jumps around and gambols. It is the same with the deer and the gnu, which immediately after birth get up and follow close to their mothers. Foals too can stand almost immediately and they very soon walk. The new-born dolphin can swim, it can remain under water and 'knows' to come up to the surface to breathe. The seal, however, cannot swim and needs to be enticed into the water.

Animals like deer which can jump and run at birth are taught to improve these skills by their mothers. Chimpanzees, orang-utans, and gorillas teach their babies to climb. Games that human children play are also played by deer and primates. Chimpanzees and deer play 'I'm the king of the castle'. Young chimpanzees play 'tag' or 'touch-last', and when they are brought up with human babies they play the pretence hiding game of 'peekaboo'; and they enjoy making towers of toy bricks and pulling wheeled toys around on string.

In man, the left cerebral hemisphere is the more important of the two for performing movements; it is the right hemisphere in left-handed people. The left hemisphere directs the right hemisphere to carry out movements needing the working together of the limbs and trunk. The right hemisphere is bad at directing the left. One would have thought that each hemisphere would have been equally good at organizing the movements of the opposite limbs; but it is not so. It may be that the movements used in emotional expression are organized by the right hemisphere.

Both hemispheres are used in planning a programme of movement. This takes place before the movement is carried out. It is as though your brain is thinking about the movement although you are not. While you are thinking what to say, another part of your brain is planning the movements of your complicated vocal apparatus so that you can produce the words.

Human beings use thought and planning, internal speech, when they learn new sequences of movements. When someone teaches you a new sequence of movements, say a dance or how to swing a golf club, he uses speech to describe and explain it, as well as showing you what to do. And then when you try out the movement, you speak to yourself; you say something like 'I have to move the right foot forward and then bring the left one up to the right one' or 'I must remember to follow through after I have hit the ball'. We use inner speech throughout most of our activities.

Certain kinds of movements develop only under the influence of hormones. Nest-building, sitting on eggs, copulating—these occur only when the correct hormones have their influence on the brain and spinal cord. Under the influence of the hormone prolactin, birds go through all the movements needed for constructing nests, though they may never have seen a nest or known what the finished product would be like. In species less developed than primates, the movements of copulation are inborn and do not have to be observed or learned; but they become more efficient with practice. They are inborn but they do not develop till puberty, when certain neurons react to the influences of hormones secreted by the ovaries and testes. No doubt those pretty movements of mother cats as they gently pick up their kittens in their teeth by the loose skin at the back of their necks are not learned but are inborn, though needing the secretion of hormones to come into play. And incidentaliy the kitten shows an inborn reflex, present at or shortly after birth, when it is picked up in this way; its whole back is flexed, as are its hindlimbs; the forelimbs remain moderately extended. Thus its hindlimbs are lifted from the ground, it tucks itself into a small space and when it is dropped back into its basket, its forelimbs are already extended to stop its head hitting the ground.

The effect of hormones on certain sorts of movements can be seen in such an everyday occurence as a dog passing urine. As we all must have noticed, male puppies do not cock a leg when they pass urine; they crouch a little, round their backs and lower the pelvis. The adult male dog's way of urinating is a secondary sexual characteristic; and it can be induced before the onset of puberty by the injection of testosterone. Bitches also acquire it if they are given this male hormone. If male puppies are castrated soon after birth, they do not develop the adult male posture for micturition; but they acquire it if they are given this hormone. It does seem curious that the position taken when passing urine should be a secondary sexual characteristic. Doubtless this is associated with the male dog's way of marking out its territory by means of urinary signposts. How the hormone affects certain neurons within the central nervous system to make them work in such a way as to produce a certain posture of the body, we do not yet know.

Movements organized at lower levels tend to remain intact when disease strikes the nervous system. A common kind of paralysis in man is hemiplegia. The movements controlled by the opposite damaged hemisphere no longer occur, though a few reflex movements organized lower in the brain remain. The patient automatically moves the paralysed arm when he yawns or sneezes though he cannot do so when he wants to pick up a book.

It is no mere figure of speech to say that we are weak with laughing; laughter brings the flexor muscles of our lower limbs into activity. Fear can also bring us to our knees. With these emotions, the body tends to crumple up, bending at the hips and the knees, the trunk flexes, the head and neck bend forward a little. Such movements occurring without our intending to do them show us that the higher levels of the brain, those we use when we intend to do something, are not necessary for all movements.

There is a rare disorder called cataplexy, in which the pathway from the parts of the brain particularly concerned with movements associated with emotion becomes abnormally easily available. Patients with this trouble fall to the ground when they experience a strong emotion. Laughing may weaken them so that they fall; you can fell them with a joke. If a patient with cataplexy gets so furious that he wants to hit you, as soon as his emotion gets the better of him he will fall limp to the ground. I once saw a mother of some young children who had this disorder. When she got so annoyed with them that she wanted to hit them, she just flopped down, unable to move.

12 Awake and exploring; relaxed and sleeping

Selection and paying attention

> For from this proceeds the passing quickness of his attention.

If one were to design a nervous system, one might have had the receptors signalling all events to the central nervous system and have left the brain to sort out this mass of incoming messages. The ear might report every sound, the eye everything to be seen, and the nose all smells floating in the air. A million impulses would reach the nervous system every second. If this input were not reduced, there would an overloading of the lines and the whole system would get clogged up. If much of it did get through, we would be too preoccupied to act and incapable of responding.

Selection is necessary as so much is going on. The sun is shining, there are long shadows on the far side of the wood, there are pine-needles on the ground, and a robin is threatening just inside his territory. But none of this matters to the deer, sniffing the wind and pricking up its ears. It selects the unexpected, the new smell arriving on the wind and it listens for the sounds that may come with it. The animal is alert, seeking information. It is also neglecting the great bulk of stimuli that arrive. Only some aspects of the environment interest us. If we are thirsty, we have to be looking out for water; when hungry, we must be searching for food. Our attention and our interest are arranged by our needs; and the need that is predominant at any time will make us attend to those aspects of the environment likely to satisfy it.

By using a tape-recorder, we can easily observe how well the nervous system selects what it wants to know. When we play back what we have just been recording, we will be astounded to hear a clock strike in the middle of it. We would have sworn that at the time we were recording, no clock struck; yet there it is on the tape. The tape-recorder does not select; it records everything.

What the brain needs to have is news, and news, as it says, is something new. The input has to be reduced as to allow important news to come in. This means selection. The nervous system needs to control its own input, to play up one input and to play down another. The first problem is how to reject the vast number of impulses arriving from the receptors so as to notice those that could be important. One has to bring out the signal from the background noise. This has to be done—as far as we know—by just two mechanisms, excitation and inhibition. Taking note of the important messages starts at the receptors. Nerves go from the central nervous system to affect the cochlea, the receptors of the vestibule, the olfactory receptors and the muscle spindles. The input from the skin is controlled as it enters the spinal cord. We are all familiar with the first element of selection of the visual sense organs, our eyelids. We can cut off the visual input merely by shutting our eyes. Marsupials can do the same with their outer ears when they go to sleep. Hippopotami can also close their ears like this and they use these muscles when they go underwater. Apart from shutting the eyes, we can adjust the amount of light that reaches the retina by altering the size of the pupil.

Inhibition is used to highlight an important input. It can reduce the number of impulses coming in so effectively that it can block out the message together. Inhibition can also be used to bring out contrasts. We discussed this occurring in the retina. This mechanism of surround inhibition is used throughout the central nervous system.

A pain will wake you and demand attention. Our various sensations are usually accompanied by feelings—surprise, familiarity, pleasure, or aesthetic appreciation. Touch and hearing are liable to alert you. If you are lying dozing out of doors, the smallest of flies has merely to alight on your forearm and you suddenly wake up and pull your arm away before you know what is happening; and how much more alarming it is when the fly crawls up your nose or into your ear. If we tread on a nail, one level of the central nervous system causes us to feel pain, to make us have an unpleasant emotion, and to localize the pain to the lower surface of the foot. Other levels receive the message and deal with it according to their needs, interpreting the information as demanding action, such as raising the blood pressure, constricting the blood vessels of the upper limbs, stabilizing the body on the unpricked limb and withdrawing the pricked limb from the ground. At a higher level in the central nervous system, the input arising from treading on the nail has more complicated effects. It not only is sent on to parts of the cerebral cortex for further analysis, so that the animal feels pain in the foot and can try and work out what has caused that pain. It is also sent to sensory areas for other inputs, hearing, vision, vestibular sensation. It may inhibit these other inputs, so that attention is focused on the foot; or it may heighten these inputs, so that all afferent channels become more important and attention is focused on every sort of sensation.

The distribution of the input within the central nervous system needs to be a changing one, continually capable of being redistributed. For instance, the passage of food along the alimentary canal does not usually need to occupy our consciousness. Our consciousness—what we call 'we'—must be left free to enjoy music. But if something goes wrong, if there is a traffic block in the alimentary canal, an obstruction, then the usual afferent impulses coming in from the canal are increased and finally the neural substratum of consciousness is made aware of what is happening. If we then get colicky pains, we can use the tools of consciousness —knowledge, reasoning, planning—to take steps to get rid of the obstruction.

Important work on the selection of the input was carried out by Hernández-Peón in Mexico and California. He found that if an animal's attention is distracted from one kind of stimulation and is turned to another, the size of the electrical response being recorded is decreased. One of the first experiments he published was done in this way. He recorded the nerve impulses coming along the visual pathway while a light was repeatedly flashed in front of a cat's eyes. Then he brought a tin of sardines up to the cat's nose or else he whispered something in its ear. When he did this, he found that the nerve impulses coming in from the flashing light ceased to arrive at the visual region of the cerebral cortex. When the smell of sardines was removed or the whispering was stopped, the nerve impulses due to the flashing light returned to their original number. These experiments could also be done the other way round, the visual, odorous, or painful stimuli obliterating the auditory input. When Hernández-Peón showed the cat the sardines or a live mouse in a glass, the auditory input from the repeated clicks was suppressed. It was also suppressed by the smell of the sardines or by a painful stimulation of one of the paws. From these experiments it was concluded that when a cat's attention is focused on one sort of stimulus, a regularly repeated and unimportant stimulus into another afferent channel is not permitted to reach the primary receptive area. There are also neurons of the cerebral cortex that react only when the animal is paying attention. If a light is shone in front of a monkey and he is not interested, some neurons of the cortex scarcely react; but if the monkey becomes interested in the light, these neurons become very active.

Hernández-Peón later carried out some of these experiments in man. He found that the nerve impulses coming in from the eyes were greatly reduced when the person was engaged in conversation, when he was solving an arithmetical problem or when he was asked to remember something. And what is more interesting, he found that when he suggested to the person that the brightness of the flashing light was being altered, the action potential he was recording from the brain was correspondingly altered. If he said the light was being made brighter, the action potentials got far bigger and when he suggested that the intensity of the light was being reduced, the response became less. All this was done without actually changing the intensity of the light. Similarly it was found that the volleys of impulses arriving at the primary tactile area or primary auditory area could be reduced by giving the person problems to solve or just by engaging him in conversation. Also the number of impulses arriving at the higher centres of the brain diminished when the stimulus is continued regularly and becomes monotonous, as had previously been observed in the cat.

When an event stops being new, it becomes less important and loses priority; the lines must be cleared for new events. For the nervous system, an event is new if it is changed in any way. If a click is repeated, the nerve impulses caused by each click gradually fade away. But if the pitch of the sound of the click is raised or lowered, if the click is suddenly made softer or louder, then the response in the cochlear nucleus is immediately brought back to its original size for this is different from the previous input. It may be important and so it constitutes the kind of information the brain wants. When this occurs at the higher levels of the central nervous system, it is familiar to us all. A monotonously repeated sound may not keep us awake and it may even help us sleep; we soon cease to hear it. But if it changes in any way—by dropping a beat, or by changing its pitch—our attention is involuntarily turned to it again.

With practice one can learn to neglect a sensory input. Everyone who uses a microscope learns to pay no attention to the input coming in from the eye that is not looking down it; one does not close that eye. I have already mentioned how one does not hear extraneous noises when recording something with interest. Similarly one can learn with practice to neglect a lot of nearby noise and to attend to what one is doing. It could be that the brain inhibits the particular input when we are concentrating on something else. If this is so, it is not that we take no notice of the neglected input; it actually would not come into the brain or spinal cord. Ballet dancers learn to suppress the input coming in from the vestibular apparatus when they keep turning rapidly. They use their eyes instead and avoid a conflict between the inputs from the vestibule and from the eyes and in this way they cease to feel giddy or to have nausea.

We have talked of descending control of afferent pathways to the higher levels of the brain without saying what parts of the brain exercise this control. Each primary receptive area of the cerebral cortex is able to control its own input, its own afferent pathway. For instance, the visual area of the cortex can control the retina and the relays on the visual pathway, and the auditory area of the cortex can control the inner ear and the relays on the auditory pathway. The sensory area of the cerebral cortex controls the input to the spinal cord arriving via the nerves from the skin, muscles, and viscera.

Throughout the centre of the brainstem there is a specialized mass of neurons called the reticular formation (Fig. 17.1). It goes upwards through the midbrain into the hypothalamus and thalamus and downwards into the grey matter of the spinal cord. This mass of intertwining neurons forms a part of the brain from the earliest vertebrates onwards; in fact, in the lower vertebrates, the central nervous system consists of little else than this structure. In the reticular formation, the neurons are short with short axons, and the dendrites overlap and intertwine. There are enormous numbers of these neurons, so that this neural formation is like a net, and so it is called reticular. It is a very slowly conducting system; faster conducting systems evolved later.

The reticular formation is concerned with the basic functions of living, with breathing, with controlling the heart and the blood pressure, with sleep and waking, with being vigilant and resting. To keep the animal alive in a world full of creatures eager to eat it and at the same time to keep it eating and drinking is the function of the reticular formation. It can influence what comes into the spinal cord and what is transmitted on to the brain. One of its main functions is the organization of sleeping and waking. It stops messages reaching the neural elements that underlie consciousness when the animal needs to sleep, and it allows them to wake the animal and then gives priority to inputs related to what is most important at the time. All incoming pathways, such as those for touch and hearing, send in messages to the reticular formation, so that it can fulfil these functions. In experiments in the cat, it has been possible to divide the fibres ascending into the reticular formation. The cat then stays asleep; only the strongest stimulation can wake it and it returns to sleep as soon as the stimulation ceases.

The incoming sensory input is distributed to the reticular formation in two ways. In one way each kind of input goes to general neurons so that any one neuron receives impulses coming from, say, auditory, tactile, and visual channels. In the other way, private lines predominate; a group of neurons receives only visual or only auditory input. It may be that the neurons receiving many different sensory inputs are a part of the mechanism for making the animal attend to everything happening or about to happen and that neurons receiving single sensory inputs form a part of the mechanism for focusing attention on one kind of sensation. The reticular formation of the brainstem and hypothalamus and thalamus (see chapter 17) excites the cerebral hemispheres and keeps the cerebral cortex active and alert. It also brings about relaxation and repose and prepares the animal for sleep. These two regions work reciprocally. When there is an increased input to the brain, the alerting system is activated, and as the input diminishes, the reposing system comes to the fore. The reticular formation also receives masses of nerve fibres from above, from the cerebral hemispheres. Presumably this is how thoughts, ideas, and emotions take control of both parts, either arousing our interest or letting us relax.

When the alerting system of the reticular formation is active, impulses are rushed down to the spinal cord. They go to the motoneurons of the muscle spindles, making all the spindles tense. This is like tuning the strings of a violin. They are then ready to be played upon.

This action of the reticular formation on the muscles of the body is present throughout waking life and also to a certain extent during sleep. People who are psychologically tense unconsciously keep their muscles active and tense; and those who are relaxed allow their muscles to relax. The activity of muscles in people about to be executed has been investigated in the United States. As would be expected, these people have most of their muscles actively contracting. Many anxious people are in the same state all the time. They feel that most conditions of living threaten them; and they react like those facing death, being anxious and apprehensive.

Sleeping and waking

For there is nothing sweeter than his peace when at rest.

Nearly all animals sleep; and no one knows why. Fish have periods of inactivity akin to sleep. The sea-mammal, called the porpoise in

England and the bottle-nosed dolphin in America, submerges when it sleeps but it comes up twice a minute for air, waking at each breath. When asleep, it keeps one eye open, scanning its environment. Snakes and lizards sleep with their eyes open, having no movable eyelids. Bats and flying foxes sleep when they are hanging with their heads down. Man spends about a third of his life asleep.

Sleeping habits differ greatly between the various species of vertebrates. Deer sleep for only very short periods, and then, they are deeply unconscious and can be touched without being woken. Sheep and domestic cattle sleep very little. It is usually thought that they sleep so little because they have a stomach designed to digest cellulose. For this purpose they have a special stomach called a reticulorumen, which is the first of their stomachs. For this to work properly and to empty, it must be kept in an upright position; and to keep it upright the animal has to keep its thorax upright. It must not lie down. If it went into deep sleep, the thorax and head would fall onto the ground, the rumen would not empty properly and the gas formed during digestion would not pass up the oesophagus and be belched out of the mouth. As domestic cattle spend so much of their time eating and the rest of their time ruminating, there is almost no time left for lying down and sleeping. Calves and lambs still at the breast do sleep, and so do very old cattle and sheep.

Hediger, from his great experience of animals in the wild, in zoos and menageries, concludes that animals which eat vegetation and which are the prey of the carnivores sleep very deeply but for a short time; they also copulate quickly, and their young can stand and walk at birth. Antelopes copulate merely for seconds, and their offspring can run within half an hour of birth. Bears which have no natural enemies, except for that universal enemy of all living creatures, man, copulate for hours, and their cubs are born in an immature state. The punishment for people who kill animals, one hopes, is that they will be reincarnated as antelopes and not as bears.

Even when asleep, an animal must be alive to danger; and so animals choose places to sleep where danger is least. And when asleep, they must be prepared to wake suddenly. The cry of her baby in the night must waken the mother, while the radio blaring across the street should not waken her, otherwise she will be tired and tense in the morning. Even the true lord of the jungle, the elephant, is very sensitive to anything moving at night. Hediger spent a lot of time studying elephants asleep in Africa, and in zoos and circuses in Europe. He found he could never creep about quietly enough not to waken them. When elephants sleep, they put their heads on the bodies of their comrades and even rub their hindquarters hard against each other without waking each other up; but they would always wake immediately a human being made the slightest noise. Many herbivores are woken so easily by noise that that is why, Hediger says, there are no photographs of ante-lopes sleeping; no one has been able to get close enough without waking them.

Horses normally sleep about seven hours of the twenty-four. They lie down flat for deep sleep but they can doze off while they are standing. The European swift can sleep while flying. Appar-ently soldiers can sleep while marching. This means that the neu-rons working innumerable muscles are active, as well as neurons of the labyrinths and the neurons co-ordinating these activities.

Sleep is not just passive relaxation of wakefulness. There are neural structures in the brain that actively cause sleep. When certain neurons are electrically stimulated the animal goes to sleep; when others are stimulated, it wakes up. The sleep-inducing and awakening neurons are scattered in many regions of the brain. They are in the most primitive parts of the cerebral hemispheres, that is in the front parts of the temporal lobes, in many parts of the hypothalamus, in the thalamus, and in the reticular formation throughout the central core of the brain. When the neurons con-cerned with sleep in the front part of the hypothalamus are destroyed, the animal no longer sleeps. In the epidemic of encephalitis lethargica that occurred after the First World War this part of the brain was damaged. These patients had strange disturbances of waking and sleeping. The normal rhythm was upset, and sometimes they would stay awake for hours, being unable to fall asleep. If these neurons are destroyed in experiments to find out their function, the animal becomes sleepy. It looks around for somewhere cosy, becomes quiet and relaxed, curls up and goes to sleep. It stays asleep for hours without these neurons being stimulated again. When the waking centre is active, it activates the cerebral cortex; the animal becomes lively and ready to face the world.

A Russian surgeon, Burdenko, reported a case of a soldier on whom he operated during the war against the Germans. A metal fragment had entered the patient's skull, and had lodged in the hypothalamus. When the surgeon, operating under local anaesthesia, tried to pull the piece of metal out, the patient immediately fell asleep. The surgeon then stopped as he thought the patient had gone into a state of shock. After a few minutes the patient woke up, and when questioned said he had had an irresistible desire to sleep. The surgeon finally removed the metal fragment on the third attempt; on each occasion when his forceps moved the piece of metal in the hypothalamus, the patient went to sleep.

Waking and sleeping still occur after the entire cerebral hemispheres have been removed or are not working; and they occur too in babies born without hemispheres and in patients in whom the hemispheres have been destroyed.

In the nineteen-fifties, a great step forward was made in our knowledge about sleep when Kleitman and Dement in the United States recorded the electroencephalogram throughout a whole night's sleep. It then became clear that only parts of the brain are inactive during sleep. Some parts are inactive during some stages of sleep, others at other stages. There are two kinds of sleep, rapid-eye-movement or r.e.m. sleep, and slow-wave or non-r.e.m. sleep. The name r.e.m. sleep comes from the fact that at this stage of sleep there are rapid irregular movements of the eyes behind closed eyelids. In this phase, heart-rate and breathing are fast and not regular, and the brain gets a greater blood supply than during waking life. Erection of the penis occurs in four-fifths of males, though not if there are dreams of anxiety. During slow-wave sleep, the heart beats slowly and regularly and breathing is slow. The deepest phase is reached after about half to one hour. After we have spent about one to one-and-a-half hours in this phase, the first phase of r.e.m. sleep arrives. During a night there are four to six periods of r.e.m. sleep, each lasting between ten and thirty minutes. Young adults spend up to a quarter of their sleep in the r.e.m. phase; babies spend far longer and old people far less. Old people spend less time in the phase of slow-wave sleep. These two phases of sleep depend on different transmitters in the brain: r.e.m. sleep depends on acetylcholine, and slow-wave sleep on dopamine.

An interesting experiment was carried out in the United States showing that the r.e.m. phase is related to higher cerebral activity. A group of people wore inverting spectacles all day long. Inverting spectacles make the whole world appear upside down. This extraordinary change in the experiencing of the environment demands constant adaptation and learning. During this time of learning, these people spent a longer part of their nights in r.e.m. sleep.

If people are woken during the r.e.m. stage of sleep—this is recognized by continuous recording of the electroencephalograph —they nearly always say that they were in the middle of dreaming. It is not known whether this means that dreaming occurs mainly during r.e.m. sleep, or if it means that dreams are remembered during this stage and forgotten during deeper sleep. In either case, it is obvious that we remember only the merest fragments of our dreams, the parts occurring just before we wake up.

Talking in one's sleep, the night-terrors of childhood, and sleep-walking occur during non-r.e.m. sleep. Lady Macbeth was not alone in seeming to be looking for something nor in talking when she walked in her sleep; both are common in sleep-walkers. If the sleep-walker is woken, he is not dreaming at the time and he can recall nothing.

Cats have more r.e.m. sleep than man; but reptiles do not have r.e.m. sleep. Birds have r.e.m. sleep for about a second and spend less than one per cent of their sleeping time in r.e.m. sleep.

R.e.m. sleep is not an equivalent of visual dreaming even though rapid eye movements are such a conspicuous feature. For r.e.m. sleep is most developed at birth, and at this time there is no visual imagery. New-born kittens have a lot of r.e.m. sleep before their eyes are open. And men who have had their entire cerebral hemispheres damaged by head injury or disease have r.e.m. sleep.

One can be certain that other mammals than man dream. They show the same r.e.m. sleep. Before the electroencephalograph was used to investigate sleep, many experiments had been done on animals' dreaming. For example, sausages were put in front of the noses of sleeping dogs, in Germany, of course; the dogs would then make chewing movements and wrinkle the skin around their mouths. Records have been kept of the movements sleeping puppies make from the moment of birth. At the end of the first week, they made lip-smacking and sucking noises; later they snarl and utter minimal barks; later still they make running movements.

Sleep is upset in many diseases, but there is one disease that is really a disorder of sleep. This is narcolepsy; it occurs with cataplexy, which was mentioned at the end of Chapter 11. Patients with this complaint have to go to sleep during the day; this may happen for periods of five to fifteen minutes six or seven times a day. From each little nap they wake up quite restored. These patients fall off to sleep very quickly and their sleep is restless and disturbed. They may walk in their sleep. And some of them have short periods of waking during the night just as they have periods of sleep during the day.

There is another rare disorder of sleep called sleep paralysis. Nurses on night duty occasionally have this. When the person with this disorder is tired, tending to fall asleep, or if they suddenly wake up, they go to move and find they are quite unable to move even a finger. This total paralysis lasts from a few seconds to a few minutes. During this time, they may be very frightened and can have visual or auditory hallucinations, like dreams.

One of the tortures used by governments of all civilized countries is to deprive their victims of sleep. If one is prevented from sleeping for three days and nights, one tends to get a temporary psychosis, hallucinations, and paranoid delusions. This state is induced on purpose by brainwashers.

Most people wake every morning at about the same time. At this time sleep is light, and it may be that the daily visual and auditory stimuli wake us. But this is not the whole matter; for these stimuli have all the insignificance of familiarity. In winter it may be dark, in summer light. Most remarkable is our ability to wake ourselves automatically at some unusual early hour, say five o'clock. This is not a perfect mechanism, for usually we wake before this set time and keep waking ourselves up several times before five; and then the final waking may occur after five. It is likely that the parts of our brains concerned in the waking are the cerebral cortex and part of the reticular formation concerned with alerting the brain. But how one sets this mechanism going, no one knows.

13 Needs, desires, and emotions

For he will not do destruction, if he is well-fed, neither will he spit without provocation

During the last quarter of a century, a new science has been evolved: ethology, the study of animal behaviour. It is related to the anatomy and physiology of the nervous system, as any science of psychology has to be.

Just as, a hundred years ago, Freud had uncovered his ears and listened to his patients, so Konrad Lorenz opened his eyes and looked at the animals around him. What he saw was animals imbued with energy, inquisitive, active, always busy, and each one preoccupied with the others of its group. That is all obvious to anyone who looks at animals without having had any training in a psychological laboratory. But at the time Lorenz began observing the animals among whom he lived, psychologists regarded animal behaviour as consisting of chains of reflexes or as being responses to stimulation. In reality, motivation comes from within. The brain leads the animal to seek from its environment the things that are necessary for its survival. The brain gives the animal its appetites and makes it carry out acts of behaviour designed to satisfy them. It translates needs into desires. People think of the brain as the organ of the mind, as the source of the intellect, of thinking, of ideas. It is all that, and it is much else besides. It is mainly the organ of motivation, the part of ourselves that makes us do everything we do.

Lorenz thought of animal motivation in the following way. There are certain basic instincts, each with energy at its disposal. The energy mounts up until it is discharged; after it has been discharged in the consummatory act, it gradually builds up again. And this cycle of damming and discharging of instinctive energy makes animals spend their time seeking the stimulation that will discharge the energy. The necessity for discharging instinctive energy is what makes animals active and inquisitive, so that they move around the world exposing themselves to danger. There are cues that serve to make them discharge this instinctive energy in an act, named 'releasers'. As the fulfilment of desires is pleasant and the inability to fulfil them is unpleasant, animals learn by a natural system of rewards and punishments.

The animal's desire or need to perform certain acts of behaviour differs at various times. One factor causing the difference is the amount of hormones circulating in its body and affecting its tissues, including its brain. Depending on the presence of hormones, features of the environment may stimulate the animal or they may evoke no interest. From the animal's point of view, the stimulus is not the same on every occasion; it depends on its internal state. If we present a male trap-door spider to the female, we might imagine that this stimulus is always the same, being the male of the species. However, the response of the female spider to this constant stimulus varies a great deal. She may live contentedly with him for several months, she may live with him for only a day or two, or she may eat him straight away, rather than await the inevitable tedium of married life. The male never knows what sort of reception he is going to get; he may be invited to the marriage bed or he may be invited to a supper, not to eat but to be eaten. The same stimulus—male trap-door spider—releases different behaviour in the female, depending on factors within, such as whether she is ready to mate or whether she has recently mated.

The more important the stimulus from the world without, the less motivation there need be from within, and vice versa. When there is much motivation, an otherwise inadequate stimulus from the environment will suffice. Or if any kind of releasing mechanism fails to be found in the outside world, the total innate reaction can be manifested spontaneously without being triggered off by stimulation. This behaviour, reaction to a stimulus which is absent, is called vacuum activity or reaction to deprivation. Such vacuum activities have often been observed in birds and other animals reared apart from their fellows, and so there is no question of them having been learned. The existence of vacuum activities shows us that such acts of behaviour are innate and inherited.

Lorenz has reported instances of whole episodes of behaviour being manifested in the absence of the essential stimulus. He had a starling brought up in captivity and accustomed to receiving its food from a dish. This bird would fly up and carry out the complete motions of catching a non-existent fly; it would focus on it, swoop on it, apparently catch it, and swallow it. It had never seen another bird catch an insect. Waxwings have been seen catching non-existent insects during frosty weather, when no insects are around. Similar *in vacuo* behaviour has been seen in hummingbirds. They fasten non-existent materials for nest-building to non-existent twigs. Whether the birds are actually experiencing hallucinations of the missing objects, we do not know. We do know, however, that humans under conditions of maximal deprivation often do have hallucinations; these are a sort of mirage, supplied by the imagination, driven by need. It may be that dreams should be considered as such hallucinations. Hallucinations satisfy to some extent, and that perhaps is their purpose and the reason for their existence.

When a drive has recently been adequately satisfied, the stimulus must be ideal in every respect to serve as a releaser of behaviour. Even then, only a token reaction may be produced. A correct stimulus no longer works when the need for it is absent. Once the need has been satisfied, the animal will not respond to the very stimulus that previously evoked the response. For instance, a stimulus that gives rise to certain behaviour during the breeding season is meaningless and causes no response when it occurs at other times. This is common observation. When we have just finished eating a meal, another excellent meal placed in front of us evokes different behaviour from when we were hungry. Sexual stimulation that would evoke copulation in the male when he has not copulated for a long time does not do so when it occurs shortly after several copulations. Thus satiety reduces or stops the drive and the desire; but only for a time.

Among human beings, consciousness is used in the continuous seeking to satisfy needs. How far it is used in other animals, we do not know. Obviously it is used by the animals we know best, dogs

and cats, tigers, lions, and elephants. Because we use consciousness, we tend to overvalue conscious awareness, thought, and
planning; and we find it difficult to imagine how an animal acts
effectively without this conscious thinking.

Professor Richter at Johns Hopkins University in Baltimore
devoted many years to the study of animals choosing a correct diet.
He deprived rats of an essential ingredient, for example vitamin
B1 or calcium. The animals were then put in a kind of self-service
shop. He and his colleagues would observe what foods and how
much of them the rats chose. From these investigations we have
learned that animals choose those foods that supply the elements
that they need. If a rat is deprived of a certain vitamin, it would
choose foods rich in that vitamin. Female rats would take a lot
more fat when they were lactating; the amount reverted to average
when the litter was weaned. When rats were provided with pure
protein, starch, sugar, fats, and vitamins, all substances previously
unknown to them, they chose a well-balanced diet. Richter also did
experiments in which he upset the animal's metabolism by removing some endocrine glands. When the parathyroid glands are cut
out, the body loses its calcium and retains too much phosphorus.
Richter found that those rats in which the gland had been cut out
had a craving for calcium and a diminished appetite for phosphorus. Pregnant rats choose a particular diet; they take an
increased amount of calcium, phosphorus, protein, and fat, all of
which they need to build the foetus and to produce milk.

In these examples, we are observing how the animal's need
induce its desires. We do not know how this comes about; but we
know that it does so through its taste receptors. If the nerves
coming to the brain from these receptors are divided, the rat no
longer makes these life-saving choices in its diet. In the case of salt-
depletion, brought about by removal of the adrenal glands, Richter found that the rats had a lower threshold for the taste of salt;
they were able to taste salt dissolved in water when the concentration was fifteen times less than that which normal rats could taste.

If a rat gets nausea from any taste, it will always avoid that taste
in the future; one trial is enough to put it off. If can even be put off
tastes that it usually likes, such as sugar. It is therefore difficult to

kill rats by poisoning them. Richter found that rats could be poisoned only when the poison was so well mixed with the food that its taste was masked or when the poison was insoluble in saliva so as to be tasteless.

Similar mechanisms, whatever they are, operate in human beings; or rather, they tend to until they are altered by implanted social influences. That untrammelled human infants act like this is known from a few cases reported in the medical literature. A particularly striking case was reported by Richter and Wilkins in Baltimore. A little boy, aged three and a half, had been born with a great deficiency of the adrenal glands. This had the effect of upsetting the body's control of its salts so that the child was constantly deficient in sodium, the most important element of all. The boy had a natural craving for sodium chloride, common salt. From the age of one, he had always taken large amounts of salt. At this age, the little boy started licking the salt off pretzels. He would chew salt biscuits and bacon; after he had got the salt out of them, he would spit the rest out. He eventually discovered the salt in the salt shaker, and then showed a great appetite for it. His mother reported to the doctor what had happened when the child was eighteen months old. 'When I would feed him his dinner at noon, he would keep crying for something that wasn't on the table and always pointed to the cupboard. I didn't think of the salt, so I held him up in front of the cupboard to see what he wanted. He picked out the salt at once; and in order to see what he would do with it, I let him have it. He poured some out and ate it by dipping his finger in it. After this he wouldn't eat any food without having the salt too. I would purposely let it off the table and even hide it from him until I could ask the doctor about it. For it seemed to us like he ate a terrible lot of plain salt . . . After we gave it to him all the time he usually didn't ask for it with his dinner; but he wouldn't eat his breakfast or supper without it. He really cried for it and acted like he had to have it.' All the foods the boy liked were salty ones. And interestingly enough, the first word he learned to say was salt. He took a lot of water too, which he also needed. The sad end to this tale is that when the little boy was taken into hospital, he was given an ordinary diet, with no extra salt; and he died.

The behaviour of this little boy, not only so sensible but so necessary, comes as a surprise. We think of the brain as being able to plan the future, making use of its experience of the past. But that the brain should possess this kind of intuitive or instinctive knowledge comes as a surprise. We always overestimate consciousness. It is unnecessary for animals to know the purpose of their activities; all that is needed is that they should behave in the right way.

How the animal's needs come to cause its appetite is a large subject which is still being investigated. The physiological mechanisms differ for different needs and among different species. In higher mammals both hunger and the sensation of feeling full depend on receptors in the stomach and on the concentration of glucose in the blood. If blood from satiated rats is transfused into hungry rats, these rats will stop eating. A substance, glucagon, secreted by the pancreas, also plays a role in providing the sensation of satiety. Another and different mechanism is that of osmoreceptors in the hypothalamus. They are sensitive to the osmotic pressure of the plasma of the blood, and they can make the animal eat or stop eating.

Hormones (to be discussed in the next chapter) also play a role. Before an animal goes into hibernation or migrates, it needs to eat more; and so it needs to have a bigger appetite. More of what it eats at that time is converted into fat, for that is a better fuel than carbohydrates. A hormone secreted by the pituitary does both these things; it increases the appetite and it converts carbohydrate and protein into fat deposits. In birds, it is probable that the hormone prolactin makes the animal have the need to move off on its long journey of migration.

An animal's needs are not only the obvious ones, eating, drinking, and avoiding enemies who prey upon it. Depending on the species, the baby animal may need to cling to its mother, to push its behind up against the side of the nest, as does the baby cuckoo, it may need to skip and jump, to strengthen its leg and learn to use them. In species akin to ourselves, such as the anthropoid apes, we can see the distress of the young animal if it is prevented from satisfying its basic needs.

As the young animal gets older, the needs and the consequent desires becomes more complicated. Again, depending on the species, it has general social needs. It may need companionship; without it, the animal cannot develop normally and will never function as a proper member of its social group. Yerkes, who knew chimpanzees better than anyone did in his time, has written of them:

The need for social stimulation, such as is provided by companions, becomes so strong during late infancy and early childhood that isolation causes varied symptoms of deprivation. In addition to overt behavioural expressions of distress, there is general physiological dysfunction. Taken forcibly from companion or group and left alone, the ape cries, screams, rages, struggles desperately to escape and return to its fellows. Such behaviour may last for hours. All the bodily functions may be more or less upset. Food may be persistently refused, and depression may follow the emotional orgy.

Monkeys have been brought up in complete isolation in order to find out what effect this has on their psychological health. These monkeys became psychotic; they had the kind of psychosis called catatonia, in which there is no emotional expression and probably no feeling of emotion. In their brains there were abnormalities in the activity of neurons of the sensory part of the thalamus and the septal region, a part of the brain concerned with experiencing pleasure.

Chimpanzees are very ready to accept other animals as companions, human beings, orang-utans, gorillas, dogs, or cats. It is the same with the young gorilla. Hediger has related how a child gorilla in a zoo succeeded in tricking its young lady keeper into its cage one evening. The latch of the lock clicked shut and so she had to spend the whole night being hugged and loved by the poor lonely young gorilla. The social needs of animals in zoos are not considered; and in the arguments for and against having zoos, this inevitable deprivation is one of the reasons against imprisoning animals.

After puberty, reproduction demands that the animal should mate and found a family. After mating, the animal experiences the needs and emotions associated with preparing a home for the young. This brings about nest-building in birds, rodents, and sticklebacks. After the birth of the babies, there follow the emotions associated with the succouring and protection of the young, retrieving them and bringing them back to the nest in the case of rodents, teaching the fledgelings to fly in the case of birds, and for man all those thousand things from changing the nappies to teaching them the knowledge acquired in their culture.

Some emotions aid the satisfaction of desires. They add to the energy provided by each basic need and drive. All emotion can be totally removed by cutting out certain parts of the brain. When this state is induced, the animal is inactive. A man will just sit or lie wherever he happens to be and he does not bother to feed himself or get up to get himself something to drink.

Emotion increases the energy of drives; or it may be that emotion provides the energy of our drives. The emotion of aggression is needed to make the animal establish its territory, to provide enough food for itself, its mate, and its young brood-to-be. The painful emotion of fear is needed to make animals flee from their enemies. Painful emotions result from being unadapted to the environments; their purpose is to make the animal adjust better.

If the environment provides no stimulation, most animals experience boredom. This is a negative emotional state, though its unpleasantness is different from that associated with an inability to satisfy a strong internal need, such as hunger or thirst. Boredom is commonly seen in animals kept captive in zoos and in animals under domestication. In the zoo it may be seen in members of the cat family, showing itself in their compulsive pacing up and down and ritualized turning movements, to a psychiatrist so reminiscent of the behaviour of some human compulsion neurotics. If boredom occurs in animals under natural conditions, it may act as a spur in the search for necessary stimulation. In man, we know from introspection that it can lead to satisfaction in imagination, to the wish-fulfilments of dreams and daydreams, and to many kinds of substitute gratifications.

Many emotions are not for ourselves alone: they are produced for their effect on others; and they are a basic way of communicating with others. Subtle emotions are understood by other members of the same species. More basic emotions such as fear, readiness to fight, and emotions accompanying pain or pleasure are understood by other mammals or perhaps by all other vertebrates. We can tell when a dog or cat is in pain or is about to fight us; dogs can tell when the stag is frightened and about to flee and when it is about to attack them.

It may well be that some other mammals recognize the emotions we are experiencing and expressing better than we do. Possibly they detect our fear or our intended aggression towards them. I do not mean the obvious threatening behaviour, when we pick up a stone or a stick, or obvious fleeing, as we turn our backs and start running away. One has the impression that they understand the meaning of our scarcely expressed intentions before we would know those of another man. It may be that we give off smells which our poor olfactory systems cannot detect but which the sniffing dog and deer understand and which warn them of our attitudes.

Reactions to emotions are not the same in everyone; people have different constitutions. Some react to difficult situations by increasing the activity of the parasympathetic nerves to their stomachs and bowels; others cause changes in the blood vessels of the coverings of their brains and get migraine; others induce spasms in muscles and get headaches, backache, pains in their chest. Others do not express states of emotion or stressful psychological conditions physically, their bodies are not used to playing out the dramas of their lives. They deal with them in the outside world. They create emotional situations, they quarrel with all their friends, they become involved in traffic accidents; or they get depressed or neurotic in different ways.

Sometimes shocks of a psychological kind can affect the endocrine balance of the body. Horror and continual fear can cause overactivity of the thyroid gland. Some disorders result from the continual use, perhaps in an unbalanced or pathological way, of the parts of the autonomic nervous system. Nervous children frequently empty their bladders; so do elephants. Bats and monkeys pass their urine on to their assailants, using their bladders as offensive weapons. Perhaps this frequency of passing urine in children and some adults is a relic of this manner of showing aggression. Some adults, when nervous, get diarrhoea, others get constipation. Elephants and camels too are very prone to diarrhoea when they are anxious or upset. Many kinds of monkeys use defecation as an offensive weapon. Travellers in South America have reported how irritated troops of monkeys will defecate on them from above, their ability to hit the target being excellent. In chimpanzees and gorillas, micturition and defecation occur with strong emotional states. It is the same with ourselves. There is no doubt that certain chronic disorders of the lower bowel, such as ulcerative colitis, can be caused by psychological and emotional events. They have been produced experimentally by prolonged stimulation of the hypothalamus. Also when a certain region of the hypothalamus is stimulated several times a day in monkeys, the animals develop ulcers of the stomach and duodenum. In man, psychological factors can cause gastric and duodenal ulcers, and they can equally cause them to heal or not to heal. It is commonly found that an ulcer suddenly becomes worse or it starts to bleed when an upsetting psychological event occurs. There are several mechanisms known which could bring this to pass. One of the effects of adrenocorticotrophic hormone is to make the stomach secrete acid. When electrodes implanted in the hypothalami of animals are constantly stimulated, too much of this hormone is secreted, and the animals eventually develop gastric or duodenal ulcers or ulcers in the colon.

There have been one or two famous patients who have had openings made between their stomachs and the belly-wall and who have been observed by doctors aware of the importance of psychological influences on the body. Instruments could be passed through this hole, the inside of the stomach could be looked at and samples of the gastric juices could be taken. Every American and British doctor remembers hearing about such a case when he was a student. For this was a patient whose case was published by his doctor, Dr Beaumont, in 1833, and who rejoiced in the name of Alexis St Martin.

In our own time two doctors at the New York Hospital, H.G. Wolff and S. Wolf, studied another patient with a gastric fistula. They had the advantage of having the modern psychological and sociological outlook as well as quantitative methods of investigation and colour photography at their disposal. In order to study human gastric function, they employed their subject, Tom, as a laboratory worker. They also got to know him so well that they knew how any of the stresses, upsets, or pleasures of day-to-day life would affect him psychologically. Knowing how Tom would be feeling in various circumstances, they could correlate this knowledge with the state of his stomach.

Fear had the following effects on his stomach.

Sudden fright occurred one morning when an irate doctor, a member of the staff, suddenly entered the room, began hastily opening drawers, looking on shelves, and swearing to himself. He was looking for protocols to which he attached great importance. Our subject, who tidies up the laboratory, had mislaid them the previous afternoon, and he was fearful of detection and of losing his precious job. He remained silent and motionless and his face became pallid.

At the same time the mucous membranes of his stomach became pale and it secreted less than the normal amount of acid. These effects lasted for five minutes after the doctor had found what he was looking for, and had left the room. The mucous membranes of the stomach also remained pale, with diminished secretion of acid, when Tom was sad, discouraged, or was reproaching himself about anything. This effect resulting from his mood or other psychological factors would override the physiological effects due to food. For instance, beef broth would cause an increase in the blood flow in the stomach and the secretion of acid, but these would not appear if Tom was feeling depressed. If he was feeling resentful, there would be an increased secretion of acid with dilation of the blood-vessels, and a great increase in the movements of the stomach. Quite different reactions were shown by the stomach when Tom was feeling hostile and aggressive. On these occasions, the stomach was in the same state as it would be at the start of a big meal; the amount of acid secreted was three times the normal and the mucous membranes was 'turgid, engorged and much redder than usual'. On another occasion, the investigators found that when Tom's face was red with anger and resentment, so was his stomach. Anxiety also caused an increased secretion of acid, abnormal redness, and increased blood supply of the stomach; and when the anxiety persisted for weeks, so did these changes in his stomach. In Tom's case, this readiness of the stomach to receive a meal was unassociated with his feeling hungry or having a good appetite; on the contrary, he had no appetite. But in some patients, anxiety and resentment cause hunger, and these patients may eat a lot at the times when they have these emotions.

A doctor living in Chicago has recorded his own case. He had the interesting habit of examining his own gastric juices by sucking them up by means of a stomach tube every morning. One day thieves entered his house and killed his landlady. On that day, his gastric hydrochloric acid was double its normal strength. For the following ten days, he expected to be shot by the gangsters in revenge for helping the police track them down; during this time the concentration of his gastric acid remained very high. After he had moved to what he considered a safe place, his acidity returned to normal.

The actual feeling of emotion is a mixed mental and physical experience. Fear and anxiety are felt in the pit of the stomach. When certain parts of the cerebral hemispheres are stimulated in conscious patients, the patients experience this feeling, and they cannot say if the sensation they feel is a physical one in the centre of the abdomen or if it is a mental or psychological one. When the same parts of the cerebral hemispheres spontaneously discharge, as they do in epilepsy, patients experience before the actual fit this sensation of fear or anxiety in the pit of the stomach.

Emotion will suddenly send up the blood pressure and this may cause a cerebral haemorrhage and death. Aubrey has recorded that when the Earl of Dorset was Lord Treasurer, he was giving evidence at a trial.

The Lord Treasurer had in his bosome some writings, and which as he was pulling-out to give in evidence, sayed 'Here is that will strike you dead!' and as soon as he had spoken these words, fell down starke dead in the place.

Aubrey comments:

An extraordinary perturbation of mind will bring an apoplexie: I know several instances of it.

14 Pain

Sleep and pain tend to inspire poets and philosophers; urination and defecation do not. With psychoanalysts, it is the other way round.

There have always been two different theories of the mechanism of pain, one usually called the quantitative theory and the other nowadays called the stimulus-specific theory. The quantitative theory goes back to Aristotle. The stimulus-specific theory was developed when the scientific investigation of sensation began in the last century.

The quantitative theory considers pain to be the result of excessive stimulation: too hot a stimulus, or too cold, too hard a pressure or squeeze, and pain results. The same peripheral nerve fibres are thought to be conducting impulses with the ordinary stimulation as with the painful stimulation; it is just that they are conducting far more impulses per second with the stimulation that causes pain. According to this theory, hot and cold are two extremes of a single temperature-sensing system. A lot of stimulation of the receptors is thought to cause the sensation of hot, little stimulation that of cold, and very intense stimulation causes pain to be added to the other sensations.

The stimulus-specific theory proposes that pain is an independent form of sensation, just as touch, warmth, and cold are. Each of these sensory systems is thought to be independent of the others, each having its own receptors and each system finally ending in different regions of the cerebral hemispheres.

At present, it seems that both theories are right. There are stimulus-specific receptors and nerve fibres, responding to only one kind of stimulus; and there are receptors that respond to more than one kind. Receptors of the muscle report the tension put on the muscle or developed by the muscle itself and nothing else. There are nerve fibres of the skin that are activated only by mechanical events, such as deformation or movement of the skin. No matter how frequently these receptors are excited, they never give rise to pain. There are different warm and cold receptors; they are not the two ends of a spectrum, as is required by the quantitative theory. One lot is activated by rising and the other by falling temperature. There are different nerve fibres reporting stimulation that is damaging or threatening to damage the body, and these nerve fibres are the basis of our feeling pain. When nothing damaging is affecting the body, these fibres are silent.

In the case of the viscera, the quantitative theory fits best. Pain occurs when a large number of impulses are sent to the spinal cord by nerves from the alimentary canal or the bladder. When a moderate number of impulses per second are sent in, one feels the sensation causing the desire to empty the bladder or the rectum.

A sensation is the result of activation of neurons of the cerebral hemispheres. Sensation is not the same thing as the input to lower levels of the nervous system. For this reason one speaks of mechanoreceptors and nociceptors, and not of touch fibres or pain fibres; one talks of a noxious or nocuous input, and not of pain. Apart from theoretical reasons, this usage is right because some stimulus that is painful to one person may not be so to another, or it may be painful on one part of the body and painless on another. One can have pain without damage and damage without pain. Cancer is noxious and can be painless. Phantom limbs that occur after amputations can be painful though innocuous.

Sensations are usually accompanied by emotion. A sudden new sensation in the skin is accompanied by surprise and the emotion of being startled. Sensations can be pleasant or unpleasant. Tickle causes pleasure to young children and it makes babies laugh. Certain rhythms of tactile stimulation or rubbing may be accompanied by pleasure. The right balance of warmth and cold is pleasant, the wrong amount of either is unpleasant. One supposes that the purpose of the accompanying emotion is to teach the animal correct behaviour: correct means tending to aid it in continuing to live and to give birth to the next generation; incorrect is the opposite.

When the operation of leucotomy (discussed in Chapter 23) was introduced, it was discovered that the sensation of pain could be separated from its associated unpleasant emotion. When the brain was cut so that the frontal lobes were separated from the thalamus, the patient no longer complained of the pain of cancer and he seemed to be indifferent to it. He could feel pain when he was pricked or when he burned himself, but he no longer suffered from the previous constant pain. Most of the patients said, unemotionally, that pressing on the tumour was still painful, but they were obviously not disturbed by the pain. There was a chasm between the affective emotional aspect of pain and the pure sensation of pain.

The kind of pain we feel depends largely on the tissue that is being damaged or irritated and also on what is causing the pain. Blood itself causes pain when it is in the wrong place, that, is when it has leaked out of blood-vessels. A lack of vital blood-supply in the right place can cause pain. This happens when a muscle is working and its blood-supply is reduced or cut off. It is the cause of the pain of coronary thrombosis. Suddenly one of the arteries that supplies the heart muscle gets blocked. The heart goes on beating (it may not, and then the person dies of a heart attack) with insufficient blood to bring it oxygen. That causes pain. There is similar pain when any muscle goes on working without enough blood supply. It happens in old age when the arteries get furred up, like old pipes. Then the old man has to stop walking to give the muscles of his legs a chance to get more blood while they are resting.

Any kind of stimulation of the pulp and the dentine of the teeth is painful. That is why it hurts when the dentist blows hot or cold air into your teeth. I am hoping that one of two dentists will read this book, and blow air on our teeth at the same temperature as our mouths. Damage to bone causes a deep, aching, gnawing pain. Irritating chemicals injected into muscles cause a similar deep, aching pain. The brain can be cut or burned without there being any kind of sensation. But damage to the peripheral nerves is painful; and the pain of cancer is often due to the growth invading these nerves. The kind of pain caused by damage to the skin depends on which layer is being involved: damage to the most superficial layer causes itching and burning pain; damage to the deeper layer causes an ache.

Pain in the viscera feels altogether different from pain in the skin, the muscles, or the bones. The lungs, liver, and spleen do not give rise to pain, no matter how they are stimulated. Usually the activity of the intestines and the ureters goes on silently (well, relatively silently) and automatically without giving us any sensation. When this activity becomes more vigorous, we have the sensation that the viscera need to be emptied. When the stomach contains a lot of fluid and is working hard, we may be able to feel as well as hear the gurglings and splashings. When the intestines are contracting hard to push their contents past an obstruction, we get the pain of colic. This is a rhythmical waxing and waning of pain, as the intestines contract and relax. Some viscera tell us that they exist only when they give us pain; there are the ureters, the urethra, the biliary, and the pancreatic ducts. People are surprised to hear that the intestines can be cut through or even burned without this causing any sort of sensation. But this is not really surprising, because it is unlikely that they will ever meet these fates and so they have not evolve any defensive mechanisms to deal with such unlikely events. If they are pulled on, that causes pain. For that is something that is likely to occur a few times during a life; when they are working hard to push through an obstacle, then they do pull on the tissues that hold them in place, and they are pulled in return.

Some pains make you move; colic of a ureter trying to pass a kidney stone is an example. Others make you lie still; this happens with peritonitis and when there is bleeding in the abdominal cavity.

Although one can cut and burn the brain without causing any sensation, severe pain can arise within the central nervous system itself: this is called central pain. It is liable to come on after a stroke affecting the thalamus or the neighbouring regions. With central pain there is continuous pain, and excessive pain when any stimulus strikes the body. At its worst, this pain affects a half of the body, the opposite half to the damaged thalamus. So far, no drugs have been discovered that have any effect against this sort of pain.

When a part of the body gets inflamed, substance are made in the tissues that excite nociceptor nerve fibres and cause pain; they also make the nociceptors more sensitive to other kinds of stimuli. In an inflamed area, warmth and touch stimuli cause pain. It is likely that some of the neuromodulators of the nerve fibres within the inflamed area are put out into the local tissues, and that that aggravates the inflammation. One of the substance formed is prostaglandin E. Aspirin and related drugs stop this substance being produced; that is how they relieve certain kinds of pain.

One pain can obliterate another. I once saw a patient who had constant pain following shingles. Shingles in medicine is called herpes (Greek for creeping), and the dreadful pain that follows this virus infection is called post-herpetic neuralgia. One day she fell and upset a kettle of boiling water all over herself and had severe burns. From the moment she had the worse pains from the burns, she ceased to have the pain of the post-herpetic neuralgia; she could not even feel it if she tried. After about eight months, her burns recovered sufficiently for the pain to go off; then the pain of the post-herpetic neuralgia came back.

When a nerve is damaged or cut through, as occurs when a limb is amputated, nerve fibres grow out of the cut nerves into nowhere. These sprouting fibres are abnormally sensitive to pressure or to being moved, squeezed or stretched; they are also sensitive to noradrenalin which is emitted all around them by the accompanying sympathetic nerve fibre. And so they fire off impulses to the spinal cord, impulses that cause pain. In some patients, repeatedly blocking the sympathetic nerves going to the damaged or cut nerve can stop the pain.

When we have pain, we may wish that man were not born to suffer and we are likely to think that pain is all bad. But that is not true. There are a few rare congenital conditions in which the person does not feel pain. In one of these, congenital non-progressive sensory neuropathy, the nerve fibres and their connections in the spinal cord necessary for feeling pain are defective or absent. In another condition, wrongly called congenital indifference to pain, it appears there is an excessive amount of endorphin circulating in the body. This is a peptide with actions similar to morphine, which will be discussed below. Or it may be that the neurons of the spinal cord that receive a noxious input are being continually inhibited. Patients having either of these conditions do not reach adult life without scarring large parts of their bodies, damaging their joints, and biting their tongues and the insides of the mouths. Pain is protective. It protects against damage from the surrounding world, and also against damaging oneself, over-stretching the bladder, biting oneself, or swallowing liquids which are too hot.

So far, we have been discussing acute pain, the pain one feels when one treads on a nail or when a cigarette touches the back of one's hand. Chronic pain is the pain that goes on for days, weeks, or years. With inflammation, substances are made in the inflamed tissues that excite the non-myelinated afferent fibres running to the spinal cord. They set up an excitable state in the local grey matter. Once this state has taken place, it continues, whether more impulses arrive in the nerve fibres or not. The neurons of the excited region of grey matter send axons up to the brain, and so the state of excitability is passed on to certain regions of the brain.

Pain going on for a long time can affect the central nervous system for the rest of the person's life. Two examples of a severe and lasting pain affecting neurons permanently are reported in Chapter 22. In these cases, certain groups of neurons retain the pattern of firing together just as they did when the pain first occurred; if they are excited again, they reproduce the whole of pattern firing. This is a kind of basic memory. Memory implies learning; and so, in some cases, neurons in the brain can be shown to have learned pain. Something similar may be happening when someone develops tics, those involuntary screwings up of the corner of the mouth or movements of the face; once learned, almost never forgotten. But learning these movements and learning pain, these are rare. Why this sometimes happens, we do not know.

When some pains have been going on for a long time—and I don't know what length of time a long time is—the behaviour of certain neurons of the thalamus and cerebral cortex becomes changed. This has been found out by operating on the brain under local anaesthetics. We may take an example of a painful phantom upper limb that has come on after amputation. At one time neurosurgeons tried to cure the pain by operating on the opposite cerebral cortex and removing the arm area. The arm area, as will be seen in Chapter 17, is a region of the cerebral cortex in the parietal lobe which receives impulses causing sensation of touch and pressure in the opposite arm. Above this region is the same region for the leg and below it the region for the face. In some of the patients with a painful phantom upper limb, the cortical arm area enlarges and spreads out onto the areas of the face and the leg. The constant pressure of the painful phantom is also associated with something else abnormal. When the surgeon stimulates this area electrically, the pain from which the patient is suffering is reproduced. Normally stimulation of this part of the brain never causes pain; it causes a feeling of numbness or pins and needles. But now the electrical stimulation of this part of the cerebral cortex reproduces the patient's pain. This operation of trying to remove a constant pain by cutting out part of the cortex had to be give up, as the pain invariably returned.

Over the past twenty years, important advances have been made in the understanding of pain. This subject is more complicated than has been realized for many centuries. Pain and all sensation used to be thought of as being only afferent, as being messages delivered to the cerebral cortex. In 1969 a Canadian psychologist, D.V. Reynolds, reported that he had been operating on rats, burning, cutting, or pinching them, and that the rats felt nothing, provided he electrically stimulated a certain part of the midbrain deep to the collicoli. During this stimulation the animals seemed to feel touch or pressure, but they gave no indication of feeling pain. They had no reflexes suggesting that something painful was going on, there was no change in blood pressure, no change in breathing, no squeaking. Nothing quite like this had been seen before. Usually the electric stimulation of the brain causes something obvious, a movement, a change in breathing, or, if the animal is awake, it shows some sort of behaviour, it looks, listens, or moves. Although inhibition of neurons of the spinal cord was already known, a complete absence of the pain and the manifestations of pain from stimulating parts of the brain was something surprising. Eventually, many regions of the brain were found whose stimulation stopped pain being felt. They were all in the central reticular formation of the brain; this is the oldest part, already developed in ancestral fish. Stimulation of various neurons in this region excites inhibitory neurons in the medulla oblongata. These neurons have long nerve fibres that descend throughout the spinal cord and block the input from the peripheral nerves that would otherwise cause pain.

When this electrically induced analgesia had been explained as activating an inhibitory system of nerve fibres, the thought occurred to many research workers that morphine and the related opiates might work by activating this system; could it be that morphine is an effective drug against pain, an analgesic drug, because it excites the neurons that had been stimulated electrically? If this were found to be so, then morphine would be working by inhibiting the incoming impulses caused by noxious stimulation. This could not be the whole explanation of morphine's action against pain, because it was known already that it acted at two levels, on the spinal cord and on the brain. Some research workers then injected morphine in minute amounts into the region of the midbrain from which electrical stimulation caused analgesia. The morphine produced the same effects as the electrical stimulation. If the neurons of the medulla oblongata were previously destroyed, then morphine no longer stopped pain; and if this tract of inhibitory fibres had already been cut, then morphine no longer worked. If the tract had been cut on one side of the spinal cord, morphine did not stop pain on that side of the animal; and if the tract had been cut on both sides, then morphine did not work on the lower limb, below the level of the cut. This evidence showed that morphine, whatever other actions it has, works as an analgesic drug by activating this descending inhibitory system. It also acts directly on the spinal cord. It causes pre-synaptic inhibition of the nerve fibres coming in reporting noxious stimulation, so that their message does not get through to the spinal cord.

It is curious that morphine and other opiate drugs are fixed on to the membranes of neurons of animals, for they are substances formed in plants. If morphine molecules fit into the membranes of certain cells of the body, there may perhaps be some chemical substances in the body that normally fit these sites on cell membranes. Many workers then began searching for what are called endogenous opioids. At present, more than ten substances, all peptides, have been found in the body that have similar actions to opiates. It is probable that only four of these are of importance, beta-endorphin, dynorphin, leucine-enkephalin, and methionine-enkephalin. These peptides are not only used to stop pain, they are important as neuromodulators throughout the body.

One wonders if we are using this pain-suppressing mechanism all the time: are we constantly inhibiting transient and not very important inputs that might be causing us pain? The answer appears to be yes. People who have some chronic painful condition, such as arthritis or backache, are making use of this mechanism. If they were not doing so, presumably their pain would be worse.

This pain-inhibiting mechanism is also turned on by pain itself, by stress, by sexual stimulation and activity, and by training. It may be that stress was the basic factor that caused the development of the mechanism.

Rats can learn to turn on this pain-reducing mechanism and raise the threshold for pain; and presumably not only rats. If a rat is given shock to its foot every day, as is done when analgesic drugs are tried out on these animals, it rapidly learns to raise the threshold for pain by Pavlovian conditioning. After a few trials, as soon as the rat is placed on the electric grid, it raises its pain threshold before it is given a shock.

Perhaps the most important factor causing this inhibition of pain is pain itself. One hopes that poor deluded martyrs, such as Joan of Arc or Guy Fawkes, were able to inhibit this terrible input and not feel the pain inflicted on them. This may also be the explanation of people who run swords through their tongues, dance on red-hot coals or hang themselves up with hooks through their skins. When these people have been investigated by physiologists, they have been found to be able to induce slow waves in their electroencephalograms. Without training one cannot do this. Zen Buddhist monks also learn to go into the same state, and they induce the same slow waves in their brains. Those who pierce their skins with nails or swords do not bleed. The only other physiological fact we know about the state needed for these feats is that the sympathetic system is very active at the time. This may cause closing down of the blood-vessels of the skin, and prevent the bleeding.

In the last few years everyone has been astounded to watch operations on television being performed on wide-awake Chinese patients, acupuncture analgesia being used instead of a general anaesthetic. Although acupuncture is 5000 years old, its use to stop the pain of surgical operations is new to the Chinese, just as it is to us. Like most things in medicine, it was discovered before it was understood how or why it works. The method consists of putting needles through the skin into the deeper tissues in two regions of the body. Needles are put near the operating site and electrically stimulated at a rate of about 100 per second. Fewer needles are put in at a distance from the site of operation. Common sites are in the muscle between the big toe and second toe or in the similar site in the hand or in the ears. These needles are stimulated irregularly at a rate of 3 per second. This is now done electrically but it used at first to be done by hand. Relays of assistants would twiddle the needles throughout the operation. The stimulation needs to be started 20 minutes before the operation.

It is probable that acupuncture analgesia—not acupuncture for the treatment of disease—depends on three mechanisms. Local presynaptic inhibition is called in by a fast rate of stimulation. It reduces the reception of a noxious input. The stimulation at a slow rate activates the various nuclei of the reticular system. These are in the central grey matter of the midbrain and in the medulla oblongata. These are the nuclei that send inhibitory nerve fibres to the posterior horns of the spinal cord so as to decrease a noxious input. One of the neuromodulators used in this inhibition is beta-endorphin. Chinese research workers showed some years ago that twenty minutes of acupuncture stimulation carried out on a rabbit produced some changes in the cerebrospinal fluid that could be transferred to another rabbit. Having given the first rabbit the acupuncture, they took the cerebrospinal fluid, and infused it into the cerebrospinal fluid of the second rabbit. This rabbit then had its threshold for pain raised. Thus the experiment showed that the acupuncture stimulation had caused some substance to appear in the cerebrospinal fluid that acted on the nervous system to raise the animal's threshold for pain. From our knowledge acquired some years later, this substance would be an endorphin. Thus the mechanisms of acupuncture analgesia appear to be inhibition occurring at spinal level, descending inhibition from the medulla oblongata and other regions of the brain to the spinal cord, and emission of endorphin in certain parts of the brain and spinal cord. These parts are near the cavities containing cerebrospinal fluid in the centre of the brain, and so some of the endorphin seeps through into the fluid, where it can be detected.

The physical part of morphine addition can be cured by acupuncture. What happens when someone takes morphine continually is that this morphine stops the emission of the body's natural endorphins, as it replaces the natural substances at their nerve-endings. It was discovered in Hong Kong that people having acupuncture as surgical analgesia did not suffer from the terrible manifestations of withdrawal when they stopped taking opium. This good news was brought from China to England by Dr Margaret Patterson. She started treating addicts of all kinds by using electro-acupuncture applied to the head. It was later found by research workers in the United States that this electric stimulation in the rat activated certain neurons in the brain that normally emit endorphins. Thus, acupuncture makes the brain produce its own opium-like substance or opioid; and so the withdrawal of the morphine or heroin that the addict takes can be done without the usual upsetting reaction. The addict no longer gets a craving for the drug, as his own naturally occurring opioids are being mobilized.

We are beginning to see the connecting links between acupuncture analgesia used in China for operations, acupuncture done by twiddling or electrically stimulating needles for the treatment for some diseases, the treatment of some chronic pain by electric stimulation with electrodes on the skin, and the treatment of drug addiction, smoking, and alcoholism by electric stimulation of the head. The body reacts differently to slow and fast rates of stimulation, fast being impulses arriving at 80 or more a second, and slow being at rates considerably less than this. Fast rates of stimulation activate the neurons in the medulla that inhibit the messages in the afferent nerve fibres reporting noxious events. Thus they can stop pain. Slow rates of stimulation increase the amount of β-endorphin in the cerebrospinal fluid in patients who have constant pain. These are the rates used in acupuncture and in electric stimulation for chronic pain.

15 The centre of the brain: the hypothalamus

The hypothalamus is in the centre of the brain; this is shown in the drawing of Fig. 15.1. It is immediately above the pituitary gland and below the thalamus, as its name indicates; and it is surrounded by the massive cerebral hemispheres.

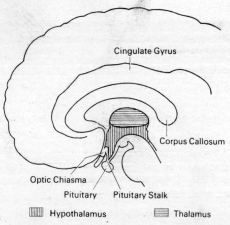

Fig. 15.1 The brain has been cut through from front to back to show the position of the hypothalamus and thalamus.

The hypothalamus organizes all the functions of the body and acts of behaviour that are needed to perform these functions. Part of the way in which it carries out these fundamental acts is by arranging the output of controlling hormones by the pituitary gland, and by regulating the autonomic nervous system.

The first physiologist who conceived of the idea of investigating the anatomical basis of animal behaviour was W.R. Hess of Zurich, and he spent most of his life doing this. Hess brought an altogether fresh way of thinking about physiology and anatomy; he has provided all research workers too with a most useful way of investigating the nervous system. This technique consists of introducing very fine electrodes into the brain, the leads of which come out through the skull; they are left in place for ever. After the operation, the animal recovers rapidly and goes on living its normal life, unaware of the electrodes in its brain. We know this, as the identical procedure has been carried out in human patients. When the animal is living its usual life, the electrodes can be stimulated; this excites the neurons among which the electrodes are placed. The effect on behaviour of stimulation of these neurons can then be observed; and thus one can learn about their function.

Nowadays the stimulating is done by remote control; no wires are fixed to the electrodes. When enough data have been collected, a destructive current is passed through the electrodes, which destroys the little block of brain tissue lying between the two electrodes. This is painless too; the animal feels nothing. Then the effect on the animal's behaviour of life without these neurons can be observed. When the animal is finally killed, microscopic examination of the brain is carried out to find out exactly which neurons were destroyed. In these, as in all experiments on animals, the way of killing is absolutely painless. The animal is given a large dose of a barbiturate drug, which sends it to sleep, and it never wakes again.

Hess's work was greatly extended by von Holst and his colleagues at the Max Planck Institute for Physiology of Behaviour near Munich. They implanted electrodes in various parts of the brain in domestic chickens, and stimulated them by ultra-short radio waves. In this way they were able to produce about the whole repertoire of chickens' behaviour. According to the site stimulated and the strength of current, a chicken would stop pecking at food and suddenly go to sleep. Or it suddenly looked apprehensively into the distance as though it felt that something threatening was approaching. Chickens at the bottom of the pecking order would begin to strut proudly along and peck at animals that were normally their bosses. A chicken doing nothing in particular may, when stimulated, suddenly show interest in what is or is not happening just below. It first seems to look at its feet. As the current strength is increased, it stretches its head down from its perch to have a good look, and then jumps down to the ground. From stimulation of other regions of its brain, the acts of picking grain off the ground and of drinking are performed, all with no grain and no water. It may behave as though it is confronted by a chicken higher in the pecking order when no other bird is there. A hen will gather her non-existent chicks, and act to defend them from a non-existent predator in the sky. There is little doubt that in all these situations the bird has the hallucination; she experiences the absent predator or the threatening hen.

The general hierarchical way in which the central nervous system is constructed is like this. The more fundamental a function is, the more completely it is organized at lower neural levels. The hypothalamus organizes whole entities which we see as acts of behaviour. Lower neural levels control various components of an act of behaviour; each higher level then adds its contribution, in accordance with what it has received from all the neurons connected to it. For example, the rhythmical movements of breathing are arranged at the level of the spinal cord and of the basal part of the brain. The hypothalamus alters the basic rhythm, the rate and depth of breathing, when it is organizing acts of behaviour, such as running away, fighting, sleeping, or waking up. Breathing has to be altered in accordance with various states of emotion; and when bosoms heaved, as they did in Victorian novels, it was presumably the hypothalamus that did it.

The hypothalamus controls body temperature, and it does so by using the sympathetic system. It can dilate or constrict the blood-vessels of the skin; it dilates them to lose heat and constricts them to keep the body warm. It can raise the hairs of the skin, trapping a layer of warm air to surround the skin. When the body's temperature starts to fall in a cold environment, the hypothalamus makes the muscles do work in shivering. This increased metabolism of all the muscles tends to raise the body's temperature again.

Hess conceived the hypothalamus as organizing two opposite kinds of behaviour: relating oneself to the external world, and attending to the needs of the body. The first uses mainly the sympathetic nervous system and the second the parasympathetic system. The second aspect of living is restorative; it includes digestion, elimination from both ends of the alimentary canal, elimination of urine, and sleep; and also hibernation for those who hibernate and aestivation for those who astivate.

The basic physiological acts are organized by lower levels of the nervous system. At the higher levels, they become complete acts of behaviour. An instance of this is the organization of the acts of urination and defecation. When these acts are ordered by the hypothalamus, it is not merely a matter of emptying the bladder and rectum. The animal performs these acts according to the way of its species, the whole skeleton and musculature being organized, the adult male dog urinating on three legs while cocking the fourth. Although these acts are performed in a normal manner, they are not fitted into the programme and circumstances of the animal's life unless the cerebral hemispheres are in control; for these highest levels of the brain are necessary to take stock of a total situation and to organize behaviour accordingly.

One can observe the hierarchical organization of the brain by comparing the behaviour of an anencephalic baby with a normal baby. Whereas the deformed baby with only a medulla oblongata is able to suck and swallow when something touches its lips, a baby with a hypothalamus can demand food from its parent. By opening and shutting its mouth, and making sucking sounds and movements, it makes its needs clear.

Reward and punishment

For he purrs in thankfulness, when God tells him he's a good cat.

We know that in art and science discoveries are often made by mistake. The worker may be investigating one problem and he finds something different of greater importance. In 1954 in Montreal, Olds and Milner were studying the physiology of the reticular formation by means of electrodes implanted in the brain of the rat. One day the electrodes were put in the wrong part of the brain, in a region in front of the hypothalamus. Milner and Olds noticed that after this animal's brain had been electrically stimulated, the rat would return to the place where the stimulation had occurred. The rat seemed to be seeking the stimulation, just as a hungry animal looks for food in the place where it has previously been fed. The conclusion was that this stimulation was giving the animal pleasure. Since their observation, this work has been confirmed in cats, dogs, pigeons, monkeys, dolphins, goats, goldfish, and man.

The regions of the brain that give the animal pleasure when they are electrically or chemically stimulated are now called pleasure or reward centres. Olds spent the rest of his life doing experiments related to this discovery. He connected the implanted electrodes to a circuit incorporating a lever that the rat could press with its forepaws; when it pushed the lever, it stimulated its own reward centre. Rats got such pleasure from doing this that they would keep on pressing until they fell asleep or dropped from exhaustion. In some other experiments, he put very hungry rats in cages with stacks of food; these hungry rats preferred pressing the lever to eating. Rats would run mazes and solve puzzles or even put up with a painful electric shock to a paw, all for the pleasure of pressing the lever and stimulating the pleasure centre. Unlike conventional rewards given in training the animal, this reward never reached satiation level and never ceased through habituation. In normal life rewards lose their potency; enough is enough. But animals with electrodes implanted in reward sites in their brains tend to continue stimulating themselves. Destruction of the reward centre at operation makes animals indifferent to whatever happens and incapable of showing any emotion.

One of the reward centres is the septal area situated just below a thin membrane called the septum pellucidum. It is around the anterior commissure shown in Plate 13. It is connected with the temporal lobes above it and with the hypothalamus below. There are also reward centres in the hypothalamus and temporal lobes connected to the septal area, in the thalamus, and in the midbrain.

Olds went on to find other parts of the rat's brain that the animal obviously disliked having stimulated; he called these aversive centres. However, the idea of aversive centres is less definite than reward centres; for a region electrically stimulated might have caused the animal to have pain or anxiety, fear, or any unpleasant emotion. In man parts of the brain can be electrically excited that cause pain, fear, or anxiety; but one might not think of the area as being an aversive centre. The aversive areas were found to be around the ventricles in the hypothalamus and midbrain.

We do not know, then, if connections to aversive centres give the animal punishment when it does the biologically wrong thing, but we think that the animal learns correct behaviour by being rewarded with pleasure. Once an animal has some experience of living, it will remember from previous occasions that the discharge of energy in the instinctive act is associated with relief and pleasure; or it will remember that a certain conjunction of circumstances was accompanied by unhappiness or pain. In the nature of things, the animal is forced to avoid pain and discomfort; and so it is taught to avoid the state associated with these emotions and feelings, and to seek the opposite state.

It seems probable that it is the same pleasure centre that rewards hunger as rewards sexual stimulation. Eating enough food excites the pleasure centre. How eating too much excites the aversive centre or inhibits the pleasure centre, we do not yet understand.

Professor Robert Heath of Tulane University in New Orleans had the idea that, as schizophrenics show and seem to experience no pleasure, stimulating the region of the pleasure centre in these patients might be a good form of treatment. He put electrodes into the septal region, stimulated it, and then instructed the patients to carry on stimulating themselves. The manifestations of pleasure were not striking. But some neurosurgeons have implanted electrodes in the septum in patients with severe pain in cancer and allowed the patient to stimulate the area. During stimulation, and for a long time afterwards, the patients no longer feel pain; instead, they get a contented or a happier feeling than mere contentedness. Heath continued his work on schizophrenia by introducing transmitter substances to the septum down a fine tube. This did have good effects, and brought about a remission of the illness for many months in many patients.

Fighting and fleeing

> For when he takes his prey he plays with it to give it a chance.
> For one mouse in seven escapes by his dallying.

Hess discovered when he stimulated certain regions of the hypothalamus in the cat, the animal would become aggressive and attack, or else it would be submissive and run away. Hess called these two patterns of behaviour, fighting and fleeing, the defence reaction. The reasons for putting them together was that the neurons producing both kinds of behaviour were next door to each other, and both ways of behaving are used for saving the animal's life.

Physiological experiments led Hess to conclude that these two reactions must be closely linked. Many years later ethologists concluded from the observation of animals behaving in the wild, that aggression and fear are two aspects of one kind of behaviour. Both aspects of defence are manifested by animals as far apart as fish, birds, and mammals; and they occur in social animals living in groups. If an animal is seeking a territory and it happens to enter a territory already occupied, it may let itself be chased off. When it is the proud owner of a territory, it favours the law that says 'Trespassers will be prosecuted', and it will do the prosecuting itself. Which aspect of the defence reaction the animal manifests depends chiefly on the location of the trespasser. If the trespasser has intruded well into the property, its intrusion will be met by aggression. If the intruder is only on the boundary, aggression will take the form of threat. In either case, the intruder is likely to flee. When neighbours meet at their common boundary, both animals show mixed pictures of flight and fight.

Animals living in packs, like wolves, also show both manifestations of the defence reaction. When a wolf threatens another one, it will either go on threatening or else it will submit, depending on the behaviour of the animal being threatened. Similarly, household hens show both aspects of the defence reaction in the establishment of pecking order.

Which aspect of the defence reaction is shown depends, according to Hediger, on the critical distance between the animal and its enemy. When this distance is considerable, the animal will go off, either by walking away or by fleeing; when the distance is small, the animal will attack. The actual distance differs from species to species, and in the same animal from time to time. Hediger's concept covers the general observation that an animal when cornered will fight; and naturalists know that this applies also to timid animals, such as small antelopes, rabbits, and mice. Before attacking, all or nearly all vertebrates threaten; they prefer to scare an enemy rather than fight.

The kind of behaviour induced by stimulating electrodes in the hypothalamus differs in some ways from similar behaviour arising naturally. Under normal living conditions, the defence reaction is integrated into the animal's total activity. Aggression or flight is preceded by preparatory behaviour, and is followed by slow cooling off. Before attacking, the cat threatens. When it attacks, it direct its attack well, aiming at the face or the eyes of its enemy. The aggressive behaviour of a cat being stimulated artificially by means of electrodes in the hypothalamus is directed at any living creature near it. The behaviour is carried on somewhat like that of an automaton.

In experiments of this type, when no human being or other animal is in the laboratory, the stimulated animal behaves as if it sees another animal; as far as one can judge, it behaves as if it has an hallucination. When these experiments are done on pigeons, the pigeon circles round a non-existent animal, preparing either to attack or flee.

If the neurons of the flight reaction region of the hypothalamus in a rat are destroyed, the animal no longer runs away from a place where it has been hurt. One can put a rat in a cage in which part of the floor is electrified; if the rat steps on that part it gets a shock. A normal rat immediately gets off this bit of floor. But if a rat in which these neurons have been destroyed is put in the cage, it will remain on this very spot.

From experiments such as these one learns that a certain region of the brain organizes totalities of behaviour. One then has to find out how this region plays a role in the behaviour of the intact and living animal.

When a person feels the emotion of fear, there is neural activity in certain parts of the cerebral hemispheres and in the hypo-thalamus; these two regions are connected together. The parts of the cerebral hemispheres concerned are some large masses of grey matter in the front part of the temporal lobes; they are called the amygdala, as earlier Greek-speaking anatomists thought they looked like almonds. The neurons of this region can excite and inhibit neurons of the hypothalamus; they can cause fear or stop fear; they can induce rage or prevent it.

Hess found that when he stimulated certain neurons with mini-mal electric current, the animal would show a state of vigilance. As the current was increased, the reaction would become more intense, finally becoming an actual attack, with all the manifesta-tions of fury. The usual bodily changes which are a part of fight or flight occurred. The cat would look for someone on whom to vent its rage; it usually found the experimenter, one is pleased to note. Its fur would stand on end, its ears would be laid back on its head, it would arch its back or crouch ready to spring, and then jump at the experimenter, biting and scratching him. If another cat were placed in the cage, the stimulated cat would attack it, even though it was normally friendly or perhaps even afraid of the other cat. When the current was switched off, the animal quickly calmed down and went on doing what it had been doing before. When other nearby regions of the hypothalamus were stimulated, the cat showed typical signs of fear and tried to run away.

Probably, in real life, the display of the rage reaction is organized by the hypothalamus. It may be that the amygdala brings subtlety in the reaction, modifying it according to the rap-idly changing circumstances resulting from aggression. The high-est levels of the brain provide the animal with consciousness and memory, enabling it to organize these acts of behaviour in accor-dance with its previous experience.

Mating

For having consider'd God and himself he will consider his neighbour.
For if he meets another cat he will kiss her in kindness.

The total act of copulation is organized in a part of the hypothamalus, the septal and preoptic regions which are just in front of the hypothalamus, and a part of the thalamus. Cats with the cerebral hemispheres removed can still perform sexual intercourse if they are placed in the right position. The parts of the hypothalamus concerned are not the same as those organizing the defence reaction. In fact, these two functions are opposed. For a sexual act to take place, fight and flight have to be prevented. Females have to cease to be aggressive and become receptive. The neurons of the hypothalamus concerned with sexuality perform their function only when they receive gonadal hormones in their blood supply. The hormones change these neurons in some way, though in what way we do not yet know.

Patients with lesions here sometimes get an increased libido and a strong sexual appetite. This is about the same region of the brain as causes a strong feeling of pleasure when it is stimulated. One patient had this part of the brain disturbed by a clot of blood. When she was in hospital waiting for an operation to remove the clot, she would ask any man who was visiting to come to bed with her, then and there, in the ward. After the clot had been removed at operation and the lady was again behaving normally, she was most embarrassed when questioned about her unusual conduct.

This part of the brain can be ruined in less skilful boxers, as it is particularly vulnerable to the trauma of repeated head injuries. Some of these men become placid and indifferent; they lose all interest in sex, and may become impotent.

Also in epilepsy originating in the deeper parts of the temporal lobes, the sex drive may be abnormal. The commonest defect is a much diminished libido compared to that of healthy people; these patients have diminished sexual responsiveness, and they do not experience orgasm. If their kind of epilepsy is treated by the surgical removal of the damaged temporal lobe, the sexual drive becomes normal or even excessive. One concludes that many epileptic saints and holy psychopaths may well have had an abnormally low sex drive and no interest in sex; hence their antagonism to sexuality and their failure to understand the behaviour of normal human beings.

When electrodes are implanted in the hypothalamus of the

rabbit and the activity of the neurons is recorded, it has been seen that sexual intercourse creates a great deal of activity among the neurons concerned with sexual behaviour. When these neurons are excited into activity, they stimulate the pituitary gland to secrete the luteotrophic hormone that causes ovulation. Once the amount of this hormone in the circulation reaches a certain level, chemoreceptors in the hypothalamus stop the hypothalamic neurons stimulating the pituitary gland. In this example of the sexual activity of the female rabbit, we can see how one act follows another. A certain activity, in this case copulation, is caused by the actions of hormones on neurons in the hypothalamus. This activity in turn excites related neurons in the hypothalamus, and they act upon the pituitary to cause ovulation. Once this has been achieved, the balance of hormone secretion is again altered, so that no more ova are discharged, and the nest stage in reproduction can be prepared with the implantation of the ovum in the uterus.

Although grooming and care of the fur are not sexual activities, they may be mentioned here. When cats were stimulated by Hess in the front part of the hypothalamus and in the septal region, they stopped doing whatever they happened to be doing, and groomed themselves in that thorough manner typical of cats. They would usually go on till they had finished the task although the stimulation had ceased.

Eating and drinking

For tenthly he goes in quest of food.

Eating and drinking are so essential that people do not realize that the brain has anything to do with such activities. In fact, the hypothalamus controls the intake and output of water and the metabolism of fat and carbohydrates. It makes the animal aware of the need to eat and drink, and it is essential in making it feel replete when it has had enough. What an animal chooses to eat is the concern of the cerebral hemispheres. They retain the knowledge of what is edible, they remember where it is to be found, and

they direct their possessor's steps in search of it
experimentally cut out, the animal will chew and
thing put into its mouth.

There are neurons of the hypothalamus that, when sti
make the animal go around investigating everything to find
it is edible or not. When the current is strong, the animal will
anything, even chewing sticks. In certain experiments, male rats
with electrodes implanted in this region were put in cages containing both a lot of food and some females on heat. The males
immediately showed interest in the females. When the current was
turned on to stimulate the neurons organizing eating, the rats all
left the females alone and started eating. When the current was
turned off, they would stop eating and again take an interest in the
females. Thus the desire to eat could be induced and made pre-
eminent by stimulating these neurons. If the electrodes are left in
permanently and are frequently stimulated, the animal goes on
eating and eating, eventually becoming exceedingly fat. If it is
allowed to stimulate the neurons itself, the animal will go on
rewarding itself with food continually for twenty-four hours or
more. Two research workers in Warsaw have proved that the
animal actually feels hunger. They trained a goat by means of the
conditioned reflex technique to raise its foot whenever it felt hungry and wanted to eat. They then implanted electrodes into this
animal's hypothalamus. Whenever they stimulated these neurons,
the animal raised its foot.

Electrodes have been implanted in this region in monkeys. The
neurons become active when the monkey is looking at food, but
they are inactive if it feels satiated. The timing of these events
reveals how quickly it all happens. It takes a fifth of a second
between the monkey seeing the food and the hypothalamic neurons becoming active; it takes 150–200 msec for the activity of
these neurons to be transferred to licking movements. It thus takes
half a second for the transmission of information to the visual
cortex, to other visual areas in the temporal lobe, then to the
amygdala, and from there to these neurons of the hypothalamus.

There are neurons in this region that are excited by glucose
reaching them, but only when the animal is hungry; satiation stops

When they are
swallow any-
mulated,
out if
eat

normally, the animal goes on eating
eact.

of reciprocal innervation, there are
lamus which, when stimulated, stop
n of these neurons makes the animal
ruction of the eating-excitatory neu-
ing-inhibitory neurons stop the ani-
ll then die of starvation in the midst

ings. There are glucose receptors in the hypothalamus that sense the amount of glucose in the passing blood; when it goes down, the animal feels hungry. But it is not only a question of glucose; fatty acids and amino acids in the blood also play a role. There are also hunger contractions of the stomach. People when they are hungry get an almost painful sensation in the pit of the stomach due to the contractions. But this is not an essential mechanism for feeling hungry, for patients who have had their stomachs removed still feel normally hungry. Experiments undertaken on rats have shown that stress may make the animal either reduce or increase the amount it eats. This seems to be the same for man.

There are also neurons in the hypothalamus that control the animal's drinking. If they are destroyed, the animal loses the urge to drink, but it will go on eating normally. Stimulation of this region makes the animal drink. The right amount of fluid to be taken in is governed by osmoreceptors in the hypothalamus. These receptor cells are activated by a minimal increase in salt content when the cell loses fluid. Thus, when we lose fluid, the cell fluid decreases, the salt content of the cell increases, the osmoreceptors are activated, we feel thirsty, and we drink. Also dryness of the mouth caused by reduced saliva is noted by receptors in the lining mucous membrane (a mucous membrane is the equivalent of the skin for internal cavities). In actual fact, we don't wait to feel thirsty before we drink.

Feeling that one has had enough to drink also depends on receptors in the stomach wall which report that the stomach is full. The glucose receptors and osmoreceptors of the hypothalamus also react to the temperature of the passing blood. When the temperature starts to rise, one feels thirsty but not hungry; cooling the blood makes one hungry.

These are the basal mechanisms of thirst and drinking at the level of the hypothalamus. The mechanisms are fitted into the circumstances of living by various parts of the cerebral hemispheres, and in particular by the amygdala of the temporal lobe (see Fig. 15.2).

However, choosing a correct diet is more complicated than that. For animals not only come to eat a right amount of food, they eat a proper variety. Nearly all animals have to take varied diet; and they do so by stopping eating a certain food, even when there is a lot of it available, and by eating something else, even when there is less of that food around. One factor is the availability of the food; another and important one is whether they want that food or not. And this is determined somehow by internal needs.

There are other neurons in the brain of the rat that, on being stimulated, make the rat hoard food. Perhaps there are similar neurons in the brain of man. Hoarding is one of the actions that is not stopped by a consummatory act. Other actions of this kind are playing and exploring.

There are also needs to eat and drink unrelated to hunger and thirst. Babies need to carry out a certain amount of sucking, however much fluid they get; indeed, experiments have shown that the amount of sucking is more important than the amount of milk. This is an inborn drive, a need to carry out the sucking act.

Circadian Rhythms

The universe is orderly, and there is an eternal recurrence of events. In this universe living organisms have become adapted to the regular changes. They live according to day and night, the warm and cold seasons where these show periodical changes in temperature, dry and wet seasons in other parts of the world. As the first periodic behaviour to arouse interest among biologists was the alternation of sleeping and waking with night and day, these rhythms were called circadian rhythms (Latin *circa*, about: *dies*, a day), and this term is used for rhythms of other durations. These rhythms are basically endogenous, built into the nervous systems of animals.

What is curious is that many circadian rhythms of human beings have a 25-hour cycle. This has been learned by putting people in underground rooms or caves where daylight does not penetrate, and where factors such as humidity, temperature, and atmospheric pressure can be kept constant. This 25 hours varies a little from person to person, but it is almost always more than 24 hours. If a person in such an experiment usually got up at eight in the morning, after twelve days he would be getting up at twelve in the evening, thinking he was getting up at his usual time in the morning. This independence of the usual 24-hour cycle shows us that we have an intrinsic oscillator, independent of the earth's rotation. Yet in normal living this intrinsic rhythm is changed to a 24-hour rhythm. Aschoff and Wever in Germany have done extensive and very long-lasting experiments to find out what changes the intrinsic 25-hour rhythm to the usual 24-hour rhythm. Although the periodicity of light and dark is important for certain species, it plays no role in man; keeping man under varying periods of light and dark does not alter his circadian rhythms. The factor that does govern the 24-hour periodicity is the earth's magnetic field. This field changes in a 24-hour cycle as the world turns on its axis.

When in experiments people are isolated from the magnetic field of the earth, they have the circadian rhythm of 25 hours. When they are returned to the earth's magnetic field, they have the usual 24-hour cycle. In these experiments the subjects are totally unaware of being influenced by any outside agency; they do not know that their internal clocks have changed from 25 to 24 hours, and they do not know when they are living within this field or when it is excluded. We have no idea what part of the body senses the magnetic field, nor whether it is all the cells of the body or some particular sensory receptors.

The earth's magnetic field is influenced by the sun. The possible effects of solar activity on ourselves and other living organisms could be observed better if cyclical events were noted in relation to the 27-day period of revolution of the sun around its axis, instead of in relation to lunar months or to the arbitrary calendar.

The internal clock that sets off our sleeping and waking, rest and activity, is a nucleus in the front end of the hypothalamus, the suprachiasmatic nucleus. This nucleus is just near the two optic nerves, and receives nerve fibres from the retina. These nerve fibres report the hours of light and dark, and this information adjusts the internal clock in certain species of animals. The nucleus has been destroyed experimentally in the hamster, in which animal it can be destroyed without there being much damage to other neural structures. When it is destroyed, rhythms of general activity, sleeping and waking, drinking, changes in body temperature, and endocrine secretion, are all upset.

The suprachiasmatic nucleus is active in the day time and quiet at night. What is amazing is that when the nucleus is cut out and kept alive in a dish, its neurons continue to manifest the rhythm for 12 to 18 hours.

The suprachiasmatic nucleus forms an essential link in the annual reproduction of many animals. It has connections with the septal and preoptic region at the front end of the hypothalamus; the preoptic nucleus is important in causing the oestrous cycle. This region of the brain is connected to the pineal gland. In many animals the pineal acts on the pituitary gland and the hypothalamus, influencing the production of sex hormones. In this case, what the suprachiasmatic nucleus is taking note of is not so much the duration of night and day as the total amount of daylight. For this is the important factor in deciding when sexual activity is wanted so that the next generation gets a good start in life.

The intrinsic rhythm generator has been studied in *Aplysia*, a large snail. In this animal there are neurons in the central nervous system that fire off volleys of impulses at the end of every 12 hours. If the neurons are dissected out and put in a dish surrounded by necessary nutrients, they continue to fire off with their 12-hour rhythm. Thus, this rhythm of firing is a property of the cells; it seems to depend on their biochemical characteristics.

The autonomic nervous system

In the second century AD, Galen described and named the sympathetic nervous system. He called it sympathetic because the word meant harmonious in those days; and he considered that this system of nerves acted to keep the various parts of the body acting in harmony. In addition to organizing the body so that the hands of the two sides of the body have the same temperature and the same degree of dilation of blood-vessels, and the same for the feet and two sides of the head, the sympathetic system is hyperactive when one is manifesting the defence reaction, and feeling either rage or fear. The obvious physical accompaniments of these states were first investigated physiologically by Walter B. Cannon in the early years of this century. Cannon described the effects of strongly activitating the sympathetic system as follows: 'Respiration deepens: the heart beats more rapidly; the arterial pressure rises; the blood is shifted away from the stomach and intestines to the heart and the muscles; sugar is freed from the reserves in the liver . . . The key to these marvellous transformations in the body is found in relating them to the natural accompaniments of fear and rage—running away in order to escape from danger, and attacking in order to be dominant.'

When the crisis is over, one can relax, eat and drink, digest, secrete saliva and digestive secretions throughout the alimentary canal; this is what the parasympathetic system organizes.

The automonic nervous system is built on different general principles from the central nervous system. The central nervous system has all synapses within the spinal cord and the brain. In the autonomic system, there are synapses collected together in minibrains called ganglia outside the central nervous system. The nerves of the peripheral nervous system break up into a few branches, each one supplying a muscle fibre. The autonomic nerves break up into a multitude of small branches, and each branch is able to affect many cells as it passes between them. The transmitter substances are put out at little swellings along the nerve fibres, the varicosities. There are hundreds of them per millimetre of nerve fibre.

The sympathetic system is that part of the nervous system by means of which the blood-vessels and blood flow are governed. When one is getting cold, the blood-vessels of the hands and feet are constricted, so as not to lose heat. When one is hot, the sympathetic nerves are quietened and the blood-vessels dilate. In animals with large ears, like the elephant, the sympathetic system stops constricting the blood-vessels of the ears, and heat is lost. The sympathetic system also makes our hair stand on end. This happens all over the body, as we see in cats and dogs. It is used to keep warm by trapping a layer of air around the skin, and to strike terror into the adversary by making the body appear larger.

When we are sleeping, the sympathetic system is inhibited by neurons in the reticular formation of the medulla oblongata. The sympathetic system wakes up when we wake up.

The same pattern of physiological behaviour occurs when we wake up as occurs in the defence reaction, though in a milder way. When emotions of fear or aggression are aroused, this pattern increases in degree. A mere token of these emotions increases these activities; even talking does it. A sudden shout or driving a car speeds up the heart rate. In motor racing, heart rates of 200 a minute have been recorded. If something is startling enough, the pupils dilate, eyelids retract, showing the white of the eye above the pupil, and the hair stands on end, all due to the sympathetic nervous system.

Some species of animals possess chromatophores, cells containing pigment, to enable them to camouflage themselves and sink into the background. There are two ways used to bring these cells into activity: the circulation of melanocyte-stimulating hormone and the autonomic nervous system. Chameleons, so famous for their colour changes, organize their chromatophores entirely by the autonomic system; this enables them to change colour rapidly.

The salivary glands are supplied by parasympathetic and sympathetic nerves, the main supply being parasympathetic. The parasympathetic system is quietened during anger and excitement: the mouth is dry owing to less activity of the salivary glands. It may be difficult to swallow, as the chewed-up food is insufficiently lubricated. Weeping is also a parasympathetic activity, and so is defecation and urination. Most of copulation is also parasympathetic. Erection and ejaculation depend on parasympathetic nerves. Sympathetic nerves play a small part; they close off the

the bladder at the start of ejaculation to stop the semen going into the bladder.

Most acts of behaviour are not just sympathetic or parasympathetic. It is more complicated and subtle than that. Although the skin has to have a good blood supply to evaporate sweat, the immediate and first action of sympathetic activity is to constrict the blood-vessels of the skin. Anxiety and anger both make one pale. Facial pallor can also be due to a fall in blood pressure accompanying fear. In 1870, an American physician recorded the case of 'a travelling mountebank, who exhibited a wonderful control over the hue of his face, becoming flushed or deadly pale as he pleased'. And he mentioned another case, this time of a gentleman, who could 'produce at will contracture and roughness of the skin with prominence of the papillae and erection of the hairs—gooseflesh—with apparent loss of heat and visible paleness of the surface'. Thus it is possible to control the autonomic nervous system voluntarily.

One sees in animals that behaviour is very different according to whether an animal is bravely attacking or slinking away. In most cases it tends not to run away, as that provokes pursuit. But there are no general principles here. A small antelope surprised by a lion runs for its life, because the lion is a poor runner, and so it may well escape. The lion kills by hiding in the bushes and then leaping on the antelope which it kills, with luck, before the antelope knows what has happened. The pattern of an animal's behaviour is different for enemies swooping from the skies and those approaching on land, for enemies of one's own species and those of other species. A good picture of sympathetic activity associated with aggression and fleeing is given by Professor Yerkes, who spent many years of his life with chimpanzees.

When a cow approached, the apes would retreat in alarm; but when the potential threat to safety chanced to walk away it was boldly chased and threatened. There were corresponding sudden changes of bodily attitude and appearance in the apes and indications of secretory and excretory processes. When it is aggressive the chimpanzee is likely to march or run forward erect, swinging its arms and seeming to swell in size, partly because its hair rises. It stamps or beats the ground and bangs anything near that will resound. Often it screams, barks, or shouts, with its mouth wide open and the lips drawn back to expose the teeth. A chimpanzee retreating is an entirely different creature. Its hair lies flat, its body seems to shrink as if to escape attention, and it runs away quietly. Unless, indeed, every hair stands on end with terror and the challenger becomes a capering ball of fur. In all these cases and apparently correlated with the strength of the stimulus, frequent defecation may occur, or, less commonly, urination and vomiting.

All sorts of sudden events and chronic stresses alter the balance of the two parts of the autonomic system. Both parts are continuously played upon by the emotions. In man, anger causes the secretion of noradrenalin, anxiety the secretion of adrenalin. And adrenalin itself causes a feeling of anxiety.

The hypothalamus has four principal ways of using these two parts of the autonomic nervous system; it can diminish or increase the activity of the sympathetic system, and diminish or increase the activity of the parasympathetic system. Only in extreme circumstances does it both decrease the one system and increase the other. Normally both systems are active all the time, their activities being harmoniously balanced according to the needs of the moment.

In addition to the general activation of the sympathetic system, there are local sympathetic reflexes. Every harmful and painful stimulus brings out two sympathetic reflex responses: a local spinal response; and a longer supraspinal response in which impulses are sent up to the medulla oblongata and others return to the spinal cord. This second response is more general, and brings in sympathetic activity over the general region of the body that has been stimulated.

The alimentary canal is controlled by sympathetic and parasympathetic nerves. The sympathetic quietens it, for general activity within the world demands peaceful internal action. The parasympathetic activates it, for you can digest at your leisure when you are relaxed. Throughout the alimentary canal, parasympathetic nerves excite all the glands into activity so that they secrete their enzymes and lubricants to digest the food. In many carnivores, the smell of blood activates the parasympathetic nervous system so that their mouths water and enzymes are secreted throughout the alimentary canal. Evidence of parasympathetic activity can be observed in one's cats. When you take them on your lap and stroke them and they sit in relaxed security, they often dribble. Salivary glands are mainly activated by parasympathic nerves.

The parts of the hypothalamus in which parasympathetic centres are located are the same as those that contain the rewarding or pleasure centres; these are the parts that the animal will endlessly stimulate in itself by pressing the lever. The parts where the sympathetic centres are located are parts that the animals do not stimulate if the permanent electrodes are implanted in them. It appears then that the parasympathetic centres give a feeling of contentment and pleasure, whereas the excitement or agitation of sympathetic activity is not welcomed.

The transmitters of the sympathetic and parasympathetic systems, adrenalin, noradrenalin, and acetylcholine, are not the only chemical substances used in the alimentary canal. There are also local hormones, produced by cells of the alimentary canal called paracrine cells. Many of these local hormones are produced by the food as it passes along. For instance, fat in the food passing through the duodenum induces the secretion of cholecystokinin. This hormone acts on the gall-bladder, making it contract and pour out bile; the bile is needed for digestion of fat. Paracrine cells of the pancreas also produce this hormone; here it makes the pancreas secrete insulin, and insulin is needed to digest carbohydrate.

Over and above the hypothalamus

The hypothalamus does not initiate behaviour. That is the function of the cerebral hemispheres. The hemispheres collect information from all input channels, make a total and meaningful picture from it, supply the picture with suitable emotions and memories, and then organize a programme of behaviour.

Certain parts of the cerebral hemispheres are closely related to the hypothalamus. For example, the orbital cortex, which is the part of the cerebral hemispheres lying above our eyes, connects to the front part that commands the system. Many parts of the temporal lobes are connected to the region of the hypothalamus which controls the pituitary gland and the secretion of hormones.

The earliest parts of the cerebral hemispheres to develop during evolution are called the limbic lobe. This lobe is made up of various parts, which are shown in Fig. 15.2. These are the cingulate gyrus (*cingulum*; Latin, a girdle, as it engirdles the corpus callosum), the hippocampal gyrus, the uncus (Latin, a hook, as it looks a bit like a hook), and the amygdala. They are closely related to the hypothalamus and the septal area.

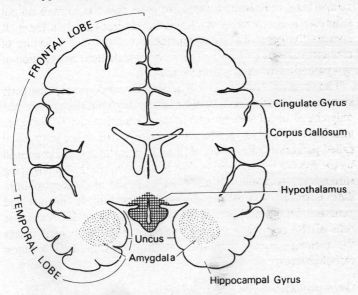

Fig. 15.2 The human brain cut from side to side to show the position of the hypothalamus and the parts of the limbic lobe, amygdala, and uncus.

When the temporal lobe is dissected away, one can see the amygdala and hippocampus. In Fig 15.3. the nerve fibres can be seen passing forwards to the septal area and the hypothalamus. These fibres connect the earliest parts of the cerebral hemispheres with the centres organizing the many functions discussed in this chapter.

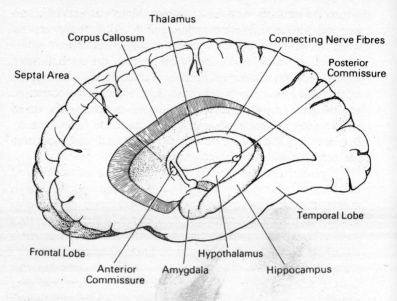

Fig. 15.3 The amygdala and the hippocampus in the depth of the opposite temporal lobe. The three commissures, anterior, posterior and corpus callosum, are shown.

One notices incidentally from the names that these nomenclators lived around the Mediterranean: they were in fact Romans. A part of the brain was called the olive; here we have the amygdala, an almond, and hippocampus, a sea-horse. The amygdala was developed in fish, perhaps to interpret the inputs of taste and smell. In higher animals, all sensory inputs are relayed to this grey matter.

What the hypothalamus receives has already passed through the cerebral hemispheres. The animal behaves by responding to the situation in which it find itself. Before it can respond to this situation, all the inputs have been integrated and assessed. This is the function of the cerebral hemispheres. What is occurring is related to past experience, and in the higher vertebrates it may also be related to a probable future. Only when the situation has been interpreted and judged is a line of behaviour ordered, and the hypothalamus called upon to organize this behaviour.

It works similarly with regard to more simple aspects of behaviour too, such as defecating, eating, and drinking. It appears that when we imagine a delicious a meal or see, smell, or start tasting food, we are activating the insula; this part of the cerebral hemisphere is closely connected with the hypothalamus. And so, the smell, taste, or just the thought of food activates the hypothalamus and the parasympathetic system. This makes our mouths water; farther along the alimentary canal, other digestive juices are similarly secreted, and the movements of the stomach and duodenum are increased, all ready to receive the meal.

It is possible that the cerebral hemisphere-hypothalamus circuit can be short-circuited at every level. For instance, the foot is pulled off the thorn of the cactus before the cerebral cortex knows what is happening. Something sudden and potentially dangerous alarms the animal before it knows what it is. The alarm reaction is set off by certain regions of the mid-brain. The whole nervous system is alerted, and the cortex is made vigilant to find out what has happened. The cortex does not need to find out and then spread the alarm throughout the central nervous system; though things can also happen in this order.

There is one other situation in which it may be that hypothalamus behaviour is in control, the cerebral hemispheres being short-circuited: fleeing in panic before an unknown horror. Many people in a panic-stricken crowd have no idea why they are fleeing. They are wholly taken up in terror, imitating the behaviour of everyone else, and the urge to flee, and that organizes their behaviour. The contributions of the cerebral hemispheres, reasoning, memories of past experience, planning play no role.

It is likely that the same occurs in boxing or other fighting when one loses one's temper; and the skilful boxer may try to make his opponent do so if he can. For the man who has lost his temper may be wilder but he has lost his cunning. All that he has learned and remembers, all his strategy and his planning, has gone. These are the contributions of the cerebral hemispheres. It may be that when one loses one's temper, one short-circuits the cerebral hemispheres, and acts with the hypothalamus alone.

The relationship between the cerebral hemispheres and the

hypothalamus is not merely one of inhibition. In normal life, it could be that the hemispheres call upon the hypothalamus to produce the patterns of behaviour organized in this structure when the total situation of the animal demands them. Now that the patterns of behaviour obtainable from experimental stimulation of the hypothalamus have been observed, it appears that such acts of violent behaviour are almost never seen in pure form in natural conditions. For what was seen in these experiments was somewhat different from what is seen in normal life. When the cerebral hemispheres are in control, the animal is capable at all times of reviewing the situation. It is not merely a wildly fighting object or a wildly fleeing animal. Its behaviour is related to the total situation. A bird will be aggressive when it is on the border of its territory; it will flee when it is attacked in someone else's territory. Hypothalamic behaviour is adjusted and graded by the hemispheres. Using its cerebral hemispheres, the animal can appreciate the whole situation and is able to choose. The cerebral hemispheres provide a means of delaying direct responses. Above all, they integrate the basic ways of behaving into the whole situation.

16 Broadcasting information: hormones

Hormones are substances released by endocrine glands and by certain neurons into the blood stream and extra-cellular fluid in order to have effects on other cells. The neurons that put out hormones are mainly certain neurons of the hypothalamus that act on the pituitary gland.

If the obvious analogy for nerve fibres is the telephone or telegraphy, then the analogy for hormones is radio. There are then two broadcasting systems, a local radio station serving just a few houses, and a general station for the whole country. The control of the general broadcasting station belongs to the central authority of the brain. Just as there are many broadcasting stations, so there are many different hormones. The programme is broadcast far and wide, but it can be picked up only by those with sets tuned to receive it. So it is with hormones. They are poured into the bloodstream and sent all round the body; but they bring meaningful messages only to those cells tuned in to receive them.

Hormones might be thought of as drugs manufactured in the body. The chemical constitution of most of them has now been worked out, and they are also manufactured by the pharmaceutical industry. The practical result of this is that if our own bodies give up making them, we can take them artificially, by swallowing them or having them injected.

The terminology is rather unsatisfactory as it was worked out a long time before much of our present knowledge had been acquired. The result is that one and the same substance can come in different guises and is labelled according to its mode of secretion and its receptor cells. If a substance is made by one cell and acts on the surrounding cells, it is called a paracrine substance. If it is passed into the bloodstream to affect many target cells in the body, it is called a hormone, and the gland that forms it is an endocrine gland. Other glands, such as tear glands or salivary glands, pour their secretions through little pipes or ducts into the cavity designed to receive them. If the same substance is put out by a nerve-ending, it is a transmitter or a modulator, depending on its action.

The brain organizes behaviour, the total growth of the body, and the changes in growth that occur at puberty and after sexual activity runs down and when old age arrives. This overall control is dealt with by the hypothalamus; and the hypothalamus carries out most of its general functions by emitting hormones and by controlling the pituitary's emission of hormones. The correct amount of hormones is adjusted by self-regulating servo-systems. 'Correct' often means correct for the whole group of the animals rather than correct for that individual.

Hypothalamic hormones affecting the pituitary are brought to its anterior lobe in veins in the pituitary stalk, called portal veins; they are shown in Fig.16.1. Each of these substances is named in relation to the pituitary hormone that it releases or inhibits.

The first one to be discovered was thyroid-releasing hormone. It makes the pituitary emit thyroid-stimulating hormone, which activates the thyroid gland. For sex the most important hormone is gonadotrophin-releasing hormone. It makes the pituitary put out the two gonadal hormones, luteinizing hormone and follicle-stimulating hormone. The releasing hormone is put out in bursts and not continuously. Two pituitary hormones, prolactin and growth hormone, are controlled by releasing and inhibiting hormones. The growth hormone-inhibiting substance is called somatostatin. Corticotrophin-releasing hormone acts on the pituitary to make it secrete adrenocorticotrophin.

Hormones have obvious effects on behaviour. They give the animal desires in order to make it perform those functions that are needed for its survival and that of the group. The environment in which it lives also stimulates its desires and satisfies them. Potential sexual objects generate desire. In rats maternal behaviour can be kept going far longer than normal by the presence of the young. If, as fast as the rat's babies are being weaned, they are replaced by a

Hypothalamic neurons emitting
inhibitory and releasing hormones

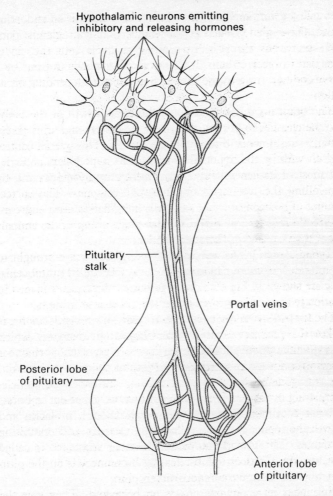

Pituitary
stalk

Portal veins

Posterior lobe
of pituitary

Anterior lobe
of pituitary

Fig. 16.1 The hypothalamus sends hormones to the pituitary gland in the portal veins.

new litter brought to the mother, the mother rat will continue to show maternal behaviour for several months instead of the normal period of a few weeks. She build nests and retrieves the wandering young; and without being fanciful, one may presume she feels the emotions related to these maternal acts. It is the same for most kinds of mammals and birds. It has often been observed that a childless woman, soon after adopting a child, conceives and starts to produce children of her own. Whether this is really so or not has not been examined statistically, as far as I know. It may well be true. The presence of the baby acts as a constant stimulus to parts of the brain, altering the balance of secretion of hormones, and this may allow fertilization to take place.

Changes in the tissues of the animal and changes in its behaviour brought about by the secretion of hormones are obvious to bird-watchers and owners of cats. The cock bird's change in plumage, together with its change in behaviour, appear in spring with hormones causing mating, nest-building, and bringing up the young. The bower bird of Australia and New Guinea collects its favoured coloured objects, arranges them in its bower, and then dances before this backcloth. The weaver-bird of Africa, obeying its inner compulsions, makes its hanging nest. In our own islands at the end of winter, birds such as the peewit and the bunting, which had lived contentedly together in flocks, go off on their own. Every male acquires a territory; and with it he acquires a new personality, and a new kind of behaviour towards his former friends. He becomes aggressive and eager to fight anyone entering his domain. In the few species in which this subject has been investigated, it is the increasing length of daylight that starts off this new behaviour.

Hormones are not the only instigators of total behaviour. Thoughts and imagination can bring about the secretion of hormones. Thoughts come from the activity of cerebral and hypothalamic neurons, and these neurons connect to others controlling the pituitary. Thus imagination can call forth the hormones that can then re-stimulate the very same neurons in the brain. This is a positive feedback mechanism; it can cause an ever-increasing demand made by the animal on its fellows and its surroundings till this cycle is broken by the factors that satisfy the desires and bring the relief of satiety. Similarly, the secretion of hormones can be stopped by thought. Grief suppresses lust far more effectively than religion.

To such questions as do hormones form behaviour, or does

behaviour produce the hormones, the answer is that both are true. Hormones produce needs and desires which do not occur until the hormone reaches the brain. In its turn, behaviour influences the brain, and this affects the secretion of hormones.

The brain is not to be thought of as loftily surveying all that is going on. It is itself a part of the body and subjected to all those influences that affect the rest of the body. It receives the same blood that circulated through the muscles, liver and alimentary canal. This blood contains the last digested meal. And one wonders what will happen when that hot chocolate sauce eventually gets to your brain. The neurons of the brain receive the alchohol you take, the hormones you secrete, and drugs. One must remember that everything the pregnant mother eats, drinks, and experiences will reach the foetus within her womb.

The brain, like all the tissues of the body, is either male or female. Like the reproductive system, the brain is basically female. It has to be made male by the action of gonadal hormones during development of the embryo. When the testis is formed from the germ cells, it secretes the male hormone, testosterone. In fact, testosterone is also secreted in the female embryo, but there is less of it than in the male. This secretion of testosterone has to be done at the correct time during embryonic development. At this sensitive period the hormone affects the neurons of certain nuclei just in front of the hypothalamus. These differences can be seen with the microscope. The male preoptic nucleus is much larger than the female, and the pattern of the dendrites of its neurons is different from that of the female. These nuclei, when the time comes, have the functions of organizing the pituitary to put out the correct hormones for male or female reproduction.

Thus, hormones already play a role in the formation of the embryo. The testes of the foetus secrete testosterone, and that hormone makes the undifferentiated tissues become the male reproductive organs. Without the hormone, the tissue becomes female organs. When parts of this development go wrong, various kinds of intersexed people result.

There are also hormones passing from the mother's blood across the placenta into the bloodstream of the baby. There they reach the brain, and have a permanent influence on certain developing neurons at a particular and important time.

The right or the wrong balance of hormones the baby receives when it is in its mother's womb can later affect the sexual anatomy, physiology, and psychology of the child, and then of the adult. We have learned this from giving pregnant women progesterone or similar substances in order to prevent a threatened miscarriage or to treat toxaemia of pregnancy. The few studies of the children of such mothers showed that the girls were more intelligent than the average and had more masculine interests. They liked to play with boys' toys, were more athletic than other girls, and were not interested in caring for babies and putting on feminine clothes. On so-called intelligence tests, these children got a mean IQ of 125 (the average of ordinary children being 100), and 6 of the 10 scored above 130; only 2 per cent of the average population have this score. In one other series, in which the controls were the neighbouring baby in the labour ward and also children of mothers with toxaemia of pregnancy, the children of the mothers who had had progesterone did better than the other in verbal reasoning, English, and arithmetic. The best results were obtained when the progesterone was given the mother before the sixteenth week of pregnancy and for a period of eight weeks. The boys of such mothers, on reaching adolescence, did not go out with girls so often, did less day-dreaming about girls, marriage, and family life, and they were more likely to cause disciplinary problems in their schools. Both the boys and the girls were more studious and less socially orientated than the controls. In the follow-up of one group of such children, 11 of the 34 adolescents from the progesterone mothers obtained university places. This was 32 per cent of the children. The percentage of normal 18-year-olds entering universities at the time was 6 per cent.

There are no comparable children whose mothers received oestrogens during pregnancy. But when they are given certain mammals experimentally, the male offspring are less self-assertive and aggressive than their mates.

One of the surprising general facts learned from many thousands of experiments on rats is that the pattern of behaviour of each sex is built into both sexes; and yet under the normal circumstances of their lives each one manifests only its own sexual pattern. That each sex has in its brain neurons capable of organizing the sexual activities of the opposite is shown by the injection of male hormones into females and female hormones into males. In rats each sex then shows the behaviour of the opposite sex so successfully that it is treated by other rats as if it were of the sex belonging to the hormone injected; for instance, castrated males injected with female hormones are treated by other males as females. These injected males build nests, an activity normally carried out only by females after puberty; they retrieve the young and bring them back to the nest, behaviour normally shown only by females after the birth of their young. It is remarkable enough that a female rat, raised in isolation, knows how to build a nest. It is extraordinary that male rats, who are never normally called upon to do such a thing, also know how to do it, once they have been injected with the female sex hormone progesterone. Male canaries sing; females do not. But if a hen canary is injected with the male hormone tostersterone, it starts singing. This male behaviour is associated with an enlargement of nuclei in the front of the hypothalamus, mentioned above.

Bird-watchers also have seen evidence that the behaviour of each sex may be built into the nervous system of both sexes. Sometimes among those birds in which the male normally feeds the female in courtship, the opposite has been witnessed; the female will feed a male or other females. Aristotle recorded in his book on the generation of animals that two female doves will form a pair if there is no male available; this has frequently been corroborated for many other birds.

The sex of a person may be uncertain. There is sex according to the chromosomes, sex according to the kind of gonads possessed by the person, testes or ovaries, sex according to the internal organs that are not seen, such as the uterus or the seminal vesicles, or sex according to the obvious external sexual organs; and the whole body can be influenced towards a feminine or masculine form and behaviour in accordance with the secretion of hormones.

In a sense, feminine sexual organization is basic. It requires certain hormones during a period around birth to cause masculine sexual behaviour at and after adolescence. If they are absent, both sexes will show feminine behaviour. This has been found in experiments in small animals that can be kept in laboratories; but it may not be so important for humans. Experience indicates that for human beings, social factors are the most important determinants. Studies of human hermaphrodites show that the sexual role assigned to the child and in which it is brought up determines its adult behaviour. If the child is brought up as a boy, it will prefer girls when it reaches puberty, and if brought up as a girl, it will prefer boys. According to the dictates of some religions, males have to be circumcised. Occasionally the penis is cut off along with the foreskin—by mistake. These children are usually brought up as girls, and they behave as girls in all respects. Incidentally, human homosexuals of both sexes have normal amounts of pituitary and sex hormones.

The cells that are affected by a hormone are called its target cells or receptor cells. Certain cells of the brain are the target cells for sex hormones. When these cells unite with the hormone, they instigate sexuality. There are cells in the septal area, the amygdala and hippocampus, and the hypothalamus that are the targets for the female sexual hormones, the oestrogens. These cells, in the cat, when stimulated by the oestrogens, change the female cat's behaviour towards the male from aggression to acceptance.

It is amazing how quickly hormonal effects on behaviour are produced. One example of rapid action comes from the world of insects. The singing of the male grasshopper attracts the female who, hearing it, arrives post-haste and ready for copulation. But when the act is finished, the very same song no longer attracts her. It has been found that the reason for the female's changing her mind is that during copulation the male has injected a hormone with its sperm; and this hormone suppresses the activity of certain neurons in her brain. When these particular neurons are active, this female longs to hear the serenade; but when they are inactive, either this music is not heard or noticed, or it means nothing to her.

How hormones act on certain cells so as to cause such effects is still being investigated. So far, two different mechanisms have been discovered. The hormone either acts on the cell membrane or it passes through it and enters the cell. Amino acids, such as noradrenalin, and peptides, such as prolactin and adrenocorticotrophic hormone, unite with the target cell membrane. Steroid hormones, such as oestradiol, pass through the cell membrane and unite with a receptor within the cell. This combined hormone and receptor enters the nucleus of the cell, uniting with the DNA; and then the cell manufactures a different kind of protein.

Hormones also act on the intellectual and mental functions of the brain. They affect one's concentration and attention; and, at least in rats, they affect the ability to remember.

The pituitary consists of an anterior and a posterior lobe; in many species there is also an intermediate lobe. Human beings do not have an intermediate lobe, except when the female is pregnant; after the birth of the child, it regresses. When it is active, it secretes proopiomelanocortin. The anterior lobe secretes corticotrophin, alpha-melanostimulating hormone, beta-endorphin and beta-lipotrophin, growth hormone, thyrotrophin, prolactin, and two gonadotrophin hormones, follicle-stimulating hormone and luteinizing hormone. The posterior lobe of the pituitary does not make any hormones but it receives two from the hypothalamus, vasopressin and oxytocin. These substances are also put out by many nerve-endings throughout the brain and spinal cord.

There are always two factors interacting, the intrinsic data of the body and the environment in which the body lives. The duration of daylight affects the pineal gland. In summer the amount of the pineal hormone, melatonin, goes down, for light suppresses the gland. Darkness increases the amount. Its secretion is maximal at midnight and minimal with the morning light. These effects depend on its sympathetic nerve supply.

Melatonin inhibits those pituitary cells that produce the hormones which organize sexual activity. Thus, the length of daytime influences sexual life. In many birds, this relationship between daylight and reproduction seems to have been developed so that the parent birds have enough time during the long days to collect insects to satisfy the voracious appetites of the young. In their case, the rhythm of life, the onset of puberty, the times of mating and producing young, as well as the time of migration, are all set by the length of daylight, reported by the eyes to the pineal gland.

If a young rat is kept in constant light, the pineal gland is damped down and its inhibitory effect on the pituitary is decreased. What happens then is that puberty arrives early. The opposite also occurs. A rat constantly in the dark reaches puberty late.

Young Syrian hamsters have to be born in the spring. The animal hibernates during the winter, and while it hibernates, its testicles are atrophic and no spermatozoa are produced. As the duration of daylight starts to be more than half the twenty-four hours, the secretion of pineal hormones decreases, and the gonads respond to the hormones emitted by the pituitary. Then things happen rapidly; the young are born sixteen days after hibernation stops. The connections between the eyes, the suprachiasmatic nucleus of the hypothalamus, the sympathetic centres in the spinal cord, the pineal gland, and back to the hypothalamus were described on pages 23 and 179.

The effect of the pineal gland on the pituitary is shown up when a tumour of the pineal gland develops. The hormones produced by the tumour can stop the pituitary secreting its own hormones, and the patient comes to the doctor with all the manifestations of absence of pituitary function. If the tumour stops the pineal gland forming the hormones that inhibit the pituitary, then puberty comes on abnormally early. The same state can occur with a tumour of the hypothalamus. The young girl may develop breasts and start menstruating. In boys the changes that occur produce such well-developed muscle that the condition has been called Infant Hercules, where boys of 4 years old have big muscles and their voices break; their genital organs enlarge, and they can successfully perform sexual intercourse. However, the suppression of the pituitary by the pineal is not a one-way street; oestrogens suppress the pineal gland too.

Melatonin taken by mouth makes one sleepy. There seems to be a connection between darkness at night, sleep, and melatonin. Melatonin counteracts jet-lag.

Melatonin has another role, related to light and darkness. It contracts certain cells in the skin, called melanophores, those containing melanin. Contraction of these cells makes the animal's skin light, and dilatation of the cells makes it dark. Thus, the skin of some becomes darker in the sun, and troglodytes have an unearthly pallor.

A quite different factor causing the circulation of more melatonin is stress. Stress stimulates the adrenal medulla; more adrenalin then enters the circulation; it arrives in the pineal gland, and there it is changed to melatonin.

Growth depends on the hypothalamus, which makes the pituitary secrete growth hormone. If the hypothalamic neurons controlling growth are experimentally destroyed in an animal, the secretion of growth hormone stops, and the animal stops growing. Children who are very small usually have normal amounts of growth hormone; but some people with gigantism (the opposite of dwarfism) have excessive amounts of the hormone. Heredity is a main factor in determining a person's size; no doubt it acts through determining the amount of growth hormone.

Children who are miserable may not grow, and they remain abnormally small. They have a deficiency of growth hormone. It soon becomes normal when the child is taken from its unhappy home; growth then starts again.

When too much growth hormone is secreted before puberty, gigantism results. In this condition growth is normal but excessive, that is to say the person is big, though with normal proportions. Such people are usually very strong.

After puberty, the ends of the bones, or epiphyses, are fixed to the shafts of the bones, and no further growth in length is possible. When there is an excess of growth hormone after puberty, acromegaly (giant extremities) results. In this case the proportions are abnormal. The bones become thick and deformed, particularly the bones of the hands, feet, and face. The sinuses in the face enlarge, and that makes the voice deeper. The soft tissues also overgrow. This condition is associated with diminished secretion of gonadal hormones. Evidence is now appearing showing that in these people there is an excessive amount of growth hormone releasing factor. They have therefore been given growth hormone inhibiting factor, but unfortunately this also has effects on insulin secretion and on the hormones of the alimentary canal; and that stops it being useful.

There was a famous giant in Russia early in this century called Machnov. He was said to have been more than 9 feet (254 cm) tall.

The two hormones that act on the gonads are follitrophin and lutrophin. Follitrophin makes the ovaries produce the female hormone, oestradiol. In the male, it acts on the tubules of the testicles which produce the spermatozoa. Lutrophin acts on the interstitial cells of the gonads. In the female it causes the expulsion of the ovum from the ovary; in the male its effect is to produce androgen. In both sexes, lutrophin makes the gonads grow at puberty. Recently it has been discovered that young men with mania have a greatly excessive amount of lutrophin.

The secretion of gonadotrophins, no doubt like that of all hormones, is influenced by psychological factors. In those animals in which smell is a guiding sensation, the presence of the smell of the opposite sex influences the amount of the hormones. Female mice do not produce gonadotrophins when they live among a lot of other females; they need the smell of male mice. It has been found in experiments that the presence of one male is enough to negate the effect of the smell of thirty females.

What is more surprising is that infant female mice, exposed in infancy to the smell of the adult male mouse, come to choose adult male mice as sexual partners when they reach sexual maturity. But if they are reared only with other females or with males daily sprayed with perfume, then later they show no preference for males. The period during which the presence or absence of male odour has this lasting effect is very short. This is an example of imprinting (see page 244). In this case, it is olfactory imprinting; in most other cases investigated so far, imprinting is visual.

It is thought that what starts puberty off is that neurons of the hypothalamus become less sensitive to testosterone and oestradiol. These neurons then put out the demand for the secretion of more gonadotrophins, and so more testosterone and oestradiol are produced. These hormones then act on the spinal cord and brain, particularly on the anterior nuclei of the hypothalamus. Their obvious effects are on the size of the genital organs and a growth of hair on certain parts of the body. There is enlargement of the larynx and sinuses in both sexes; this is more marked in the boy, and accounts for his voice breaking. Bass and baritone singers have more testosterone in their blood than tenors. Testosterone enlarges the muscles and the sebaceous gland of the skin. With this increase in sebum there often goes acne, which upsets the adolescent's confidence in his appearance.

Prolactin is not well named, for males also have the hormone. Indeed, it is very high in male babies just after birth. After puberty, females have more. After its birth the baby sucks the nipple; this stimulus sends impulses to the spinal cord; they are relayed to the hypothalamus. The hypothalamus makes the pituitary secrete prolactin, which fills the breasts with milk. This is another servo control system; the baby stimulates milk secretion by sucking; when he ceases to suck, the milk supply dries up. Prolactin alone is unable to supply a good enough milk supply. Adrenocorticotrophic hormone is needed, and also oxytocin to eject the milk.

Prolactin makes females maternal. Prolactin injected into virgin female rats or castrated male rats makes them behave like mother rats. They retrieve baby rats, bringing them back to the nest. Without this injection, both are indifferent or even antagonistic to the young. When prolactin is injected into cocks, it makes them behave towards chicks as hens do, instead of showing the usual superior male indifference. In virgin hens, it causes broodiness; in certain virgin fish, it produces nest-building. In the human male it seems to have no function. In some birds it acts in both sexes, preparing them for migration by putting on fat before the long journey.

To come back to the case of man, there are some tumours that prevent the pituitary from developing normally. Gonadotrophins are not made, and puberty never comes. In these people, the growth of the skeleton continues for longer than usual, and so they have abnormally long limbs. The voice does not break; the man has fine, soft hair, and does not need to shave. With the enormous population nowadays, there must be quite a number of such eunuchs around. It would be a good idea to train some of them as alto singers. Instead of castrating infants for the Pope's choir as used to be done for the greater glory of God, we could now obtain singers in a normal way. The female counterpart of a eunuch does not seem to have been studied or have aroused as much interest as the male—another example of injustice to women.

There are two hormones formed in the hypothalamus and passed down the pituitary stalk into the posterior lobe of the pituitary. They are neurophysin-oxytocin and neurophysin-vaprosessin. They leave the posterior lobe of the pituitary by passing into the veins. Oxytocin is essential for many aspects of reproduction, vasopressin is for maintaining the osmotic pressure of the tissues and the blood. These hormones are also passed into the anterior lobe of the pituitary through the large portal veins. They also enter the cerebrospinal fluid, which circulates throughout the brain and around the spinal cord.

Oxytocin also occurs in males, though it is not yet known what function it fulfills. In females, stimulation of the genital organs causes its secretion. When the hormone reaches the uterus, it makes the muscle undergo rhythmical contractions; these movements help the spermatozoa reach the ovum. The violent movements of the uterus during labour also make the hypothalamus secrete large amounts of the hormone; this again helps the uterus make rhythmical contractions, thus helping the expulsion of the baby. After the baby is born, sucking the breast stimulates the same neurons of the hypothalamus and more of the hormone is produced. In this phase it aids the expulsion of the milk. Thus it is seen that each subsequent step in reproduction is induced by the previous step.

The speed at which this occurs is surprising. In the rat, neurons in a nucleus in the hypothalamus fire off volleys of impulses. They make the posterior pituitary release oxytocin; the oxytocin works on the smooth muscle of the mammary gland, and that causes milk let-down. From the time of the volley of nerve impulses sent off to the ejection of milk is 10–15 seconds.

Vasopressin suppresses the formation of urine; this may be

needed in order to keep the osmotic pressure of the blood plasma correct. It also controls the amount of water taken in from the alimentary canal. Various kinds of stress increase the amount of vasopressin put out by the hypothalamus. At the same time it puts out adrenocorticotrophic hormone, which is also useful in times of stress.

If some injury or disorder stops the hypothalamus from sending vasopressin around the body, then there is a condition called diabetes insipidus. What is usually called diabetes is diabetes mellitus, in which the urine contains glucose and so is sweet, hence mellitus. Diabetes insipidus, with insipid as opposed to sweet urine, is also characterized by the patient drinking a great deal of fluid and passing large amount of urine. In this case, it is due to the kidney being unable to reabsorb sufficient amounts of water when it is not supplied with the antidiuretic hormone.

Vasopressin and oxytocin are formed in the hypothalamus, and yet they are hormones eventually passed into the circulation to have a general effect. There is in many cases no difference between transmitters and hormones. Both may be formed in neurons. Usually the transmitter is formed in very small amounts and acts locally on the next neuron or on a muscle. But in some places the amount of transmitter is large enough to be sent throughout the body to act as a hormone.

The adrenal or suprarenal gland caps the kidney, hence the name. There are really two quite separate glands, medulla and cortex. The cortex produces three different steroid hormones, glucocorticoids, androgens, and mineralocorticoid. The medulla forms two hormones, adrenalin and noradrenalin. These hormones have the same effects on most tissues of the body. They are needed for activity, and so they put glucose into the blood to be burned for energy. It is probable that aggression makes the glands secrete more noradrenalin. Taking examinations and parachute jumping put out more adrenalin. Tense, anxious, and passive people appear to secrete more adrenalin than others. A further action of these hormones is to act on the pituitary to make it secrete adrenocorticotrophin. This hormone also affects the reticular formation of the brain. The effect of this is probably to make the animal more vigilant, more aware of what is happening in the outside environment. Other ways of coping with stress are organized by the whole brain, the higher levels of which assess the situation. They excite the relevant neurons of the hypothalamus, and the hypothalamus makes the pituitary secrete β-lipotrophin, which is then broken down into cortocotrophin and β-endorphin.

The pituitary controls the thyroid, which secretes the hormone triiodothyronine. The amount of this hormone put out depends on the animal's activity and vigilance, and the surrounding temperature. A cold environment demands more to keep the animal warm. The thermostat is a part of the hypothalamus. This acts on the pituitary, which then secretes thyroid-stimulating hormones. Stress, rather surprisingly, tends to stop the thyroid putting out the hormone.

The nervous system itself needs the secretion of the thyroid gland; without this hormone it neither develops nor works properly. Children born without thyroid glands are cretins; they are mentally defective, for their brains do not grow adequately. When the amount of thyroid secretion is insufficient later in life, the tendon reflexes become slow, and this is used as a test for diminished thyroid secretion.

The effect of hormones secreted by the testes and ovaries on the nervous system of animals, and thus on their behaviour, is something man has known about for several thousand years. For he has understood that the removal of the testes alters the behaviour of male animals. More than two thousand years ago Aristotle reported that when the ovaries of sows are removed, their sexual desires are also removed. How man discovered the effects of these operations, and how this knowledge became so general, we do not know.

Hormones secreted by the testes in males and ovaries in females have the expected influence on the animal's behaviour; nearly all animals deprived of their gonads have no sexual interests and show no sexual behaviour. Among human beings, however, women may continue to have sexual desire after their ovaries have been removed at operation or after they have atrophied at the menopause. Cats, as we can all observe, are different. Female cats who have had their ovaries removed respond to the propositions

made to them by tom-cats with hate and not with love. But if a
minute pellet of oestrogen is injected into the correct part of the
hypothalamus, their behaviour changes, and they accept the pro-
posals. In many species of mammals this reversal of behaviour
occurs naturally. The presence and absence of sexual hormones in
the bloodstream occurs in alternating cycles; it is not necessary to
remove the ovaries to observe their effects on behaviour. Those
hormones that have mainly sexual effects have effects on the
aggression-submission aspects of behaviour in some animals.
Whether they act on the parts of the hypothalamus that organize
attack and flight behaviour is not yet known. The female of the
American marten normally lives contentedly with the male, but
when she is on heat she turns on him and fights him. On the other
hand, the female short-tailed shrew chases the male away unless
she is on heat, and can be so aggressive that she may kill and eat
him.

When the ovaries of a female such as a rat or a mouse are transferred to a male or the testicles of a male to a female, the animal's
behaviour changes in the expected direction; the male behaves like
a female and the female like a male. Although in the act of
copulation, different postures and different patterns of movement
are needed from the two sexes, yet the muscles are used correctly
and in the correct order. When injections of hormones are carried
out in the correct sex before the onset of puberty, the changes in
structure and behaviour normally occurring at puberty take place
within a few days. Testosterone injected into immature or castrated males induces male copulatory behaviour. When it is
injected into male chicks, they start, fifteen days after being
hatched, to crow like cocks and to make propositions to hens. As
has been related, virgin female rats can be made both to build nests
and retrieve the young when they receive prolactin. The neurons
organizing these aspects of female behaviour do not do this unless
they are acted upon by ovarian hormones. If the ovaries are
removed before puberty, these females do not manifest the appropriate behaviour towards the male for copulation to take place. But
after being injected with female hormone, they will crouch in the
appropriate position. However, such experiments do not always

lead to the expected result. It has been found that testosterone injected into the hypothalamus of male rats induces maternal behaviour.

Among the anthropoids, sex hormones have different effects in the different species; the higher species are less under the control of hormones than lower species. Interestingly enough, the male macaque monkey is more sensitive to the hormones of the female macaque than she is herself. Although the female macaque with ovaries removed may still present herself for sexual intercourse, the male is not interested. Moreover, male macaques do not groom females without ovaries, grooming being partly a sexual activity in monkeys. The amount of grooming the male gives the female macaque is related to the amount of oestradiol injected into the female spayed macaque. We do not know what features of the female make her attractive to the male. Certainly the male's frequency of copulation is related to the female's menstrual cycle; but her own behaviour is less influenced by this cycle than his is, for she will present herself for copulation at any time.

The social rank of an animal affects its secretion of hormones and so the caste system affects the animal's metabolism and even its anatomy. This has been proved to be so for monkeys and is likely to be so for ourselves.

The effect of androgens on aggressive behaviour has been studied in many different vertebrates. In many social animals, aggression is used to obtain food and sexual partners; and those animals that are less aggressive reproduce less. Among talopoin monkeys, the level of testosterone is lower in those that are of lower social caste. And further, these monkeys are continually under stress and have the pattern of hormonal secretion that goes with stress; and they are liable to all the illnesses that occur with stress.

When testosterone is injected into farmyard hens, they become aggressive, and move up in the pecking order. Androgens injected into both sexes of the following animals increase aggression: American lizards, turtles, valley quails, rats, cocks, hens, fish. The domestic hen calls other hens to food just as the cock usually does. Presumably these hormones act on certain neighbouring neurons in the hypothalamus.

The removal of the testes tends to remove aggressive behaviour. Male rats castrated in the first few weeks of life are as aggressive as female rats, and much less aggressive than males. Normal male aggression can be restored by giving them testosterone.

Castration has less effect on man than on other mammals. One of the results of castration is, as Shakespeare tells us in *Antony and Cleopatra*, that the subject may still have the desire but lack the performance. A eunuch may have erections, and may have orgasms, but will not have seminal emission. It is said that this state may continue for years after castration. Such eunuchs were much prized in Arab and Turkish harems. The kind of eunuchs who, owing to some disease or abnormality, have never arrived at puberty can have erections; they may be capable of insertion, but not of ejaculation. In all these cases, giving androgens gives the capability of emission.

Young women who have had their ovaries removed or destroyed by disease continue to feel a need for sexual intercourse. In human beings the higher levels of the brain make up for deficiencies of sex hormones governing sexual desire and behaviour.

The effect of male hormones on those nuclei of the hypothalamus that organize aggressive behaviour is more complicated in primates than in species lower in the evolutionary scale. Among chimpanzees, the male is usually dominant; but when the female is on heat, she becomes the dominant one, the male accepting this dominance without question.

Boys with hypogonadism treated by androgens become more aggressive. They sometimes feel more self-confident; and this occurs before the development of secondary sexual characteristics. In human beings, apart from direct physiological factors, behaviour is affected by all we have learned and experienced, including the immense influence of other people in the present and, more important, in the past. And so the organization of behaviour in accordance with cultural factors has become overwhelmingly important. This means in anatomical and physiological terms that the forebrain is very important, and that the influence of hormones is correspondingly less important. That is why man is more intellectual and less emotional than other animals.

17 General Plan of the Human Brain

Western medicine was born on the island of Cos four hundred years before Christ. Hippocrates, its great originator, first understood the functions of the brain. The following lesson has come down to us.

Some people think that the heart is the organ with which we think and that it feels pain and anxiety. But it is not so . . . From the brain and the brain alone arise our pleasures, joys, laughter, and jests, as well as our sorrow, pains and griefs. Through it, in a special manner, we acquire wisdom and knowledge, we see and hear, we distinguish the ugly from the beautiful, the bad from the good, the pleasant from the unpleasant . . . By the same organ we become mad or delirious, we are inspired by dread or fear. It brings dreams, inopportune mistakes, groundless anxieties, blunders . . . The brain is the messenger for the intelligence.

This correct view of the brain was not accepted by everyone. Aristotle thought that the function of the brain was to cool the blood, and he placed the soul in the heart. Wrong views triumphed for a long time, for there is no universal principle that the right will triumph. When Christianity took over, human behaviour ceased to be based on a real thing, the brain, and was considered to arise from a wisp of nothingness, the soul. It is difficult for us to conceive of the ignorance of our ancestors in these matters. At one time in Europe, it was believed that the brain was nothing but a bag of mucus; and people thought that when one had a cold, and ones nose became filled with mucus, then a part of the brain was coming down the nose through little holes in the base of the skull.

The philosopher is the first cousin of the priest. And most philosophers continue to speculate on what they call mind-brain relationships without knowing how to do experiments to find answers to their questions. Meanwhile scientists have gone ahead

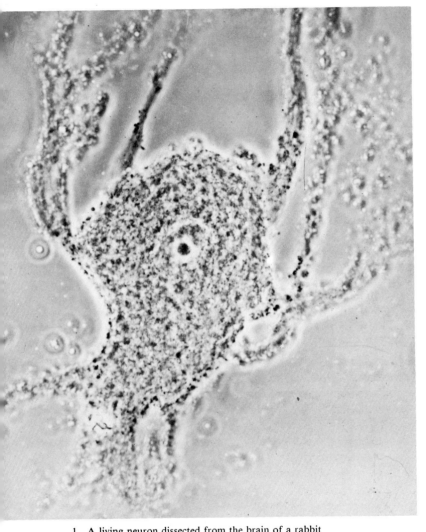

1   A living neuron dissected from the brain of a rabbit

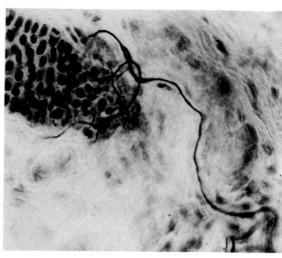

Cerebral Hemisphere

Hypothalamus
Stalk of Pituitary Gland
Cerebellum
Medulla Oblongata

Spinal Cord

Nasal Cavity

Hard Palate
Mouth
Tongue

Wind-Pipe

Heart
Diaphragm
Liver

2   Mid line section through a man

3   A nerve fibre in the skin of a man's finger

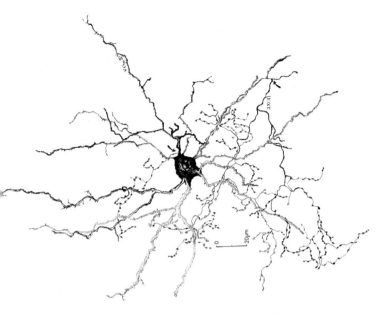

4 Several nerve fibres ending in a sensory receptor in the skin of a man's finger

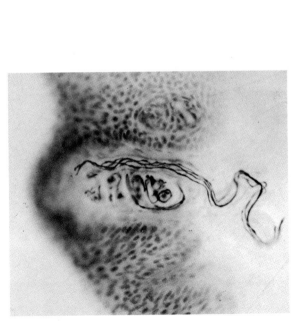

5 A neuron from the cerebellum. This type of neuron has several axons. The dendrites are thin: the axons are thick.

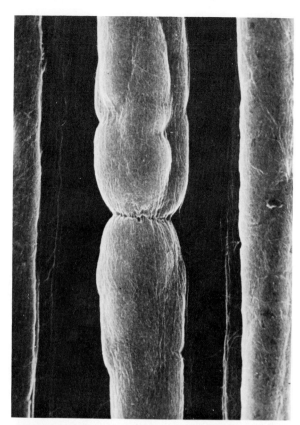

6 Scanning electron microscope study showing a node on a myelinated nerve fibre

7 Scanning electron microscope study showing a neuron in tissue culture

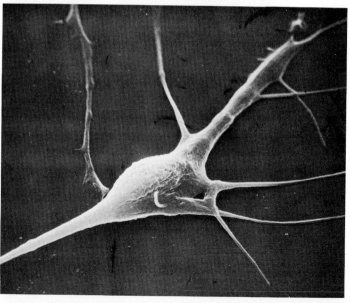

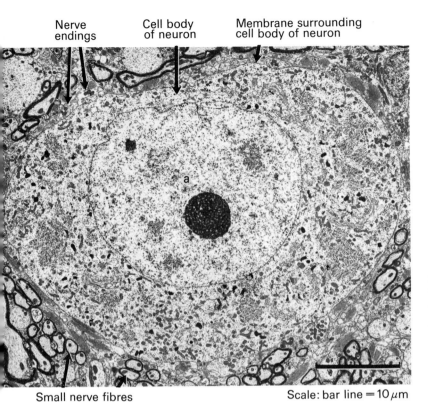

Nerve endings   Cell body of neuron   Membrane surrounding cell body of neuron

a

Small nerve fibres   Scale: bar line = 10 μm

8   Electron microscope study of a cat's motoneuron

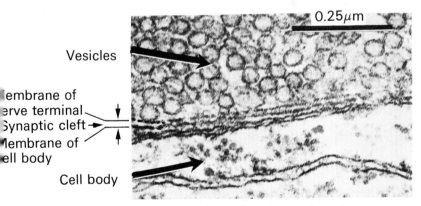

0.25 μm

Vesicles

Membrane of
nerve terminal
Synaptic cleft
Membrane of
cell body

Cell body

9   Synapses between nerve-endings and a motoneuron in a cat

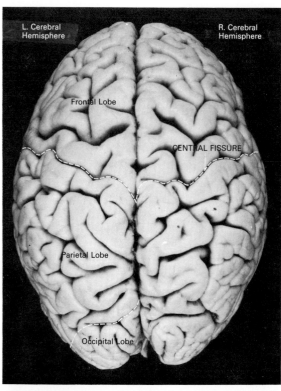

10 The brain of a fifty-year-old man from above

11 The same brain from the right side

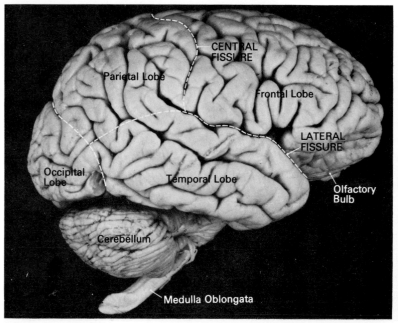

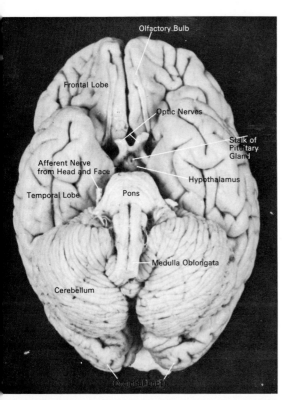

12 The same brain from below

13 The same brain from the left side

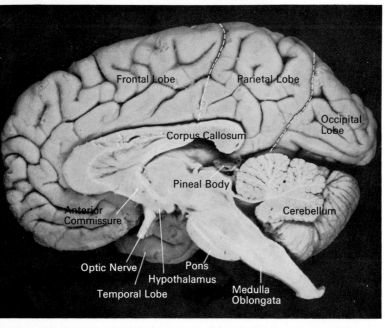

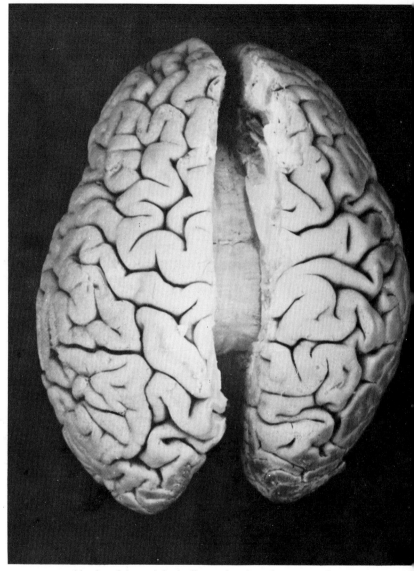

14   An adult man's brain dissected to show the corpus callosum

with their painstaking investigations, based on the assumption that the nervous system and its manifestations follow the usual laws of physics and chemistry. This approach, and no other one, has obtained results, so that we already know a lot about how the brain works. And the mysterious world of the unknowable, known only to the priests of all religions, shrinks year by year.

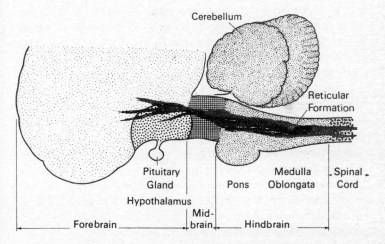

Fig. 17.1 Diagram showing how anatomists usually sub-divided the brain.

Anatomists have various ways of subdividing the brain; the usual way is shown in Fig. 17.1. The upper end of the spinal cord enlarges and opens out to become the medulla oblongata. The cerebellum originally developed out of the floor of the hindbrain; the pons, or bridge, developed in the floor of the hindbrain to take nerve fibres round the floor to the cerebellum. The three structures, medulla oblongata, pons, and cerebellum make up the hindbrain. Further forwards is the midbrain, which consists to a large extent of passing nerve fibres, those going up to the forebrain and those coming down to the spinal cord. Above the midbrain there is the forebrain. It consists of the two cerebral hemispheres with all the masses of grey matter within them, the limbic lobe with the septal area, and the hypothalamus. Throughout the centre of the brain is the reticular formation. And in the middle are the ventricles filled with cerebrospinal fluid.

Within the members of a species, size of brain is not related to intelligence. Very intelligent men and women have had smaller and lighter brains than half-wits. Brain size among human beings is dependent on height. Women have smaller brains than men because they are shorter. Dwarfs too have small brains, because they are short. Among the various mammals, difference in brain size seems to be related to the ability to learn. Man's brain is not the largest of any animal's; the porpoise's, the whale's, and the elephant's are bigger. But in relation to the animal's total size, the whale has a small brain, one of the smallest of any mammal's. The larger the brain, the less closely packed are its neurons. This may allow them to have more synapses. Man's cortical neurons are less densely packed than those of other primates; and in general he is more intelligent. Thick layers of cortex may imply neurons with more or larger dendrites, and that too means more interconnections; and they may be necessary for learning. One must remember that the bee and the ant lead astonishingly successful lives, and they have minute brains. But they are almost incapable of learning. Dealing with everything that turns up in the world by learning is a way of evolution that seems to be no longer available to them.

Although the rest of this book will be about the cerebral hemispheres, these parts of the brain are not essential for life. They are an added feature, appearing late in evolution and provided only for later models. All the essential functions had been built into the previous models for some millions of years.

Mammals made a great leap forward in developing the hemispheres. Even the first mammals had many layers, whereas most animals lower in the evolutionary scale have only one layer. In the cortex of primates' hemispheres, there are six layers. These layers provide the animal with a hundred thousand neurons per sq.mm. of cortex, and a hundred thousand million neurons in the whole cortex. Any of these neurons could be connected to twenty-five thousand others.

Brains of different animals differ according to which aspects of the world particularly concern them. Smell is a sense that we despise; there is no Royal Society of Olfactory Arts. Yet the cerebral hemispheres first developed to cope with this very sense. They developed in the ancestors of present-day fish. Smell was always related to the alimentary canal and so the chemoreceptors of taste and smell developed in the mouth of the canal. This combined sense is essential for fish to find food and regurgitate bad food, to take note of the information provided by pheromones, to find sexual partners, keep with its kith and kin and to act according to this information.

As vertebrates evolved and developed larger hemispheres, the other sensory inputs acquired end-stations in the forebrain. But the first sensory system to develop remains immediately connected with the parts of the forebrain that organize emotion. By the time the South American mud-fish evolved, more than half the sensory input was devoted to smell. The next group, the reptiles, relies less on smell and so this sensory input occupies less of the forebrain. In their brains, the hippocampus develops, the part of the cerebral hemispheres related to the hypothalamus (discussed in Chapter 16). Reptiles use their tongues as tactile organs to examine the world, and so they evolved a large sensory tactile region in the forebrain. When birds developed as an offshoot from reptiles, smell lost its pre-eminence: the sensibility of the beak and the tongue became more important. But most important was vision. Birds developed large visual areas of the brain to receive impulses from their all-seeing eyes with their large visual fields. But birds are not the main line of evolutionary development: they are out on a limb. The main line continued with the first mammals, and they used smelling rather than seeing. And smell remains the most important sense for most mammals today. It was the few mammals who took to living in trees that developed sight and neglected smell, for life among the branches of trees demands good eyesight. And so man, returning to the earth from the trees, has good sight and a poor sense of smell.

From examining the brain of an animal we can thus tell whether the animal was orientated towards hearing or smelling, whether it had big eyes or a well-developed nose. For within the phylum of vertebrates, among the various classes and species, the same parts of the brain subserve essentially the same functions. As the development of the skull is necessarily related to the size and development of the brain within, we can deduce from examining the skull of extinct animals what sort of life the owner of that skull once had. One can know whether it lived mainly visually or relied mainly on smell; just as from an examination of its teeth, we know whether it lived on meat, or vegetables and fruit.

The cerebral hemispheres do so many things that one can hardly say in a few words what their functions are. They must note whether any event is familiar or novel. Perhaps they detect those events that are always connected together or that arrive by chance. The cerebral hemispheres come to store that animal's own experience of life, all that it has learned. It learned, for instance, the geography of its environment, most necessary knowledge. This is kept in the parietal lobe of the right hemisphere. From early experience, the pain of deprivation and the pleasure of previous satiety, the animal has learned when to produce the copulating, sleeping, fighting, fleeing, eating, drinking, urination, and defecating organized by the hypothalamus. These patterns of behaviour are integrated into the animal's life by the cerebral hemispheres. They choose the moment, the occasion, and the place for the right behaviour.

It may be that cerebral hemispheres evolved in higher vertebrates so that the animal could be aware of its own activities. Being aware of oneself and of what one is doing is a kind of feedback. It may help to know what one is doing so as to monitor its effectiveness. Awareness of one's behaviour is called consciousness. It occurs in all higher vertebrates; perhaps it is present to some degree in all animals. It could be that one has to know what effect one's own behaviour is having in order to keep on improving it; and this a feature of all animal life. If that is a part of being conscious, then all animals have consciousness. If that is not so, then biologists are presented with the question when in evolution this kind of feedback became consciousness.

Plate 11 shows the brain from below; this surface sits on the floor of the skull. The frontal, occipital, and temporal lobes are seen; the parietal lobe does not reach the undersurface of the brain, and so it cannot be seen in this view. A great deal of the temporal lobe is seen in this photograph. Within this part of the temporal lobe is the hippocampus and amygdala. Behind the hemispheres is the cerebellum with its folds and furrows, narrower than those of the cerebral hemispheres. It is at the back of the brain, situated just above the neck. Between the two cerebellar hemispheres is the medulla oblongata, which continues below into the spinal cord and above into the pons. In front of the pons, in shadow, is the floor of the hypothalamus, and in its centre is the stalk of the pituitary gland, cut through. Bordering the hypothalamus are the two optic nerves joined together. In front of them are the two olfactory stalks ending in front in the olfactory bulbs, which receive the olfactory nerves. On each side of the pons are the two afferent nerves from the face and head through which all sensation reaches the brain.

All the four lobes of the right hemisphere can be seen in Plate 13. The cerebellum is also cut across, and so its cut surface can be seen. The medulla oblongata and the pons are cut through. In front of the cerebellum the pineal body can be seen. In this unilateral, central structure, Descartes placed the seat of the soul. The large curved bridge of the corpus callosum has been cut through; this is the main structure connecting the two cerebral hemispheres. Another and more ancient bridge can be seen above the optic nerve; this is the anterior commissure. The hypothalamus is behind the optic nerve. A large mass of white nerve fibres can be seen descending into it; these fibres come from the temporal lobe of the other side.

Our bodies are bilaterally symmetrical, most structures being in pairs. We have two arms, two legs, two eyes, two kidneys. The whole body is not built on this plan of course, for we have one heart, one liver, one pancreas. If we have two eyes, two ears, two limbs, the brain has to be built on the same bilateral plan. We must have two optic nerves from the eyes, two auditory nerves from the ears, and parts of the brain related to the opposite side of the body. A brain built on this double plan runs the danger of behaving as two uncoordinated organs. This is overcome by building bridges between the two halves; in anatomy these are called commissures. They are present throughout the spinal cord, the hindbrain, and midbrain. In the later evolved forebrain, they are more obvious, as this part of the brain is more obviously constructed in two halves.

The cerebral hemispheres, when cut, are seen to be made up of white and grey matter. The grey matter is along the outside of the hemispheres and so it is called the cortex (Latin: rind or bark: French: *écorce*, which also gives us cork, the rind or bark of the cork oak). The white matter consists mainly of nerve fibres, and the grey matter of nerve cells. The surface of the cerebral hemispheres is thrown into ridges and furrows, so as to get a large sheet of cortex into the restricted space of the skull. On account of the folding, about two-thirds of the cortex is hidden from view, being folded into the depths of the furrows. The two cerebral hemispheres appear to be alike. But when accurate measurements are made, one finds that they are not exactly the same.

It was known to Greek medicine that an injury to one side of the brain caused paralysis of the limbs of the opposite side; and they deduced that the movements of one side of the body were organized by the opposite cerebral hemisphere. The rest of our knowledge was acquired from the study of patients with neurological disorders and the detailed investigation of their brains after death; from stimulating brains during surgery; and, to a large extent, from experiments on animals in laboratories.

The easiest way to get an idea of the general shape and construction of the brain is to go to the butcher's and buy one. It is unlikely that he has a human one, but a sheep's or a bullock's is sufficiently like the human one to make no difference.

Four photographs of a human brain are shown as Plates 10, 11, 12, and 13. The brain is shown from above, below, and from the right side, and the left side of the right hemisphere is shown after it has been divided from the left hemisphere.

The hemispheres are divided for convenience into lobes. The front half is the frontal lobe; it is separated by a fissure, called the central fissure, from the parietal lobe behind it. The part at the back of the skull is the occipital lobe. They are shown in Plate 10.

In Plate 11 all four lobes can be seen. The cerebellum is below the occipital lobe, and the medulla oblongata is below that. Beneath the frontal lobe, the slight projection is the olfactory bulb, which receives the olfactory nerves.

The basic anatomical organization of the hemispheres will now be considered. The afferent pathways, all of which began with sensory receptors, reach the thalamus. From here, the next relay takes them to the cerebral cortex. The general scheme is shown in Fig 17.2. Each kind of sensation has its own territory in the thalamus; though there is also some mixing, two or three kinds of sensation having their inputs going to same region of the thalamus.

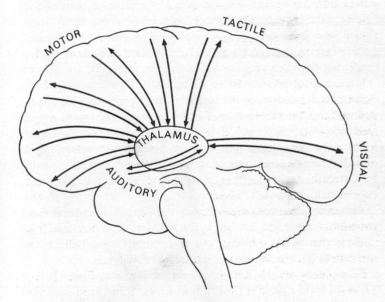

Fig. 17.2 Some connections between the thalamus and the cerebral cortex.

In the cerebral cortex are large areas serving each sense, so that we have visual areas, taste areas, and so on. These are known as the primary sensory areas. Each kind of sensation has a primary sensory area in each hemisphere. Other areas of the cortex are known as association areas. They are interconnected, and also connect back to the thalamus below. The higher an animal is in the vertebrate scale, the larger proportion of the cerebral cortex is formed by the association areas.

All sensory areas are connected to the amygdala, hippocampus, and other parts of the limbic lobe. For, in order to remember what you have just experienced, whether this is something seen or something felt, you have to send a report of it to the hippocampus. To have an emotional reaction to the experience, you send impulses to the nearby limbic lobe. This is necessary so that when you have that experience again, you both remember it and have the emotional response that you had on the first occasion. These connections are made in both hemispheres. The anatomical pathways are from each primary sensory area into the deeper parts of the temporal lobes.

The primary tactile area is just behind the motor area. This is to be expected, for feeling something means exploring it with one's fingers and hands, and thus moving them. How quickly all these connections work can be seen if someone suddenly points a revolver at you. If it took too long to know, that means to remember what a revolver was, if one had no emotional reaction to the revolver, and finally if one had no movement in response to it, one would be killed.

Above the ear and deep in the upper part of the temporal lobe is the primary receptive area for hearing. It receives from both ears, but mainly from the opposite one. Between this region and the secondary region for smelling is the primary region for taste.

From the association areas, nerve impulses are sent to various motor areas, which organize movement. What seems to be the highest-level motor area is called the supplementary motor area. The names of motor and sensory areas were given as each of them was discovered; and so we have primary, secondary, and tertiary areas, and a supplementary area, named historically and not functionally.

The supplementary area of both hemispheres comes into action while a movement is being planned, and it continues its activity during the course of the movement. The primary motor area starts working with the onset of the movement, the primary motor area of one side activating the movements of the opposite side of the body. Very simple movements, such as the repeated bending of a finger, are not planned by the supplementary motor area, but a movement such as bringing each finger in turn to touch the thumb has to be planned. The planned movements of talking are organized by the supplementary motor areas. This area has been cut out in a few patients in order to remove a tumour. Immediately after the operation, the patients could neither move nor speak; and their faces were blank and motionless.

The neurons of the cerebral cortex are arranged in layers and in columns or cylinders at right angles to the surface of the brain. The diameter of a column is about 500 μm. The columns surround a central afferent nerve fibre. Each column contains about 50–10,000 neurons. These neurons connect together up and down the column, and to a lesser extent with neighbouring columns. The central nerve fibre comes from the thalamus below, from other regions of the cortex, or from the opposite hemisphere.

18 Exploring man's living brain

It is about a hundred years since we began to learn about the functions of the different parts of the cerebral hemispheres. Before this higher level of the nervous system could be understood, it was necessary to believe that different regions of the hemispheres could have different functions. It used to be taken for granted that each hemisphere worked as a whole, the one duplicating the functions of the other. The first neurologist who had a different conception was Franz Josef Gall, an anatomist working at the end of the eighteenth and beginning of the nineteenth century. Gall is famous—or infamous—as the founder of phrenology, a subject that is usually thought to be nonsense. In fact, phrenology is not only an original conception of how the brain is organized: in many ways it is the right one. In the first place, Gall took it for granted that the physical organ of the brain engendered the mind. For this heresy in the so-called enlightened eighteenth century he was expelled from Roman Catholic Austria. Secondly, Gall proposed that higher neural functions were localized in certain regions of the cerebral hemispheres. At that time, the usual view was that the brain worked as a whole, and that there were no separate parts with different functions. Again, Gall's view is the correct one. The mistake the phrenologists made was in their choice of functions to localize in the hemispheres. This remains a difficult problem. We still are not satisfied with the functions that we at present localize in the various cerebral regions For example, the ability to draw well is not a single function, organized by just one part of the cerebral hemispheres. It needs the skilful use of the fingers, vision and visual recognition, the various cerebral functions that make up the the representation of three-dimensional space on a two-dimensional surface, the ability to form the concept of space, and many more functions of different regions of the cerebral hemispheres. But the recognition of colours is carried out by certain neurons in parts of the back of the hemispheres. The phrenologists thought they could localize within the cerebral hemispheres such functions as language, calculation, hope, and philoprogenitiveness. They were right about language. They were wrong about calculation; but until a few years ago most neurologists regarded an ability to calculate as a basic cerebral function. They were wrong about hope; perhaps they should have sought it in the human breast. As for philoprogenitiveness, they were not very far wrong for there are certain parts of the brain that do organize maternal behaviour.

The nineteenth-century thinker and physiologist, G. H. Lewes, nowadays know mainly as the husband of the novelist George Eliot, wrote in 1871: 'Gall rescued mental function from the metaphysics, and made it one of biology ... In his vision of psychology as a branch of biology, subject to all biological laws and to be pursued on biological methods, he may be said to have given the science its basis.'

The most serious mistake the phrenologists made was to think that the indentations, bumps, and dips on the surface of the skull resulted from the underlying parts of the cerebral hemisphere. Another mistake was to imagine that, if a faculty is particularly developed in someone, then the part of the cerebral hemisphere in which that faculty is located will also be large and well-developed. Gall's method of locating faculties within the brain was absurd. For instance, looking back at his schooldays, he remembered that two of his schoolmates had had good verbal memories and large eyes, and so he connected verbal memory with protuberant eyes; he concluded that the faculty of verbal memory is in the frontal lobes just behind the eyes.

During the second quarter of the nineteenth century, most large towns in Britain had their phrenological societies. Phrenology provided people with an interest in psychology, just as psychoanalysis has in our own time. And, again like psychoanalysis, it was accepted far more readily by imaginative writers and untrained intellectuals than by biologists and medical men, who were in a better position to judge it. Serious thinkers about the brain soon came to regard the subject as quackery and phrenologists as charlatans, which indeed they became, and so the contributions of phrenology to neurology have been neglected. Yet they had a formative influence on French and British neurology. In France, Bouillaud was sympathetic to phrenology as a young man; he later played an important part in getting French anatomists and neurologists to accept the idea that speech was carried out by a certain local region of the left cerebral hemisphere. Broca put forward the arguments in support of this idea; he had also been influenced by phrenology as a young man. In England, Herbert Spencer was most interested in phrenology as a boy and a young man. He had a great influence on Hughlings Jackson, the man who was one of the founders of British neurology in the last century.

The problem of what to localize is a difficult one. If the occipital lobe of one hemisphere is cut out or shot away, then the person cannot see anything on the opposite half of space, and he will never recover this vision. One may conclude that vision of the contra-lateral visual field is localized in the occipital lobe. But if the hand area is cut out of the parietal and frontal lobes, there is incomplete paralysis of the hand and partial disturbance of sensation. Both recover to some extent. One presumably concludes that these areas play a role in sensation and movement of the hand and other areas can or may play the same or similar role. If we come to ask questions concerning whereabouts higher neural or mental activity is localized, we never find the function localized to one small area of the brain. For this kind of behaviour needs the functioning of many parts of the brain.

Our knowledge of the function of different parts of the cerebral hemispheres has been acquired in three main ways. One is the electrical stimulation of the brain in living animals, including man: this is the subject of this chapter. Another has been by the removal of parts of the cerebral hemispheres, or the division of connections between parts; this again has been done in animals and man. The third way has been the correlation of naturally occurring disorders studied during life with the lesions found in the brain after death. We first learn how things go wrong, and then deduce how they work when they go right. We learn from the abnormal; we deduce physiology from pathology.

Lesions within the cerebral hemispheres can destroy the end-stations or the connecting links, or both. Destruction of the end-stations is just like destroying a railway terminus. Both sorts of termini, railway and cerebral, have afferent and efferent functions. One receives and sends off trains; the other receives and sends off nerve impulses. Destruction of the links between stations disconnects the two stations; it is the same whether the connections are railway lines or nerve fibres.

The most important neural disorder that has contributed to our knowledge of the brain is epilepsy; and the first worker to make use of this material was Hughlings Jackson. He was in a good position to study the disease as he could observe it in his wife, who had the variety now known as Jacksonian epilepsy. Jackson concluded that epilepsy was due to the spontaneous firing of groups of neurons. When fits start with visual, auditory, olfactory, or gustatory hallucinations, they do so because the neurons normally occupied with vision, hearing, smelling, and tasting are spontaneously firing off. If, after the patient's death, the lesion causing the fits is found, it will show which parts of the brain are normally concerned with these functions. When, for instance, a fit starts with a tingling numb sensation in the right foot, and a lesion is found in a certain region of the left hemisphere of the brain, it may be concluded that this region is where sensation of the right foot is organized. If neurons of the receptive area for smelling spontaneously discharge in a fit, the patient will be aware of a strange smell.

The preliminary features of the fit which the patient experiences are called the aura. An aura may be a sensation of vertigo, tingling spreading up a limb, butterflies in the stomach, an overpowering fear, or the vision of a scene from the past. When the features of the aura are correlated with the post-mortem evidence of the location of the lesion causing the fit, we learn something about where in the cortex the neurons subserving these functions lie.

Using this method, Hughlings Jackson showed that certain parts of the hemispheres are mainly concerned with movements and neighbouring parts are concerned with the sensations associated with movement. He also showed that when a part of the front of the temporal lobe is excited by the epileptic discharge, hallucinatory states appear, with strange disturbances of the awareness of reality and of oneself as a part of reality. He described this state by saying that the patients show 'dreams mixing up with present thoughts', and he called it 'double consciousness'. Now that we know more about psychopathology and about normal psychological mechanisms, we realize that sometimes repressed psychological material accompanied by strong emotion comes to the patient's consciousness during this early part of a fit.

It is interesting to find that Dostoevsky, in describing his own fits, described the kinds of epilepsy starting in the temporal lobe twenty years before Jackson did. As his kind of fits were not recognized as being a part of epilepsy at that time, both Dostoevsky and his doctors believed his attacks were partly or entirely hysterical. Dostoevsky's accounts of his fits, given in his letters, his diaries, and his novels, are so well described that one can say without doubt that they began in his left temporal lobe.

The method that has been most useful in investigating the function of the brain, electrical stimulation, was first used in 1804. A physiologist called Aldini stimulated the brains of animals in the slaughter-house immediately after they had been killed. He observed that the muscles of the opposite side of the body showed movements. He then took his investigations a step farther by stimulating the brain of a freshly decapitated man; and he observed movements of the opposite side of the face (it is unknown whether the head felt this or not). The cerebral hemispheres of living human beings were first stimulated electrically in 1874 by Roberts Bartholow, professor of medicine in Cincinnati. He was able to pass the electrodes through the skulls of two patients, as the bone had become softened and rotted away by abscesses. As he expected, he produced movements of the limbs of the opposite side.

A great step forward in the study of the brain was made in 1870 by Fritsch and Hitzig. As no facilities were provided by the Physiological Institute of Berlin for this work, they started their investigations in Hitzig's wife's bedroom. They explored the surface of the hemispheres of lightly anaesthetized dogs. From such stimulation they worked out in detail what parts of the cerebral cortex control what movements. They showed, among other facts, that Gall's main idea was right—that the brain does not work as one single organ, but that different parts of it perform different functions. Stimulation of certain parts of the cerebral hemispheres caused movements, whereas stimulation elsewhere caused nothing observable. Obviously, parts of the brain concerned with sensation, with thought, emotion, or remembering, could not show up in dogs with this stimulation technique.

The next step forward was made by Foerster in Germany and Cushing in the United States, both of whom stimulated the brains of conscious patients. By the first decade of the twentieth century neurosurgery had been developed, and operations on the brain were done with local anaesthetics, the patient being awake. Studies carried out by many neurosurgeons led to the mapping out of motor and sensory areas of the brain.

It might be thought that stimulation of the living brain in conscious patients is painful and injurious. It is neither. As has been mentioned above, the brain can be touched, cut, or stimulated without the subject feeling any pain or anything he can localize to the brain itself. When a part of the cerebral cortex is to be cut out because it causes fits, this part must be accurately located. From scanning the skull, one knows the region of the cerebral hemisphere that has to be cut out; but the exact region can be found best by stimulating the region electrically.

The technique of stimulation, localization, and excision was brought to a point where it became a routine neurosurgical procedure by Penfield in Montreal. He also applied Cushing's and Foerster's techniques to a systematic exploration of the cerebral cortex of man. The operations were performed for the removal of tumours, or scars, or for the cure of certain kinds of epilepsy. The brain was stimulated to enable the surgeon to reproduce the features of the patient's fits. When the patient reported having the same aura as he usually experienced with his fits, the abnormal region of the brain had been found. The surgeon then cut out this part; and this often stopped the fits.

It is rather surprising that such a crude investigation as the application of an electric current through an electrode should produce normal phenomena, normal movements, visual hallucinations, and the recall of scenes from the past. One might have expected that it would produce some sort of chaos or caricature of normal phenomena. But in fact it imitates normal functioning of the brain to a surprising degree. One notes too that all the phenomena caused by electrical stimulation in these patients also occur spontaneously as a part of their epilepsy. It is apparent that the stimulation of the cortex and the discharge of neurons occurring during epileptic attacks can both teach us the functions of certain parts of the cortex of the hemispheres, even though these are epileptic brains.

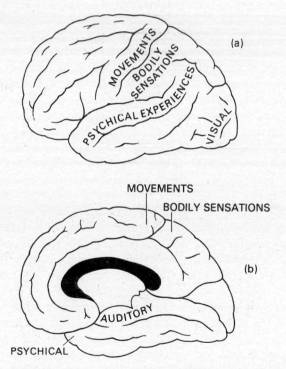

Fig. 18.1 (a) and (b). Parts of the human cerebral hemispheres which produce observable phenomena when stimulated in conscious patients.

From stimulation of the brains of conscious patients by Penfield and his successors, we have learned that the parts of the hemispheres that produce obvious responses are those parts shown in Figs 18.1 (a) and (b). Visual hallucinations occur with stimulation of the back part of the occipital lobe, and auditory hallucinations with the stimulation of the temporal lobe. Movements are obtained from stimulating the motor strip, and bodily sensations from equivalent regions of the somaesthetic area behind it. The strange experiences to be described below are obtained from stimulating the temporal lobes.

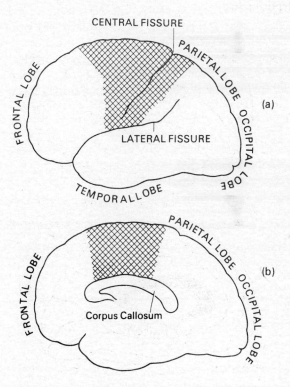

Fig. 18.2 (a) and (b). Parts of the human brain which produce movement of the body when stimulated.

Movement and sensation

When a point of the motor region of the hemisphere is stimulated, a part of the body is moved. The patient is astonished to find his arm or his leg moving of its own accord; for he does not have the feeling that he is doing the movement himself. Sometimes no movements occur but the patient feels a strong desire to move. If a part of his body is already moving when the surgeon stimulates the motor area, the movement may be stopped and the patient is amazed to find he cannot move. The regions of the hemisphere from which movements can be obtained on electrical stimulation are shown in Fig 18.2 (a) and (b).

Fig 18.3 shows the same view of the left side of the brain as Fig 18.2 (a). In front of the central fissure is the motor strip. Movements of the right side of the body are most easily obtained from stimulating this part. On the figure, the points at which stimulation causes movement of the various parts of the body are marked. It will be seen that these points on the cortex are upside down; the foot is at the top and the face and mouth are at the bottom of the strip.

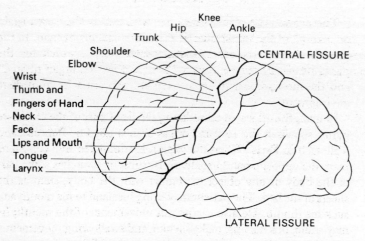

Fig. 18.3 Human brain showing the regions of the motor strip giving rise to movements of the opposite limbs.

In this part of the cerebral hemisphere, the size of the cortical region that produces movements is related to the importance of those movements in that animal. In man, for instance, the cortical region related to the mouth and tongue is large; this is because man is a great talker. In Fig 18.4 is shown the cortical area for the movements of the mouth used in speech.

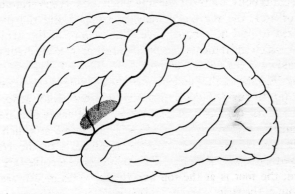

Fig. 18.4 Region of left cerebral hemisphere that organizes movements of mouth and larynx used in speech.

The region related to the fingers and hands is also large, again on account of the importance of these movements for man. In the pig, the largest region is related to the snout, which for the pig is hands, fingers, and thumbs, as well as the organ of smell and the most important instrument for exploring its immediate environment.

In man, the effects of stimulating the front part of the cingulate gyrus, shown in Fig 15.2 and 3, has been studied by Bancaud and Tailarach in Paris. When this region is stimulated in a conscious man, the opposite hand usually feels, rubs, or scratches some part of the body or any object in contact with the body, such as the sheets of the bed. The patient may bring his hand to his mouth and suck his thumb. He also carries out movements of the mouth; he may smile, lick his lips, make sucking and swallowing movements, pass the tip of his tongue round his mouth. All such movements are also seen in an epileptic fit.

Stimulation of the primary receptive areas of the cortex causes the patient to have crude sensations characteristic of each sensory area. When the somaesthetic area is stimulated, the patient gets a feeling of numbness or tingling. This stimulation does not cause pain. Sensation takes time. If the skin is weakly stimulated, and a surgeon is recording the arrival of the impulses at the somaesthetic area, it is found that there is about half a second's delay between the impulses reaching the cortical area and the patient having any sort of sensation.

When the areas surrounding the primary receptive areas are stimulated, the patient reports a change from the crude sensation to a sensation more developed and more meaningful. In the case of hearing, when the primary auditory area is stimulated, the patient hears clicks, buzzing, ringing, rumbling, chirping, or rushing sounds. He does not hear words or music. Stimulation of the surrounding area produces more elaborate sounds, as well as the buzzing and clicks. One of Penfield's patients heard a buzzing when the primary auditory area was stimulated; as the electrode was moved to the surrounding area, the patient exclaimed, 'Someone is calling.' When the surrounding area is stimulated, the patient may hear music, and he may hum what he is hearing. More than one patient has heard an orchestra playing. As long as the electrode stimulates, the orchestra continues playing. In one of Penfield's patients, whenever that particular spot on the cortex was stimulated, the patient heard the orchestra playing a certain popular song. This music was so real to her that she was convinced that a gramophone was being turned on in the operating theatre, and still believed this when she spoke about the operation several days later. A boy who was being operated upon heard his mother talking on the telephone when this region of the right temporal lobe was being stimulated. Each time the current was turned on, he heard the same conversation. He said, 'My mother is telling my brother he has got his coat on backwards. I can just hear them.'

Very near the primary auditory receptive area is the primary area for vestibular sensations. Penfield found that stimulation of this area made the patient feel dizzy; or he might get a sinking feeling, or have the feeling that everything is swinging round him.

When the electrical stimulus was moved from the primary to the secondary visual areas, one Canadian patient of Penfield's said suddenly 'Oh, gee, gosh, robbers are coming at me with guns!' They were on his left and coming from behind him. Similar scenes were seen when the stimulating electrode was put in many places in front of the primary visual area. Stimulation in one place made the patient exclaim, 'Oh, gosh. There they are, my brother is there. He is aiming an air rifle at me.' He said his brother was walking towards him, and the gun was loaded. When he was asked where he was, he said he was at the house, in the yard.

We do not yet understand the differences between imagining a scene, dreaming it, and having hallucinations. You can imagine that here is a man in a top hat standing on your left; or you might dream the same thing. You might see the same thing in hallucinations. In this case the figure seems far more real than when he is in a dream or merely imagined. If you have an hallucination, you may or may not have insight, that is to say you may realize that this is a hallucination or you may be convinced that it is real. Hallucinations usually imply that the patient should be referred to a psychiatrist. That means that we do not yet understand the physiology and anatomy of the hallucinations. But they also occur with neurological states, such as damage to the cortex or the thalamus. Also with these neurological states, as after a stroke, the patient may or may not have insight into his seeing the figure of the man. If there is a stroke affecting the occipital lobe, the opposite half of the visual field is blank; the patient may then have hallucination. The actual content of the hallucination depends nearly always, as far as one can tell, on the patient's experiences in life.

Emotions

Electrical stimulation of certain parts of the temporal lobes in conscious people gives them particular emotions. These regions are in the temporal lobes, the cingulate gyrus, and the septal area. The emotion is in a pure form, a terrible fear, an intense feeling of loneliness, sadness, or sorrow, or intense depression. Some patients have a feeling of intense anxiety, which may mount up to panic. Some have the feeling that everything is becoming danger-ous. It is probable that anger or euphoria are due to firing-off of regions of the left temporal lobe, and anxiety or depression to the firing of the right lobe.

When these regions of the cortex become spontaneously active in epilepsy, these emotions occur in a pure state; sometimes they occur immediately after the fit, and they may continue for days. The patient is often timid about experiencing these hallucinatory emotions and frightened to tell anyone about them.

Hughling Jackson, about a hundred years ago, first understood that strong emotions could be an epileptic attack or the aura of a fit. From correlating the manifestations of epilepsy and the region of an abnormality of the hemispheres after the patient's death, he showed that this kind of epilepsy started in the deeper part of the temporal lobe.

On one occasion, during an operation for epilepsy at the National Hospital for Nervous Disease in London, the amygdala was stimulated. The patient had a terrible feeling, 'just the same' he said 'as if you looked up and found you were just going to be run over by a bus'. Another patient, who was terrified that some-thing was going to attack her, would say to me, 'Stop them, doctor: don't let them do it.' Such a patient is still in touch with reality enough to know she is in hospital and talking to the doctor whom she knows; yet at the same time she is quite convinced that her hallucinations are real. Within one second this patient would regain a little more normal conscious awareness, and then she would tell you that her hallucinations were not real but only seemed real to her when they happened, and hardly had she got these words out than the attack would return, and she would say; 'There they are again', once more under the spell of her hallucina-tions and devoid of insight.

Some patients experience a feeling of dread rather than fear; it is intense, though vague, as there is no object or event that they are dreading. Sometimes, though rarely, the emotional state is a strong feeling of guilt, of being guilty of having done something dreadful, though the patient has no idea what it is.

Dostoevsky had this feeling of guilt, the feeling that he had committed some momentous crime, associated with his fits. But far more striking was a rare aura before his fits—a feeling of ecstasy or great joy. He has described it like this:

For a few moments before the fit, I experience a feeling of happiness such as is quite impossible to imagine in a normal state and which other people have no idea of. I feel entirely in harmony with myself and the whole world, and this feeling is so strong and so delightful that for a few seconds of such bliss, one would gladly give up ten years of one's life, if not one's whole life.

The terrible depression or despair which a few patients have during temporal lobe attacks may well have been the cause of their suicide. The patients can never say why they feel depressed. The utter misery comes on them quite suddenly, without cause or reason; and it may pass off equally quickly, so that within a few minutes it has gone. Attacks of uncontrollable rage may also occur as preludes to epileptic attacks or as the manifestation of epilepsy itself. These are particularly common in children whose epilepsy begins in the temporal lobes. During such attacks children or adults may smash up furniture, put their fists through glass windows, or attack other people.

In those epileptic patients in whom the fits start in the part of the temporal lobe where emotion is organized, the normal experiencing of emotion may bring on a fit. This occurs commonly in childhood; and epileptic children often get much benefit from psychotherapy. Dostoevsky, doubtless relating to his own experience, wrote, 'Fright alone will bring one on'.

The part of the brain that produces these pure emotions is the limbic system. This region includes the hypothalamus, the oldest parts of the cerebral cortex, which are under-surfaces and most internal parts of the temporal lobes, the parts of the cortex around the corpus callosum, and the septal area. In Plates 10 and 11, the parts labelled temporal lobe form a part of this region; the cingulate gyrus around the corpus callosum forms another part, and the region beneath the front part of the corpus callosum is the septal area; this surrounds the anterior commissure.

Many patients who have a pathological condition of the

temporal lobes of the brain causing fits have the same personality features. They are said to be religiose, which is the word psychiatrists use in order not to say religious; in fact they are preoccupied with religion. They have the obsessional neurotic's concern with details. Some of them have a less than normal sexual drive, fewer have an excessive drive. They are aggressive. A strange manifestation is hypergraphia—spending hours and hours writing, everything that comes into their heads, endless autobiography. This behaviour is probably due to the epileptic focus in the left temporal lobe activating or decreasing the inhibition of the region that organizes writing. Apart from the sex drive, about which we are ignorant, all of these features occurred in Dostoevsky.

Professor Heath in New Orleans has implanted electrodes in the brains of certain patients with severe and uncontrollable epilepsy or with psychotic mental disorders, and left them in permanently, just as Hess originally did in cats. In psychotic patients he found abnormal electrical brain-waves in the septal area and in the part of the temporal lobes called the amygdala. When these patients got better, these abnormal electrical waves became normal. Patients who were given LSD had the same abnormal electrical waves in these regions. When the waves were excessive and abnormal the patients were in a dream-like state, and heard voices. The essential ingredient of marihuana had the same effects on these parts of the brain when it was injected into animals.

When the pleasure region is stimulated in man, the patient becomes more alert, active, and brighter in mood and reactions. In one patient suffering from psychotic depression, Heath reported:

Expressions of anguish, self condemnation, and despair changed precipitously to expressions of optimism and elaborations of pleasant experiences, past and anticipated. Patients could calculate more rapidly than before stimulation. Memory and recall were enhanced. One patient on the verge of tears described his father's near-fatal illness and condemned himself as somehow responsible, but when the septal region was stimulated, he immediately terminated this conversation and within fifteen seconds exhibited a broad grin as he discussed plans to date and seduce a girlfriend. When asked why he had changed the conversation so abruptly, he replied that the plans concerning the girl suddenly came to him. This phenomenon was repeated several times in the patient: stimulation was administered to the septal region when he was describing a depressive state, and almost instantly he would become gay.

Here we see clearly that one's mood and thoughts that seem to come spontaneously are due to activation of a certain part of the brain. Perhaps all sexual fantasy arises from the activity of this region.

Another patient, an epileptic, was one day agitated, violent and psychotic. The septal region was then stimulated without the patient knowing it. 'Almost instantly his behavioural state changed from one of disorganization, rage, and persecution to one of happiness and mild euphoria. He described the beginning of a sexual motive state.'

Immediate relief from intense physical pain and anguish has been obtained with stimulation to the septal region in patients with advanced and painful forms of cancer. Stimulation of any region of the brain that causes pleasure stops physical and emotional pain. It appears, then, that these regions are more powerful than those parts of the brain where pain is felt.

Many of these patients have had the electrodes left permanently in their brains so that they could stimulate the various regions when they want to. In the New Orleans group of patients, three lots of electrodes were left in, connected to three levers so that these patients could have the experience of stimulating three different structures in the brain. One of these patients would have a most pleasant feeling when he stimulated the septal region. It 'made him feel as if he were building up to a sexual orgasm. He was unable to achieve the orgastic end point, however, and explained that his frequent, sometimes frantic, pushing of the septal button was an attempt to reach a "climax", although at times this was frustrating and produced a "nervous feeling".' Another patient also found that stimulation in this region made him 'feel wonderful'; it gave him sexual thoughts. Regardless of the subject under discussion at the time, the patient 'would introduce a sexual subject, usually accompanied by a broad grin. When asked about his response, he said "I don't know why that came to mind—I just happened to think of it".' When he stimulated a certain part of his thalamus, he got the partial recall of a memory, with anger and frustration. Stimulation of a neighbouring region has made patients experience fear or rage: and stimulation of another region close by causes a strange, unreal, dream-like state. When the patients experienced rage, it was unmotivated and was not directed particularly at anyone. Stimulation of parts of the hypothalamus itself has given rise to terror, anxiety, rage, and also to 'a good feeling'.

The disorder of schizophrenia is characterized by the patient's feeling no emotion, his not being stimulated by the events of life, and having no energy and no initiative. Heath thought that the condition could be treated by putting permanent electrodes into the septal region in some schizophrenics. Stimulation of the plea-sure-inducing region did give the patients emotions of a pleasant kind. The patients felt good, they became alert, and spoke and moved faster; and like the self-stimulating animals, they wanted to continue the stimulation. But unfortunately the improvement in their disease was only temporary.

Strange experiences

The electrical stimulation of certain regions of the temporal lobes produces strange feelings about the actual situation. Penfield called them 'interpretative illusions', and Hughlings Jackson had previously called it 'a dream state', as this was the name given it by one of his patients, a doctor with epilepsy. One of Penfield's patients said: 'I had a dream, I had a book under my arm. I was talking to a man. The man was trying to reassure me not to worry about the book.'

Sometimes in epilepsy and during the stimulation of the tem-poral lobes of the brain, there may be an increased awareness of reality; the patient says that for a brief period everything seems to be more intense and more significant. One of Penfield's patient's got this 'new awareness' both before his fits and on stimulation of his right temporal lobe; on stimulation, he became unusually con-scious of the weight of his coat and of the weight of his feet upon the floor.

A commoner feeling is that of being out of touch with reality. Everything has an unreal atmosphere, which the patient finds difficult to describe. Some of the patients have an intense feeling of being outside themselves and watching themselves behaving. They may feel they are standing behind themselves, watching from a distance.

More rarely there are misinterpretations of time sense; everything seems to be slowed down, even the movements of themselves and others seem as if they are carried out in slow motion and very deliberately. Penfield observed that stimulation of the temporal lobes often caused illusions of recognition or of comparison. This also occurs with fits starting in the same region. Everything may seem strange to the patient and unreal. The patient may say that everything is unlike ordinary life; suddenly the room in which he is sitting seems unfamiliar. Jackson reported some epileptics who described this as 'I feel in some strange place', 'a panorama of something familiar and yet strange'.

The opposite sort of feeling also occurs in epilepsy. Everything suddenly seems familiar, the patient has the feeling that it has all happened before, and that he knows exactly what is going to happen next. This is the *déjà vu* illusion; and it is probably due to the right temporal lobe. Dickens mentions it in *David Copperfield*, like this:

We have all some experience of a feeling which comes over us occasionally of what we are saying and doing have been said or done before, in a remoter time—of our having been surrounded, dim ages ago, by the same faces, objects, and circumstances—of our knowing perfectly what will be said next, as if we suddenly remembered it.

That this feeling can be a part of epilepsy had already been recognized in the last century. Hughlings Jackson first reported it, and rightly associated it with lesions of the front part of the temporal lobes. The feeling that time is unrolling abnormally slowly may also accompany the *déjà vu* phenomenon.

During stimulation of the temporal lobes, some of Penfield's patients experienced *déjà vu*. One patient had the feeling that the whole operation had happened before, and that she knew what the surgeon was about to do. Another patient experienced a feeling of unnecessariness, 'a strange feeling like it is unnecessary—the craziest, doggone feeling'. In two patients Penfield obtained a pure feeling of familiarity, an unattached sensation. One patient whose brain was being stimulated told him that the feeling of familiarity had already commenced before he started speaking to her, 'as though the stage or background had been set to embrace in familiarity any concomitant perception'. One patient whose temporal lobe was stimulated had the feeling of falling over, 'something which, in fact, he had not previously experienced', and yet this sensation was accompanied by the sense of familiarity.

Epileptic patients are the commonest recipients of mystical experiences. St Teresa of Avila was an epileptic. Some of the mystical experiences of saints and holy men of all religions are due to epilepsy occuring in the temporal lobes. The relation between epilepsy and mystical experiences was well known before the arrival of Christianity: epilepsy was known as the holy or sacred malady. For before, after, or during the attack, the patient may have the feeling that he is experiencing another kind of reality, more intense and far more important than the everyday kind. What he experiences during this state is so overpowering that he continues to believe in his delusional system when he has recovered from his attack. And so, after he has seen the glory of the Lord or the power of evil, he returns to everyday life, and becomes a preacher. He knows that he saw these things during an epileptic attack, but he may regard the epileptic attack as a means of experiencing religious truth. Or he may not regard the attack as epileptic, but as the way in which the Lord God communicated with him, and that he was chosen to receive this communication from on high. Thus, he must be a very special and elevated person, and he may have delusions of grandeur. If his sincerity and his emotional intensity can persuade ignorant people of the truth of his beliefs experienced during the epileptic state, then he may found a new religion.

Sometimes when epileptic patients are being examined to see if flickering light will bring on attacks, they get the religious experience; or they may get a state of bliss or feeling of absolute peace.

This is a variant of the strong emotion of elation. When some of these patients have the psychological feeling of emotion, they may also have the feeling that they are actually elevated from the ground. Epileptic saints call this levitation, and they tell those who believe in them that they float above the earth or walk on the waves, in defiance of gravity.

Evocation of the past

Penfield classified the psychical effects of electrical stimulation of the brain in two groups, experiential hallucinations and interpretative responses. Experiential hallucinations are an evocation of the past. Penfield describes this as follow: 'The record of the stream of consciousness may be activated as though it were a strip of cinematograph film, recording the sight and sound, the movement, and the meaning which belonged to each successive period of time.' The emotion of the original scene is there when the scene is relived. Patients called these experiences flashbacks of dreams, explaining that they were similar to flashbacks used in cinematographic techniques of story-telling.

As an example, the following case is described in some detail. The patient was operated upon by Penfield when she was aged 14. She suffered from terrifying epileptic fits which always started off with 'what seemed to be an hallucination. It was always the same: an experience came to her from childhood.' With this experience, she was frightened and often screamed.

The original experience was as follows. She was walking through a meadow where the grass was high. It was a lovely day, and her brothers had run on ahead of her. A man came up behind her and said that he had snakes in the bag he was carrying and how would she like to get into the bag with the snakes. She was very frightened and screamed to her brothers, and they all ran home, where she told her mother about the event.

After that, she occasionally had nightmares in which the scene was re-enacted. At the age of 11, it was recognized that she had attacks by day, in which she habitually saw the scene of her fright. She saw a little girl, whom she identified as herself, in the now familiar surroundings. She experienced the scene with such distinctness that she was filled with terror lest she should be struck or smothered from behind . . . Sometimes this 'dream' constituted all there was of her epileptic attacks.

At operation, under local anaesthetia, I applied the stimulator to the temporal cortex. 'Wait a minute' she said, 'and I will tell you'. I removed the electrode from the cortex. After a pause, she said, 'I saw someone coming toward me, as though he was going to hit me'. It was obvious also that she was suddenly frightened . . . In a moment she called 'Don't leave me'. Thus the stimulating electrode had recalled the familiar experience that ushered in each of her habitual attacks. But stimulation at other points had recalled to her other experiences of the past, and it had also produced the emotion of fear. Our astonishment was great, for we had produced phenomena that were neither motor nor sensory, and yet the responses seemed to be psychological, not epileptic.

By this, Penfield meant that he was observing phenomena of a normal kind, and not the distorted fragments of acts and sensations that most epileptic phenomena are.

During the electrical stimulation, some of these patients no longer knew where they were; they experienced only their hallucinations. Others were aware of the situation, and knew they were having a brain operation at the time. Patients explained after the current had been turned off, 'I could see the desks, and I was there'. Or 'I had a dream'. Or 'I was listening to music from *Guys and Dolls*'. These peculiar experiences had the freshness of a real experience; they were not like events remembered in the past. During the stimulation, the patients could focus attention on any chosen feature of the episode and could answer questions on it afterwards. These scenes the patients relived were mainly visual, but the sounds and smells accompanying the original experiences were there too. All the accompanying emotions and the mood of the time were present; the patient experienced the same feeling about the event he originally had, and attributed the same significance to it as he had given it at the time. What he had thought of the situation was stored with the stored experience. As soon as the stimulation of the brain was stopped, reliving the experience ceased. When the same spot was stimulated again, the same experience was usually brought up, though this was not always so. From the surrounding region of the cortex, the electrode evokes other recollections. Sometimes stimulation of the hippocampal gyrus gives rise to jumbled-up fragments of memories. Indeed, it is more surprising that electrical stimulation does not always bring up a caricature of memory, and that it does mainly draw out a total sensible record of a previous experience. What is also surprising is that these recollected events are insignificant in the great majority of cases; they were quite unimportant to the patients.

These records are brought up from stimulation of certain parts of the temporal lobes. Penfield realized that 'there is stored away in the ganglionic connection of the brain (i.e. the neurons and their connections) a permanent record of the stream of consciousness; a record that is much more complete and detailed than the memories that any man can recall by voluntary effort'.

Automatic behaviour

The kind of fit in which the patient lies senseless on the floor, making strong jerking movements of the limbs, is not so common. There are all sorts of fits which are not usually recognized as epileptic phenomena. One of the most disturbing of these is the kind known as automatic attacks or automatic behaviour. These were first described and studied by Jackson, when in 1875 he wrote about them under the name of 'epileptic somnambulism', somnambulism being fashionable at the time. During these attacks, the patient unconsciously performs organized acts of behaviour. He is unconscious in the sense that he is not conscious of what is happening or what he is doing; and after the attack has passed he has no memory of what has happened or where he has been. During the attack, the parts of the temporal lobes needed for the recording of events as they occur are not working; for this reason the patient can recall nothing. In the attack the patient goes on carrying out the routine behaviour automatically; he is not open to new suggestions, but he may be quite capable of walking down a crowded street. Quite often the patient makes chewing and swallowing movements in the attack. This is likely to be due to the epileptic discharge spreading to the insula, the part of the cortex that controls the alimentary canal. The main place where the epileptic discharge occurs during the automatic behaviour is within the amygdaloid region of the temporal lobe or the region between the amygdala and the insula. As long as the epileptic discharge remains in this region, there will be no automatic behaviour. A total act of behaviour, like getting up and walking to the door, occurs only when the epileptic discharge spreads from this region to other parts of the brain.

Automatic behaviour is always to some degree abnormal behaviour. The patient may seize the telephone, examine it, and then put the receiver down on his desk, or he may start tearing his clothes. He may get up, murmur something incomprehensible, walk to the window and open it. If the automatic behaviour results from stimulating the brain at operation, the patient may no longer know he is being operated on. He loses touch with the surgeon and everyone else in the operating theatre; he may try to throw off the sterile towels, get up, and go off.

Sometimes, though very rarely, total acts of behaviour may be performed, carried out quite normally in all details, although the whole act is not planned and is not consciously done. The attack never lasts longer than an hour, and usually not more than five minutes. In the attack, the patient may perform an act that he wants to do anyway, but which with full consciousness he would not do. Dr Lennox, a neurologist in America who has seen a great number of epileptic patients, has reported the case of a patient who in an automatic attack went to his boss and said 'I have to have more money or I quit'. He was amazed when at the end of the week he found his salary had been raised.

19 Sensation acquires a meaning

The general problem

We have often to remind ourselves that the input to the central nervous system and the sensations we have are not the same. Sensation consists of what we feel, see, hear, taste, and smell. Perception is a higher-level process, endowing the sensation with meaning and relating it to behaviour. Seeing something is a low-level function. Recognizing what it is that you see is a higher level function, requiring the co-operation of more parts of the cerebral hemispheres.

The higher level of neural functioning is the most difficult to investigate, and so we know less about it than the lower levels. One of the questions neurology attempts to answer is, how do we know what a thing is. How do we collect all sensory impressions together and combine them to say: 'there is a white kitten lying curled up on that sofa'? How is it that the excitation of one lot of neurons gives us the sensation of something seen, of another lot that of something heard? The straight answer to the straight question is, we do not know.

We know a great deal about the underlying anatomy. The various kinds of sensory inputs go to different parts of the cerebral hemispheres. But this fact alone cannot account for our different kinds of sensation. It may be that the different neurons of various sensory inputs differ from each other in ways which at present we do not know, possibly in some physical or chemical ways. Differences in sensation might reside in the fact that the neurons have different connexions to other groups of neurons. It could be that the different sensations may be the result of the experience of groups of sensory neurons having been different. All sensory neurons may start off the same, yet it may be that, by the time the animal has lived a portion of its life, every neuron has become different from every other one.

Or perhaps, after all, there is no problem. One can equally well ask the question 'How can it be that nerve impulses cause the movements of my hand?' To someone who does not know any of the answers, this looks like a similar and almost insoluble problem. But because we do know most of the answers, and because we understand most of the physical and chemical steps involved, this question seems to be of a different order from those concerning sensation and perception, questions involving our consciousness. We now know the physical events that occur when a message spreads along a nerve fibre, how the message is passed from one nerve fibre to the next nerve cell, until finally it reaches the myoneural junction. We know the biochemical and electro-chemical reactions involved in passing nerve impulses on to the muscle fibres, and how this electrical stimulation makes the con-tractile proteins of muscle fibres contract. This makes the fingers move. If we know all the essential steps that cause a movement, it is probable that one day we shall know those for producing sensa-tion from the activity of other neurons. This seems likely as sensa-tion is a link in the chain of movement. The perception of objects is a part of exploratory behaviour. Animals examine what is new and strange—with much interest and caution. It is not so much asking what the thing is, as what to do with it. One of the questions asked is, is this thing familiar or strange? The degree of familiarity depends on the number of times it has been experienced before. Thus, a part of the answer to the question is the memory—or lack of it—of the object or event in the past. And most curious of all, the memory is not only of that individual but also of its forebears.

Inborn knowledge

For he knows that God is his Saviour.

It is surprising to learn that some animals are terrified of the animals that prey on them, even though they have never seen the predator; they are born with the inborn knowledge of their enemy. Young monkeys in India are terrified of a good picture of tigers. Chimpanzees shown a life-size moving model of a lion act appro-priately, shrieking at it and threatening it; and they are afraid of it.

Just the visual presentation of the artificial lion is enough, with no sound and no smell. And these chimpanzees have never seen or met a real lion.

Although this is surprising to us, it was known to country people in Europe in the fourteenth century. For Chaucer tells of Chanticleer, the Cock:

> And so it happened as he cast his eye
> Towards the cabbage at a butterfly
> It fell upon the fox there, lying low.
> Gone was all inclination then to crow,
> 'Cok, cok', he cried, giving a sudden start,
> As one who feels a terror in his heart,
> For natural instinct teaches beasts to flee
> The moment they perceive an enemy
> Though they had never met with it before—
> Thus Chanticleer was shaken to the core.
> (translated by Nevill Coghill)

What we have learned from the ethologists is that the young animal is born with knowledge of a certain shape or a certain sequence of sounds. When this happens, it reacts to it in a way suitable for self-preservation. Many birds already know on leaving the egg the shape and movements of the predator that is looking for them. They know the essential outline of the hawk, planing overhead. Seeing that outline, they rush off to mother, and nestle beneath her wing. The herring gull knows how to behave towards a red spot on a yellow rectangle as soon as it leaves the egg, for that is how its mother's beak will appear to it. When the little duckling breaks through the shell of the egg, it already knows the quack of a mother duck. It will follow that sound; no other sound has meaning for it. If the ducklings feel themselves deserted by her and—as Lorenz so sweetly says—peep their abandonment, then even if this is her first brood she knows the meaning of this sound. Born with this knowledge, a motor pattern of behaviour is set off by this and only this sound, and she comes back to her brood. The studies of Von Uexküll, Lorenz, Tinbergen, and their successors have discovered a large number of examples of inborn knowledge of visual and auditory patterns.

If we ask, how does a newborn duckling know the sound of its mother's voice, or how does it know that she is its mother, we put the question badly. If we ask, how does it know what to do when it hears its mother's voice, or when it sees her moving away, we are putting it in a somewhat better way, but still in a form that cannot be easily answered. When we observe a mother duck with her first brood, we see that she responds to the alarm call of her ducklings by an innate, unlearned, complex pattern of behaviour, that of defending the young. But if one of the young whose cry produced this reaction turns out, when she examines it, to have the wrong markings, she will attack it and drive it off. The correct markings produce mothering and sheltering response; the wrong markings make her drive off an intruder. Certain totalities of sensation automatically cause certain forms of behaviour. Whether it seems to the reacting animal that it has a free choice, that it chooses to react in that way and in no other way, we do not know. In fact, there is no choice. The duckling inevitably follows the adult duck's quack. Once it has been subjected to imprinting, it follows the moving object that it saw during the sensitive period.

We come nearer the mark if we think of the animal as never asking for meanings, as not formulating such a question as 'What is it?' On experiencing anything in its environment, its questions are, 'Do I eat it, do I drink it, do I copulate with it, do I fight it or flee from it, can I bathe in it or roll in it?' For its reaction is always some sort of movement, or rarely, a freezing of all movement.

Actually, of course, it does not ask question; it responds, it behaves. When the opponent squeals, it signals submission and this removes the aggression of the antagonist. Tension is reduced and peace is restored. When the ape offers itself for sexual mounting, the ape who is invited to mount knows that the other has submitted. There are hints of this in humans. Adles is right, not Freud.

Among animals, including ourselves, there is a mutual exchange of signals. The meaning is understood not only by members of the same species, but also by other mammals, other birds. Inborn knowledge provokes behaviour; it is a part of behaviour.

As animals know what to do with things rather than know what they are, at times an animal may be said to recognize something, while at other times it does not do so; its ability to recognize depends on its needs at the time. Moreover, at different times it recognizes the same object as two different things. For the female, the male is something with which to copulate on one occasion, on another he is something to eat. To the female spider, the male is never the objectively seen male spider it is to us. What meaning an animal possesses for another of the same species depends on how it behaves, on its carrying out the right social behaviour. This is, of course, the same for human beings, though in our case it has to be learned. Depending on accent, on clothes, on gestures, way of standing, sitting, and picking the teeth, we behave to another one of our own kind in certain ways, and we do not see the other person objectively (not that there is such a thing as considering anyone objectively, anyway).

We do not know the first thing about the neural basis of these inborn perceptions and the behaviour fixed to them. We must avoid being astounded by the total phenomenon as we see it in its finished complexity. It is pleasant to stand transfixed with awe and wonder before the phenomena of nature. It is pleasant too, and more rewarding, to find out how it all works, and to arrive at an understanding of what is going on around us. And this need not diminish our first feelings of wonder. When each example is finally broken down into its essential components, we may eventually find that the basic feature triggering a certain act of behaviour is quite simple. It may be that it depends on a diagonal line casting a shadow across the retina; perhaps it will be that the quacking of the mother duck will turn out to be the only frequency range of sound to which the auditory apparatus is sensitive at that stage of development.

It is best to avoid separating sensory from motor, the perception from the behaviour. This may be the traditional neurological and psychological way of investigating, but it may well make problems where none exist. In the examples we have been considering, what we have been noting is that certain patterns in one member of a mutually reacting pair constitute a sign; this sign-stimulus fires off an act of behaviour in the other member. Such sign-stimuli often occur in chains, each stimulus setting off an act of behaviour, constituting the new sign-stimulus to the other reacting animal. It has been found by ethologists that many acts of behaviour are organized in this way: this is so for mating among sticklebacks and many kinds of birds, for feeding among birds, for fighting and avoiding fighting among territorial animals. This way of organizing behaviour takes us a long way from the question, how we and other animals know what something is, or rather, it takes us a long way out of the psychological laboratory where such questions were investigated in traditional psychology.

The integration of many different sensory aspects of an object in the environment is unnecessary in unlearned or instinctive behaviour. A few sensory clues are enough; the rest is irrelevant. For instance, the male wasps mentioned in Chapter 2 needed only the smell of the secretion of the female's abdominal glands to make them carry out copulation; they would copulate with the cut-out glands, and not with the female wasp deprived of these glands. The proper clues are few that make the male attack, or the female present for copulation. In the case of copulation of the leopard frog, it suffices to put a rubber band round the female's chest; she will then lay her eggs. On the other hand, the sign-stimuli may be complicated, and they must be correctly presented. The male may have to perform a complicated dance, each series of movements being presented in the correct order, for the female to accept him.

Work on human beings on sign-stimuli is now being done. The advertising industry knows quite a lot about this without realizing it. They can present human figures so that they cause reactions of tenderness and a desire to give, or so that they cause repulsion and avoidance. They sell little furry objects which make children and women want to cuddle them, and which have no other use than that. Psychologists are now carrying out research to find out what sign-stimuli are innate in the young human and what sorts of behaviour they induce.

If we look at the whole animal kingdom, we see that every sort of sensory channel is used for signalling: emitting odours, performing dances to be looked at, making sounds, drumming on trees to cause vibration. David Lack showed that it was the red breast that made the robin attack. Whether in this case the robin is aware of other stimuli from the oncoming robin or not, one does not know. But it is clearly of no importance in the situation; it is red breast alone that determines its behaviour. The final evidence supporting this interpretation of the facts is that when the male robin see himself in a mirror, he threatens and may attack his own reflection. Other sensory clues are not so definite. When a cock-robin hears the song of another cock-robin, he seeks further stimulation from the singer. His subsequent behaviour depends on many different factors. Some of these are the actual place where the other robin is seen. Is it within, on the boundary of, or well outside the territory of the first robin? He will respond differently in accordance with the reaction of the singing robin to his own threatening display. His behaviour is also related to the time of year, for this affects his brain; the brain controls the robin's secretion of hormones; and most importantly, these hormones act on the brain itself, and influence its behaviour.

The fact that an animal's response to the same object differs at different times indicates that our philosophical questions about perceiving the real nature of an object are the wrong ones. It seems that to many animals an object has no continuity. At one time blades of grass are something to eat, at another time, the wherewithal to make a nest. It would be an anthropomorphic assumption to believe that the bird knows that it is dealing with the same object on the two occasions. It is far more likely that when it eats grass, the bird sees this as pleasant-tasting green stuff to be pulled out of the ground; and when it entwines it into the fabric of its nest, it sees it as green nest-building material that has to be pulled out of the ground, and interwined and lined with feathers from the breast. The grass is always there; but only at times do rodents and birds see it as suitable material for nest-building. Thus the meaning of sensation changes. When the season changes, the grass that was always there acquires a new meaning.

The use to which a thing is put depends on the state of the animal perceiving to it. How the same object is perceived changes with the hormones secreted by the endocrine gland. When a rat is under the influence of hormones making it feel maternal, it mistakes mice for young rats and puts them in its nest, caring for them lovingly. When it is not under the influence of these hormones, it will kill them. Hormones cause the animal's needs, needs breed desires, and desires see objects in the environment that are there to satisfy them.

As the sensory clues making up a sign-stimulus may be few, mistakes are sometimes made. Man has always caught birds by decoy. Although Chaucer's birds defied the fowler and all his wiles, the fact that there are many people among us bearing the name 'Fowler' shows that many people used to follow this profession successfully before guns were used to shoot fowl. To a young rabbit, something moving with a hoppity motion is another rabbit to be followed. Professor Otto Koehler damaged the rear-wheel of his bicycle and rode on it while it hopped regularly over a field. He found a young rabbit persistently following him and he could not frighten it away. A fawn followed Professor Tinbergen on a bicycle with the rear-mudguard painted white. This must have been so like the white hinder-parts of another deer that the young animal saw no difference. Alexander the Great thought that his sculptor was amazing because Boukephalas, his famous horse, recognized a bronze statue of itself as another horse. But we now know that this is nothing. A life-size, two-dimensional, true-to-life painting is enough; a horse reacts to it as though it is a real horse, and is clearly puzzled when he walks round to the other side of the canvas and finds nothing there. Throughout nature we find examples of mimicry based on deception of predators and enemies. Caterpillars look like sticks, the hoverfly looks like the stinging wasp. Eyes may frighten animals, and so the peacock butterfly paints them on its wings, and some tropical fish pain them on their dorsal fins.

Man also has inborn knowledge, though the catalogue of what we know without learning or imitation has not yet been made. We understand the meaning of aggressive, threatening, and submissive postures, and of behaviour of many kinds of animals; this is obvious for cats and dogs, and equally so for their more dangerous relations, lions, tigers, and wolves. We do not need to have lessons in the subject at school nor to have this explained to us by our parents; merely seeing the posture and hearing the accompanying cries is enough. We know the squealing of an animal in pain or terror without having to learn it; as some would say, we know it instinctively or intuitively.

Acquired knowledge

Although this chapter is called 'Sensation acquires a meaning', we hardly ever experience a pure sensation. Almost everything we hear, feel, see, or smell has meaning. We perceive things, we do not have sensory data. The elements of sensory data cause sensation; a lot more processes are required before a thing is seen, and still more before it is recognized. To see something moving from one part of a room to the other entails neural activity of the cerebral hemispheres that is not yet understood. We become aware of the psychological aspects of some of this activity when we recognize a melody from the separate notes spaced in time that form it. The data are the isolated notes and the sensation is what we hear; we then perceive that this is a whole, a melody, that we either know or we do not know, and we put the melody into many categories, modern music, folk music, Schubert, in three-four time, in a major mode, and in the key of C. When none of this activity takes place, a simple pure sensation occurs. We interpret what we experience as soon as we feel it. We do not think 'There is such and such a form of green on a white background'; we say 'There is a leaf on the path.' We hear music, not sound, we see objects, objects that continue in time, not light reflected from edges and angles.

That animals are born with knowledge of some of the things they are probably going to meet is a surprising fact. But for mammals such inborn knowledge as the shape of a predator seems to be exceptional. Although this innate fear is so striking, most of what has to be feared and avoided by primates—and that includes us—has to be learned.

What is innate is only a basis. Higher vertebrates have to learn to make sense of sensory images. And what the young animal has to learn must come in a correct order and within a certain time. The programme of learning is innate, it is a part of the way in which the central nervous system works. One needs to go through a long period of practice to acquire the skills of walking or of running downstairs, and so it is with perception. Whatever neural processes occur when we learn, learning is as necessary for perception as it is for motor skills. It is the same for emotional development and for the acquisition of the skill of living with other members of a group.

Some experiments on the necessity of learning for perception have been carried out in the United States. Chimpanzees were reared in total darkness from birth. When these animals are eventually brought out into the light, they behave as if they see nothing; they take no notice of their visual environment. They have certain innate visual reflexes, such as the feedback mechanism for adjusting the amount of light to fall on to the retina, but apart from such reflexes, these young chimpanzees behave just as if they are still in complete darkness. Similarly, chimpanzees reared in an environment of universal diffuse bright light are equally blind. Some of these baby chimpanzees had their heads enclosed in a translucent plastic orb, so that all the light reaching their eyes was general diffuse light, devoid of patterns and definite colours. When these orbs were removed, the young animals behaved just like the chimpanzees reared in complete darkness. These experiments show that the animal needs to experience the varied patterns of light and the changing patterns of moving objects in order to learn to perceive.

Moreover, in order for learning to be permanent, it must come at the right time. If a baby chimpanzee is reared in a normal environment and then put into darkness for two years, it is just like a chimpanzee reared always in complete darkness. The early rearing in a normal environment did not help.

From these and other similar experiments, it becomes clear that an animal must have the proper early environment in order to develop its innate potentialities. If the right opportunities for spontaneous learning are not presented during the first two or three years of life, then the child will be unintelligent, and will remain so. Freud and his successors realized that this is so for the normal development of sexuality and emotion. It is now clear that this is so for every aspect of intelligence and mental and psychological functioning. Further, the performance tests, wrongly known as intelligence tests, were designed on the premises that native and inborn intelligence was separable from what had been acquired or learned; but in fact the two are so interwined that it is meaningless to try to separate them.

The question of how much our perception of the world depends on learning has always been one of much interest to philosophers. Locke has recorded in his *Essay Concerning Human Understanding* that in 1690 he was asked the following question by his friend Molyneux, whose wife had gone blind:

Suppose a man born blind, and now adult, and taught by his touch to distinguish between a cube and a sphere of the same metal. Suppose then the cube and sphere were placed on a table, and the blind man made to see, query, whether by his sight, before he touched them, could he distinguish and tell which was the globe and which the cube? . . . The acute and judicious proposer answers: not. For though he has obtained the experience of how the globe, how the cube a..ects his touch, yet he has not yet attained the experience that what affects his touch so or so, must affect his sight, so or so.

And Locke commented:

I agree with this thinking gentlemen, whom I am proud to call my friend, in his answer to this problem, and am of the opinion that the blind man, at first, would not be able to tell with certainty which was the globe and which the cube.

Diderot, too, was much interested in perception, but unlike most philosophers, he got out of his chair, went out of his room, and made some observations on the matter. He recorded in his *Letter on the Blind* (1749) that one blind man with whom he talked said that if he were offered the gift of sight by some miracle, he would prefer to have enormously long arms instead. This most perceptive man said, 'If curiosity were not to dominate my wishes, I would like to have long arms; for it seems to me that my hands would instruct me better what is happening on the moon than your eyes or your telescopes. It would be better for me to bring to a state of perfection the organ that I have than to give me the one I am lacking.'

In our time Molyneux's conditions have come true. The very cases imagined by him and by Locke have occurred. We can answer the philosopher's questions, not only because the surgery of the eye has advanced, but also because all the known cases have been collected together and studied by von Senden, and published in his absorbing book *Space and Sight*.

Already at the end of the eighteenth century, operations had been carried out on children to remove cataracts and restore sight. When these patients came to see, it was not an unmixed blessing, as Diderot's wise informer foresaw. A lady operated upon at the age of 42 in 1826 by a surgeon, Mr Wardrop, 'seemed bewildered from not being able to combine the knowledge acquired by senses of touch and sight'. All of these patients who have had sight restored have explained how they had to learn to interpret the strange world of sight, and how difficult it has been for them to acquire a visual picture of the world.

After their operations, most of these patients have been unable to see much. They cannot distinguish between shapes which appear quite different to us. They have to train for months before they have any useful vision, and some never succeed in acquiring it. They prefer to remain in a tactile world.

Those who were blind from birth till the operation have no true conception of height or distance. To those patients who are first able to see after their operations, colours are more important than shapes and they have less difficulty in learning colours than shapes. One would probably have believed that it would have been exactly the opposite. Pictures or photographs—which are two-dimensional representations of three-dimensional objects—are at first meaningless. For a picture, like a map or a written word, is a learned symbol. In this case, the actual size of what is represented is symbolized by something much smaller (except in the opposite cases where an object is magnified in photograph). Children, after these operations, when shown a picture or a photograph, notice the frame rather than the actual picture, for visually it is more prominent. The content of the picture is prominent only to people who know that there is one, that the picture represents someone or something. Von Senden has reported that one little girl aged 8, on being shown a photograph, first noticed the wooden frame, which she called a box lid, and then added that there was something painted on it. Even when she was told it represented a human face, she could not discover any of the parts, such as the eyes or the nose. Another patient asked, when she was handed paintings or photographs: 'Why do they put those dark marks all over them?' Her mother then told her that the dark marks were shadows, and if the shadows were not put in, 'many things would look flat'. 'Well, that's how things do look', the patient replied.

One of these patients was studied for a long time by two psychologists, R.L. Gregory and J.G. Wallace. The first thing the patient saw when the bandages were removed from his eyes was the face of the surgeons who performed the operation. The patient said that he saw a blur, and knew it must be a face as a voice was coming out of it. He thought that had he not known that voices came out of faces, then he would not have known that it was a face. At first when he looked down from a window about 30 to 40 feet above the ground, he thought he could easily have climbed out of the window and lowered himself to the ground while hanging on to the window-sill with his hands. He was amazed when he first saw the moon, and thought it was a reflection of something in the window. He was fascinated by reflections in mirrors—something that he could hardly have imagined in his years of blindness; and he would pass the time looking at people in a mirror in his local pub.

Although he had always longed to be able to see, he soon ceased to be delighted at receiving the gift of sight. 'He found the world drab, and was upset by flaking paint and blemishes on things.' He often did not turn on the light in the evening, but would sit contentedly in the dark.

For these patients some objects seemed to be surprisingly large and others equally small; some objects surprised them by being too close and others by being too far away. An American blind girl explained that to a blind person 'a skyscraper is not thought of as towering into the heavens, but as indefinitely higher than a blind man can reach'. All the patients have difficulty in distinguishing two-dimensional from three-dimensional things. One of these patients could not tell a ping-pong ball from a white disk. At first, these patients cannot identify colours, and they have to learn to do this. They then do not see colour as we see it. The colour does not fill out the whole extent of the coloured object. According to Macdonald Critchley, 'in the environment there looms up a medley of colour patches, with differing tonal qualities and with properties of shininess or dullness'.

But there are differences between learning to see for the first time in adult years and learning at the correct time. To start with, there are anatomical differences. If vision is never practised, the connections within the visual pathway are not developed normally. It is probable that connections between one cortical association area and another do not develop if they are never used. Owing to these connections, we are able to transfer knowledge acquired through one sensory channel to a general store. It is then recognized by the input arriving in another sensory channel. Once we have learned to know the letter A, we can recognize it also non-visually. We recognize it tactilely, when it is traced on our skins; we recognize it kinaesthetically when we trace it in mid-air with a finger, without looking. Thus, the letter A was first learned visually; then it could be recalled to other sensory inputs, by inputs coming into the brain via sensory channels that had not been used to learn the letter.

Those who are born blind build up a kinaesthetic-tactile image of the world, whereas people who can see acquire a visual image. For someone born blind, perspective does not exist, and congenitally blind people cannot grasp what it is. Their idea of distance is very different from that of people who see. For them, objects appear smaller when they are in the distance. They have never seen an object from different angles, from above, from the side; they know the object only from feeling, smelling, or tasting it. Whereas for us, the different appearances of objects seen from various angles teach us about perspective, distance, and space. We know that an object has a constant colour, even though we see many shades which depend on the lighting and the shadows. We conclude that its shape is constant too, even though our eyes don't tell us this.

The way in which our vision gives each of us our picture of the world can be learned with much pleasure by reading Trevor-Roper's *The World through Blunted Sight*. In this book, Trevor-

Roper not only discusses the defects of vision of many painters, but also emphasizes the results of defects of vision forming the characters of children.

The comparable operation of restoring hearing to those born deaf has not yet been achieved. If ever it becomes possible, this will be a rewarding field of psychology to study, and it will not be all pleasure for those who have to learn to hear.

Perception always goes beyond the sensory data. What lies beyond is a guess, or a prediction, or a hypothesis: you may choose your word. We live in a familiar world; and perception is based on probabilities. What the child is so busy learning is the context of various inputs; it is learning probabilities, about what the sensory data in this situation probably mean. Perceiving has to be learned. If we see a black, apparently flat, apparently circular object, we say we can see a gramophone record. We will say this when we are looking at it from above, from its edge, or from an angle of 45 degrees. Yet in each of these cases our retinae are receiving totally different impressions. Seeing is believing; it is believing that the dots, lines, angles, and edges that we see do represent the objects we already know.

We never see a movement. We see something changing its position, we see it becoming larger or getting smaller. From visual clues such as these, we infer that a movement is taking place.

Because seeing entails guessing what things are, one can make mistakes. One sees what appears to be a mass of flowers in the distance; when one gets near, one finds that it is litter and paper. How strange that this seen material then arouses two opposite emotional reactions.

If a baby has good sight for the first two years of life and then goes blind, it is the same as if it had been born blind. If this child's sight is restored, it is found that the early ability to see has had no permanent effects. But if the child does not become blind till the age of 4, all that it has learned to see remains, and gives it a picture of the world. These children are quite unlike the congenitally blind. There is no doubt that the difference between the two groups—those blind by the age of 3 and blind by the age of 5—depends on structural difference in the neurons and their connections.

If seeing something is problematic or difficult, one helps with internal speech. Professor Homskaya in Russia showed how speech is used in young children presented with a difficult task. This has been reported by Luria in his book *The Working Brain*. Children who had just started school were told to make a certain movement when they were shown a pale pink colour, and to keep still when shown a darker pink. When this task was speeded up their responses 'fell off sharply, and mistakes occurred, sometimes as many as 50 per cent. If, however, the test was carried out so that the child was instructed to evaluate the shades in words at the same time (by saying 'pale' or 'dark'), and to give the appropriate response at the same time, the accuracy of discrimination between the shades was considerably increased.'

The recognition of faces is carried out mainly by the right cerebral hemisphere. If the occipital lobe of the right hemisphere is damaged by a stroke, this ability may be lost forever. A patient who has had this stroke may not recognize his wife. He also cannot tell the sex of a clothed person. In looking into a mirror, he may say he sees himself but can't recognize himself. These kinds of recognitions are normally done without the aid of speech. The recognition of faces is not so easy. It is, therefore, surprising to learn from experiments carried out in the University of Miami that babies 36 hours old can imitate the facial expressions of a person they are watching. This means that the baby already has excellent sight, for it can discriminate the facial expressions of happiness and contentment, unhappiness and sadness, and surprise. Professor Fantz, in the United States, has studied what things a young infant prefers to look at. Within two minutes of birth, babies look at faces and take no notice of other objects. By the second day of life they can recognize their mother's face. Babies prefer looking at patterned objects to plain ones, and a stylized face to a face all muddled up. The preferences occur so early that they must be innate. It is not surprising that one is born with a special aptitude to see peoples' faces; this is important as human beings spend their lives in groups and use facial movements to express themselves.

The visual input reaches the cerebral cortex

In man, the nerve fibres from the left half of the retina of both eyes connect with the left occipital lobe and those from the right with the right lobe. And so everything seen on the right is reported to the left half of the brain and everything on the left to the right half. All sensory pathways, except for the olfactory, relay in the thalamus, and then go on to the cortex of the hemisphere. This is also so for visual pathways; but in this case, the parts of the thalamus in which the relay occurs have moved from the rest of the thalamus. The relay takes place in the lateral geniculate nucleus and the superior colliculus. The fibres from the geniculate nucleus go to the primary visual cortex. This region of the cortex also receives an input telling it of the position of the eyes. This is needed both for understanding what is being seen and for directing the eyes to look at anything. During the evolution of mammals, the acuity of vision has increased. This means that there has been an increase in the number of retinal neurons and an increased area of the cerebral cortex devoted to vision. In primates, the visual area fills the whole of the occipital lobe and spreads forwards into the temporal and parietal lobes. The nerve fibres from the colliculus go to a different part of the thalamus and thence connections take this input to visual areas of the cortex other than the primary area. This pathway is for detecting movement and directing the eyes towards the movement. The nerve fibres from the retina that take this pathway are those that originated in the photoreceptors that are particularly sensitive to movement. This is the pathway designed for looking; the pathway to the primary visual area is the one for seeing.

In the primary visual cortex, a cortical neuron is excited by certain features of the visual world. For example, in one layer of the cortex are orientation-selective cells. One neuron will be excited by a line at 90 degrees to the horizontal, and does not respond to a line making an angle of 45 degrees; another responds to a line making an angle of 60 degrees, and not to a vertical line. Other neurons are stimulated by a line or an edge moving in one direction, and cease to respond when it changes direction, while others respond to the new direction. Some neurons respond only when both eyes are stimulated simultaneously and cannot be excited by either eye alone; others respond to each eye.

In the different visual areas there are different kinds of maps of the visual field. The whole of the retina is reproduced in the primary visual area in a point-to-point manner, one point in the retina corresponding to one point in the primary visual area. In the secondary surrounding area, there is also a point-to-point map, but many points that are adjacent in the retina are not adjacent in this map. In each subsequent visual area to which the input is passed, every neuron receives a larger amount of the visual field. Finally, in the front part of the temporal lobe, any one neuron receives its input from the entire visual field. In the temporal lobe of the monkey, there are single neurons that are excited only by the visual profile of a monkey, and others that respond only to the face of a monkey or human being. There are other neurons nearby that respond to auditory inputs and others that respond to both visual and auditory inputs. Others respond to tactile inputs, being excited when the animal is touched or stroked.

Professor Rolls of Oxford University asked the question what aspects of the face the monkey's temporal lobe neurons responded to. He found that different neurons responded to different parts of the face and some to presentation of a whole face. For instance, there were some neurons that responded to the eyes of a monkey or human being; if the eyes were covered, these neurons did not fire. Others responded similarly to the mouth. Neurons that are fired off by being presented with a picture of a face only responded if the drawing of the face was right. If it was drawn all wrong, say with the mouth in the forehead or the eyes low in the face, no response occurred. Of neurons responding to a face, some responded to a face near the monkey, others to a face far away, and even some to a face upside down. It is to be noted that these neurons respond to faces of various sizes, large and small; and so they are not responding to the image of a face on the retina. There are neurons that respond to different facial expressions, very important for primates.

In cats, there are some cortical neurons that are excited by objects coming towards the eyes and another lot by objects coming towards the animal but missing its head.

The visual impulses on leaving the outer part of the temporal lobes go on to the parts of the brain concerned with memory and emotion, the amygdala and hippocampus, which are nearby in the deeper parts of the temporal lobes. A case of a severe head injury has been recorded in which the pathways between the occipital visual areas and the amygdala must have been damaged bilaterally. The patient could not feel any emotion in relation to anything he saw. Everything seen became drab and uninteresting. This included no sexual interest.

In some animals, the visual system is not ready to use at birth. If a kitten is brought up in darkness, it will always be blind. The correct cortical connections develop as the animal practises looking and seeing. What the cat is finally able to see depends on the environment in which it lives as a kitten. Blakemore and Cooper raised kittens in the dark, except for daily periods of being placed in an environment in which there were only black and white vertical or horizontal stripes. One group of kittens was put in the vertical and the other in the horizontal stripe environment. Eventually neurons of the primary visual areas of these kittens responded only to vertically orientated stimulation or only to horizontally orientated stimuli, in accordance with which environment the kitten had passed its infancy.

It happens sometimes, though very rarely, that the primary visual cortex of both hemispheres is destroyed. This causes blindness, but blindness of an extraordinary kind. The patient says he is blind and that he cannot see anything; on the whole, he is right, he is blind. But when flashes or a fast-moving object are put into his visual field, he gets some sort of visual sensation, he turns his eyes towards it, and he is able to point at the light. But he still says he is only guessing and that he cannot see a thing. He certainly cannot discriminate objects nor report on their size. But he can tell horizontal from vertical bars of light; he can see the difference between Xs and Os, if they are big enough. He says that the test is ridiculous as he cannot see a thing and that he is just looking or putting out his hand at random; yet he has the feeling that there is something there in front of him, although he sees nothing. If you try to deceive him by telling him that there is a bar of light in front of him when there isn't, he is not deceived; for then he does not have the feeling that there is something.

What an incredible thing this is—that someone is seeing things, and yet has no perception of them. This shows us that perception is not equivalent to the cerebral cortex receiving an input.

After the primary visual cortex has been destroyed, the neurons of the geniculate nucleus eventually die, and later still, the neurons of the retina connected to this nucleus. But about 20 per cent survive. This strange kind of sight, known now as blindsight, depends on the input of these survivors. These surviving neurons do not finally connect to the primary visual area but to visual areas in the temporal lobes. As the visual input has not come to the primary visual cortex, the input does not give rise to the ordinary visual sensation; and consciousness says it has seen nothing.

Blindsight has been produced in experiments on monkeys. When the primary visual areas and the surrounding areas were destroyed, the animals behaved just like the patients with destruction of the main visual areas of the occipital lobe.

The monkeys were rendered completely blind only after removal of the superior colliculus pathway.

What is so interesting about scientific discoveries is that one never knows where the next advance is coming from. That there are two pathways for seeing, one going to the primary visual area, and another going to deeper regions of the cerebral hemisphere and then to other visual areas of the cortex, has been confirmed in the case of the new-born hamster. This animal is born in a rather embryonic state. At this stage, there are parts of its brain that can be removed easily. In the baby hamster the midbrain region that receives the input from the retina is large, and can be easily separated from the visual cortex. And so at this time two operations are possible. Either the midbrain visual region can be removed or else the cortical visual region. When the visual cortex is removed, it is obvious that the hamster is blind. But an analysis of the animal's vision shows that it knows where something is in its field of vision but it does not know what it is. It cannot recognize anything; but it goes straight to any object placed within its visual field. When the other pathway in the midbrain is removed, it knows what the things are that it sees; but it cannot run towards them: it is incapable of finding what it sees. In man with the primary visual cortex ruined, there is still a pathway through the thalamus and thence to other visual areas. And so this pathway provides us with information of where something is so that we can point to it with a finger, but we do not know what we are pointing to, and deny that this game has any sense anyway.

What the auditory cortex receives

Sound is heard in two regions of the midbrain, similar to vision, the inferior colliculus and the medial geniculate nucleus; they are outgrowths of the thalamus. The cerebral cortex organizes more complex aspects of what is heard, including its temporal and spatial features. The localization of a sound starts in the cochlear nucleus where the incoming nerves from the inner ear arrive in the medulla; the final and necessary part of the brain for localizing is the auditory cortex of the temporal lobes.

The primary auditory cortex is not arranged like the cochlea; it does not have neurons that respond just to one main frequency, that is, to one pure tone. These neurons of the cortex respond to many aspects of sound. Some neurons react when a sound starts, others when it ceases: these are sound-on, sound-off neurons. There are others that respond to a particular duration of a sound. Some neurons are particularly sensitive to the differences noted when a sound reaches the two ears, to the intensity of the sound, and the differences in timing. There are neurons that do not respond to a note of constant frequency but respond if the note falls or rises a semitone. Other neurons respond to the rate of change of frequency in the note. This sort of change is important for telling us whether the source of a sound is coming or going, or whether we are getting nearer or further from it. For this, the Doppler effect is used: it was described above, in the example of the echo-location of bats.

Hearing has been investigated by presenting various types of sound to the two ears simultaneously through headphones. From these experiments, we have learned that nerve impulses from the left ear end up mainly in the right temporal lobe, and those from the right ear in the left lobe. Words and sentences are recognized better by the right ear as they are sent through to the left hemisphere. The right cerebral hemisphere is the more important one for musical execution. Singing is done mainly with the right hemisphere, whereas speaking is with the left. It is claimed that the left hemisphere is essential for the temporal and rhythmical aspects of music and the right for the appreciation of pitch, chords, and melody. It seems, too, that trained musicians employ the left hemisphere for melody rather than the right; for music is more an intellectual activity for them than it is for the naif listener.

Combining sensory inputs

The two cerebral hemispheres are not equal and the same. It is probable that we are born with each hemisphere having a propensity to develop differently, and the differences are probably accentuated during childhood by learning. When we say that an ability depends on one hemisphere, this does not mean that the one hemisphere needs no contribution from the other one.

Geographical knowledge is essential for all animals, from bees to tigers. All seek the places where something satisfactory occurred and avoid those where one has just escaped with one's life: an emotional map is essential equipment for us all. In primates, a large part of the parietal lobes is devoted to this topographical knowledge, the right side being the more important. The region is connected to the hippocampus and amygdala so that what has been discovered should be remembered. If these parts of the cerebral cortex are damaged, the person cannot plan a journey because he cannot visualize the route, and when he is on the journey he has no idea which road to take whenever there is a choice. Also, the patient's orientation in space is upset. He may be unable to perceive the position of objects in relation to each other, to know if a thing is above or below something else. He therefore cannot construct any objects in space. Some of these patients, on being asked to draw something, leaves out all the left sides of things. As he cannot appreciate the right and left of objects, including his own body, he may be unable to dress himself, and he puts his clothes on in unorthodox ways, back to front or with his arms through his trouser legs. The patient cannot understand the figures and hands of a clock and so he cannot tell the time. He cannot draw or understand a map or plan. He cannot copy drawings and may not be able to copy letters, as he does not know in which direction he should make the pencil go.

The ability to add and subtract needs the appreciation of space. This is quite clear when one sees someone using an abacus, for the bobbles are arranged in columns side by side. When we add and substract using the decimal system, we are using an internalized abacus. If the relevant part of the brain has been disrupted, then the spatial aspects of adding and subtracting will be missing. Such a patient may not be able to appreciate columns of numbers, one being above another, and he cannot transfer a number from one column to the next one on the left. If he were to use Roman numerals (and one wonders how anyone could have calculated using this system), he would have no difficulty with this disruption of spatial ability, for figures are not taken from column to column.

Vestibular components are essential for our perception of space and of our own bodies in our constructed space. Both hemispheres contribute to the ability to judge distances in three dimensions and to make constructions in space, which needs an appreciation of three dimensions.

Parts of the temporal lobes and the frontal lobes contribute mood and emotion. Over the past few years one has been astounded to learn that emotion is more an affair of the right hemisphere than of the whole brain. When the frontal lobes, particularly the right, are disconnected from the parts of the brain behind and below them, a state of utter indifference occurs. We have learned this from the operations of leucotomy (discussed in Chapter 23). When this operation has been carried out in patients with terribly severe pain, the pain remains but the suffering and depression is removed. How misery, anguish, loneliness, and even guilt can accompany chronic pain is shown by Tolstoy in his masterpiece *The Death of Ivan Ilyich*.

A certain part of the brain can know an object while another part does not recognize it. The left hemisphere is likely to know the object in the sense that it can name it and put it into various categories; the right hemisphere is likely to know it in the sense that it knows what to do with it, but it cannot name it nor categorize it. It is clear that the person does know what the object is, as he knows what to do with it; but he may be unable to find the word 'razor'. This strange situation occurs (as will be discussed in Chapter 21) when some lesion disconnects two parts of the cortex. If someone cannot name the object but uses it, connections through to the speech area of the left hemispheres have been damaged.

One of the difficulties we all have in discussing and understanding the functions of the brain is due to the words we use often being inappropriate; for they have been taken over from everyday speech, philosophy, and even religion. Words such as 'know', 'understand', or 'perception' are either popular or philosophic terms; they are too vague to have the clear-cut meaning needed in science. Even the word 'I' is useless. If the right cerebral hemisphere knows something and the left does not, then where does 'I' come in?

Perception of ourselves

As well as perceiving the world around us, we need to have a perception of ourselves. Where we are in space is told to us by vision, by vestibular receptors, and from receptors of the skin and deeper tissues. These various inputs are collected together, they go to the thalamus and from there to the parietal lobes. Here they provide us with the basis of our feeling that our bodies are us, and that they are placed in such-and-such a way in the environment. With the kind of damage to the brain that occurs nowadays from wars, small circumscribed areas of the cortex of the hemispheres can be ruined without there being much damage to the rest of the brain. When a part of one parietal lobe is selectively damaged in this way, the patient no longer realizes that the limbs on the opposite side of his body to the damaged lobe are his own. He pays no attention to them, when asked to move them, he does nothing. Often when he is told to clasp his two hands together, he merely clasps one. If one then holds up the neglected hand in front of his eyes, he still does not recognize it as being a part of himself, and is unable to move it. But it is not paralysed, for it still moves adequately in automatic movements. Where there is this inability to integrate one half of one's body, the patient usually cannot conceive that side of the bodies of other people. For example, one patient with a neglect of his own left limbs, when asked to lift my left hand, always lifted my right hand and took no notice of my left. Such a patient may show little intellectual deterioration, apart from this one sort of defect. I once saw a patient with a severe injury of the right parietal lobe. When I held up his left arm in front of his eyes, he would take no notice of it; and when I asked him whose limb it was, he answered 'Oh, that! That's the arm Nurse puts the penicillin injections into'. In such cases, the patient may think that the arm on the opposite side to the brain lesion is someone else in his bed, and he may give it a name. Another of these patients used to say that the limbs were his brother. He strongly objected to their presence in bed with him, and he would try and hurl them out. Once or twice I have seen such patients throw themselves out of bed by mistake in their efforts to get rid of their right arm and leg, which they thought were somebody else in their bed.

When a patient neglects and cannot integrate half of his own body, he usually neglects the whole of the surrounding space on that side of his body as well. He does not notice that half of the face of the clock, he may walk around in a circle, turning always to the neglected side of space. He cannot localize sounds coming from the affected side, hearing them as if coming from the other side. These disturbances of perception perhaps suggest that normally our conception of the space in which we live may be arrived at as an extension of our conception of our own bodies.

The opposite kind of defect is the loss of a part of the body with retention of the part of the brain where past and present inputs are integrated. This gives rise to phantom limbs. The sensory region of the cortex is intact, and it tells us that the whole body is there, and so the absence of the limb is felt as a positive sensation. One might have thought that the loss of the part would have been registered in the sensory regions of the brain. But they do not tell us 'a part is missing', but 'a part is constantly present'; for the phantom limb protrudes into consciousness more obviously and more often than the normal parts of the body. Usually we are not continually aware of the parts, position, and shape of our bodies; and normally some effort is needed to bring them into consciousness. The main reason why the limb is still felt is that the nerve fibres from the part that was cut off are still there, and are sending off impulses all the time. This can be concluded from finding someone with an amputated limb, and then squeezing or banging the nerves in the stump. He will then get a different kind or an increase in the sensations that he usually has. He may get pins and needles running down the leg to the toes; or he may get a burning pain in the ankle. For one has stimulated the very nerves which previously went to those parts of his limb.

20 Speech and other symbols

For he can spraggle upon waggle at the word of command.

Social animals living in groups, unsocial animals meeting for sexual intercourse, parents and offspring, all need to communicate with each other. In nature there are hundreds of ways of communicating; using the voice is only one way.

The time in which we live is marvellous; for we are now reaping the harvest of a hundred years and more of the investigation of the whole universe by scientific methods. Four of man's wishes have been achieved. He is able to have sexual intercourse as often as he likes without producing children; he can fly, even better, faster, and farther than the birds; he can visit other planets; and he can understand the language of the birds and some other animals, and speak with them. Konrad Lorenz first learned to communicate effectively with birds; and in the United States, they have advanced considerably in learning to speak with porpoises and whales. Karl von Frisch has decoded the dancing language of bees, and now any of us can learn where to find nectar and honey. Lorenz and his colleagues now lead birds far more effectively than St Francis ever did by preaching at them.

Man is a typical social animal; he communicates by appealing to the eyes and the ears of his fellows. He makes use of signs and gestures; he uses his face and the rest of his body to communicate his emotional state; and he uses his voice to make exclamatory and other emotional sounds, to laugh, to cry, and above all, to speak.

If two human beings have no language in common, they can tell each other what they want by means of the language of gesture. We use this language also to add emphasis to our vocal speech. The degree to which we do this depends on the culture in which we were brought up. One can tell, even when standing behind someone talking, whether he is a Southern European or an inhibited man from Northern Europe. The Southerner not only uses his hands for self-expression; his whole trunk is mobilized as he swells and shrinks at the different points in the discussion.

We express our feelings in our speech whether we want to or not. There is the force and the tension heard in the voice. There are the accompanying expressions on our faces, smiles, usually spontaneous, sometimes politely assumed, there are expressions of horror, disgust, or disdain. Now that we know that babies 36 hours old can and do imitate human facial expressions, we cannot say that facial expressions are innate. Perhaps they are both innate and learned.

At first, we communicate with our mothers by emotional expression, by crying and smiling. Then we slowly start to acquire language. We are born innately able to acquire speech, just as we are born designed to stand on two feet and able to balance on one. But there is nothing splendidly human about associating certain sounds with meaning. All animals that can produce sound do this.

It is instructive to examine the sounds used in communication by a distant relative of ours, the squirrel monkey. According to Professor Ploog of Munich, most of its repertoire of cries is present by the third day of life. It produces its cries of communication even if it is experimentally deprived of hearing. This shows that its cries are not an answer to something heard. The young baby monkey also understands all the sounds that it receives from adult monkeys. Thus it comes to learn about certain aspects of the world by this auditory input.

One is surprised to learn that its various cries are organized by different parts of the brain. The reason for this is that the various cries are expressions of, or related to, different emotional states; and emotional states are organized by various parts of the brain, though finally they all end by using the motor organization of voice production. This could be the same for the innate cries of the human baby. Mothers recognize different cries, for instance, those of rage, of pain, and gurgles of pleasure. It is likely that the production of these early sounds used for communication is not arranged by the part of the left cerebral hemisphere that will later become the speech area but by the parts that produce rage, pain, and pleasure.

But man's speech is not just a means of communication like that of the baby and other social animals; it is something new. Even if the new features are developed from elements already present in the communication of our simian forbears, speech and language are different, something not seen before in evolution. Propositional speech has developed only in man, and only man has a brain able to use symbolic speech and to think in words.

Once man had started developing his many uses of language, his way of evolution was determined by this mode of life. Any group which made a more advantageous use of this discovery may well have had greater survival value than others, and so natural selection would have favoured the further development of language.

Man uses speech in everything he is doing and in all he intends to do. If you pay attention to your mental activity as you walk along the street, you will find that you are thinking all the time in words, something perhaps like this: 'I will go into a shop and buy a birthday card. They are on the left at the end of the shop, up at the far end. I will find one of those funny ones not one of the sentimental ones.' Then, as you enter the shop, you say to yourself: 'Ah, a glass door; smeary finger marks on it; something new at the pencil counter over there. Yes, here are the cards, pink, blue, where are the funny ones?' and so on all through the day. You can observe this use of speech clearly in young children; for up to the age of 5 or 6, their speech is not wholly internal, and they keep up a running commentary to themselves about what they are doing and thinking. And so you will hear them directing their activities by means of speech.

Using symbols

The higher levels of the cerebral hemispheres make a model of the world, based on some inborn modes of perception and on a great deal of learning. In this world of thought, certain mental events come to stand for other events. The ability to create and use symbols is the essential feature of intelligence. When this ability develops in the child has been studied by Piaget and his colleagues at the Institut Jean Jacques Rousseau at Geneva. Before the age of

2, the child begins to conclude that there are causes of the things that happen. Thus he has a sort of symbol deduced from observing an event: he can foresee the effects of a cause. Between the ages of 2 and 7 is the period of the development of symbolic function. The child then forms what Piaget calls 'images', an internal representation of the world around him, including the concept of time. He comes to be able to communicate these concepts to others; then he has acquired symbolic or propositional speech.

Symbols provide us with a kind of shorthand; and like shorthand, they are economical of time and space. They are effective because the symbol is taken as equivalent to certain things or events of the physical world. From a first set of symbols, further symbols can be evolved. Finally, all the symbols are translated back into the things and events of the real world.

There are a great many different kinds of symbols and of ways of making use of them. One of the simplest relationships is for the symbol to be a part of the whole that it represents. Instead of the total event or the whole act of behaviour, a small part is shown, and the animal who understands the symbol assumes the whole for the part.

A symbol in which the part is taken as a token for the whole is the piece of cloth or teddy-bear that baby humans, chimpanzees, or other monkeys will accept as a substitute for their parents. They take this with them when they go to sleep and will cling to it when awake, obtaining physical comfort and psychological reassurance from physical contact with this symbol. Other examples of tokens in which the part is accepted for the whole are photographs of people we love, or the hairs of Mahomet's beard, treasured in a thousand mosques.

From the point of view of communication between human beings, an important system of symbols in which the part is taken for the whole is the natural language of gesture. This is one of the ways in which most vertebrates communicate with each other. In this case, the part is usually an incomplete part of a total act of behaviour, and it signifies intention. Human gestures are usually a précis of the total act. When we point with outstretched arm and index finger, this is a part of following one's upper limb in the direction indicated. When we threaten someone, it is a part of the total movement of aggression and fighting. Much of this gesture-language is innate. Deaf-mutes who are not taught to speak make use of sign-language, mainly based on gesture.

The language of gesture is closely related to the intention-movement signs of many animals. When a bird makes movements preparatory to taking-off, the other birds understand that they should take wing, and do so. When a male monkey merely bares one or two of its upper teeth, the other monkeys take this initial sign of threatening behaviour for the total threat, and behave accordingly.

Man's distant cousin, the chimpanzee, is good at learning sign-language. A gesture language has been used for a long time in the United States, the American sign language; it is used by deaf-mutes and their teachers. This language can be learned by young chimpanzees. One of these chimpanzees had mastered one hundred and sixty signs after four years' training. Then, when she was put with some other young chimpanzees, she was able to teach a great many of the signs to them. She did this just like a human being might do, holding the other monkey's hand and fingers in the correct position. This is the transmission of culture from generation to generation. Examples such as this make it obvious that, in understanding our fellow animals, anthropomorphism is not wrong but provides correct insights. To see animals as unconscious machines is absurd.

Man's speech is not essentially different from this. His verbal speech allows him to sort things and concepts into categories, and to make use of the abstract entities. The chimpanzee can do this to a limited extent.

Symbols of other symbols allow us to create the universal symbols of algebra, geometry, and arithmetic. Such systems of symbols have their own existences and their own rules. We follow these rules and carry out operations on the symbols of symbols without having to visualize any objects represented during the process of working out. This allows us to arrive at solutions to problems which can then be translated back into the world of reality. This is a great saving in time and mental effort. Formal logic is another and similar system of symbols, underlying and providing us with symbols for reasoning. Musical notation is another system, similar to writing; indeed the clef signs were originally letters. The page of the score consists of various symbols representing the sounds the players should make. It is almost unbelievable that such beautiful music as that of Beethoven's quartets could come out of just a few dots, all looking much the same, printed on paper.

Another symbol developed by most of mankind is money; use of these tokens can also be learned by chimpanzees. This ability was studied in the 1930s in Professor Yerkes's Yale laboratories of Primate Biology in Florida, by Dr John B. Wolfe and Dr John T. Cowles. They showed that chimpanzees could learn to work for token rewards. These anthropoid apes learned to work for poker chips, which they could collect and then hand in for food. Moreover, they learned the symbolic meaning of chips of different sizes and colours. They also learned that one sort of chip was useless as currency, as no food was ever exchanged for it. It should be made clear that in these experiments the food was out of sight, and so the animals worked for money and then stored it up to exchange it for food when the time came. They even learned to work for money on one day and give it in for food on the next. Dr Geoffrey Bourne relates in his book *The Ape People* that 'the animals used to walk around clutching their earnings to their breasts, sleeping on them at night so that they would not be stolen, and getting very hysterical if any other animal came near their earnings or tried to take any of them away'.

These intelligent animals, then, are able to grasp that the act of pushing a lever is a symbol, that if they engage in this activity they will eventually be rewarded. They understand that the chips, on the face of it meaningless objects, are symbols, promising that something rewarding will come their way. Moreover, they can learn that chips of different sizes and colours have different symbolic meanings: they can learn that a white one means one grape and a blue one two grapes, whereas a brass one has no exchange value. In fact, the chimpanzees understood this coinage so well that one wonders if they would be able to cope with a real monetary system.

The ability to make use of the symbols of mathematics depends on association areas of the cortex of both hemispheres. An essential region is in the left hemisphere at the junction of the temporal and parietal lobes, in front of the occipital lobe's secondary visual area. A possible explanation of the association of mathematical symbols with this region may be that these symbols began with counting; and counting was abstracted from touching or moving the digits of the hands and perhaps the feet, this being the first and essential digital system. It is doubtless related to counting things seen, and so it is near the visual area, as well as the tactile and kinaesthetic areas.

After developing the use of his own digits for counting, man evolved the abacus, which is still used effectively in the East. With this instrument, addition, subtraction, multiplication, and division are done visually, by the manipulation of bobbles in rows. Our numeral system also depends on moving figures from column to column.

If a child is bad at mathematics but is good at most other school work, this is unlikely to be due to any defect in its brain. The reasons are undoubtedly all those factors implicated by psychotherapists and psychologists; and most important and most common of all, inadequate teaching.

Within the realm of mathematics, the most visual are geometry and the use of graphs. Here we see spatial elements coming into mathematical ability. This form of symbolization is related to the ability to envisage space, to locate things and ourselves in space, which depends on the right hemisphere. The region in the left hemisphere on which mathematical ability depends is between the regions for organizing speech and visual perceptions. This indicates that both verbal and visual symbolizations enter into mathematical thinking. Mathematical symbolization also needs the contribution from the auditory parasensory area, enabling us to use inner speech, when we make concepts in our minds. We talk about mathematical ability as though it is one entity; but it is not. It is made up of the functions of many parts of the cortex; and in different people, different regions will be used.

The ability to use symbols to represent aspects and parts of reality is one of the most advanced functions of the brain. Hughlings Jackson recognized as a general principle that when the brain atrophies, the functions most recently acquired disappear first, those longest developed during evolution remaining till the last. In accordance with this principle, we find that when the whole brain degenerates, the patient first loses the ability to grasp and to make use of symbolic thinking. The way this is usually shown up is by getting the patient to explain proverbs. For instance, when he is asked for the meaning of the proverb 'A rolling stone gathers no moss,' he will explain in detail to you that a stone that keeps on moving is not able to grow moss as it is moving. When the proverb 'A burnt child dreads the fire' is read to him, he will explain that of course the child is frightened of the fire because he has been burnt. Or 'A drowning man will catch at a straw' will obtain only the response that he does this is an effort to stop himself drowning. The symbolic meaning of the proverbs, which is their whole point, escapes him, and usually he cannot grasp it even when it is explained to him.

Memory is also based on symbols, for what is remembered is a symbol of what one experienced in the past. Remembering is not the same as throwing a picture on a television screen and reporting what one is seeing; for it is a changed version of what happened.

The ability to symbolize depends on the working of many parts of the cerebral cortex of both hemispheres. Professor Geschwind of Harvard considered that man's outstanding ability to use verbal symbols depended on the connections in his brain between all the parasensory association areas. Man is able to see a circle, to feel the circumference of a circle with his hands or feet, to draw a circle in the air with his hand or foot; on account of the connections between the visual, tactile and kinaesthetic areas, he can abstract a common circularity from these three senses. For this common feature, one verbal symbol is made, the word 'circle'. Had there been no connections between the secondary sensory areas, he would not have been able to recognize the one common feature. Seen circle, felt circle, and circle drawn in space would have been as different to him as the smell of a violet is to the feel of a cube. Indeed, it would be more different; for on account of these interconnections we are able to make meaningful comparisons, and from the different sensory inputs to deduce similarities and differences. I do not mean here the more obvious assimilation we make all the time when we create perceptions from all the sensory inputs, so that we know from the smell and the sight that this is a daffodil. I mean such facts as the ability to recognize a rhythm, for instance, in three different sensory modalities. We are able to recognize a rhythm of long-short-long heard as dash-dot-dash from a morse buzzer, we recognize it when it is tapped on our hands, and we recognize it again flashed in the visual field by lights.

The use of symbols is a great economy in the activity of the brain, and it saves time during thinking and remembering. Instead of nerve impulses having to make the complete circuit round the original paths, they need only make a smaller circuit. By this I mean that when we remember having a picnic last summer, we don't go through the whole experience again, taking as long as it took when it happened. The first symbol is the word 'picnic'; this separates that sort of event from every other sort of event. Then we have the symbols 'last summer'; these are two sorts of symbols, the symbols of words and the symbols of division of time. Again, as soon as we have though 'last summer', we have restricted the neural activity to certain selected experiences and we do not have to recollect other experiences.

Thinking

If one asks what parts of the brain are involved in thinking, one must answer that it all depends on what you mean by thinking. One uses the word to mean remembering, for trying to recall, for imagining, for solving problems in the mind or in reality, and for any other mental activities. It is thinking that a chess-player does when he works out the possible results of moving his king. It is thinking that a dress-designer does when he imagines a new dress, or when a salesman designs a plan of campaign to get the money out of people's pockets. Most of our thinking uses words, concepts, and logic. But there is thought without words. If a painter has a stroke which takes away his ability to use speech, he may still have his mental images of things visual, forms, colours, and visual relationships and memories, and he may still be able to create paintings; his originality may be unimpaired. Similarly, sculptors can still model and carve. The parts of the cerebral hemispheres that are essential for abstract thought are in the left temporal lobe; the parts needed for painting are in both cerebral hemispheres, in the occipital, parietal, and frontal lobes. Thinking that makes use of words is organized mainly by the left hemisphere, while thinking that depends on visualizing or conceiving of things set out in space is organized by the right hemisphere.

Thinking can be auditory. A composer thinks in auditory images. It is usually mixed. Thinking may be a combination of auditory and conceptual, as when a conductor plans how he will present a symphony. It may be partly auditory and partly kinaesthetic, partly tactile and partly motor, as it is for the bassoon player, remembering how to play his part in the symphony. For a ballet dancer, it is visual, auditory, kinaesthetic, and very much motor. It is the same for the footballer, and will then include a large element of spatial organization. All these aspects of thinking occur together; they are not sorted out, as they have been on this page.

Thinking about smells does not necessarily need words. If we try to remember the name of a smell, then we do use words; but we can bring an olfactory image into our minds of the smell of lavender, of the earth freshly rained upon, or of toadstools, without using words. Though the question then comes up: would we be able to think of the smell of a toadstool without first thinking the word 'toadstool'? The answer, as usual, is not simple. The smell of toadstools might come spontaneously into our minds without us having to think the word; and in that case, we would think or imagine the smell without using the speech area of the brain. Or we might get a visual picture in our mind of the toadstool, and from there the smell of it; here again, we would not need the word. But the way I arrived at the smell of toadstools just now was via the word. I thought in fact of the word and of the visual images of various toadstools at the same time; I cannot really say which came first. That is typical of how we think. We make a shorthand conglomeration of words and visual images, secondarily auditory images, and thirdly and a long way after, kinaesthetic, tactile, and olfactory images. Needless to say, the exact mixture varies from person to person. Someone who can read and write is more attached to words than someone who is illiterate. And further, their brains are different. The lives of most people have been changed by television, and so have their brains. Children throughout Europe and North America are now educated by television. Just as Osbert Sitwell wrote that he was educated during the holidays from Eton, so our children are educated during the hours spent away from school. It is disastrous that what television teaches in the West is that the correct solution to every problem is violence, and that having more money, more furs and diamonds than the Jones's is the purpose of life.

Tests show that in America children born after 1954—the children brought up to learn from television—have higher IQ's than those born before 1945. What made the difference in the IQ was a superior ability in understanding and interpreting visual sequences, and a superior ability in the perception of small differences in visually presented material. This is likely to imply that they were developing the right hemisphere more than did the children of previous generations. For the right hemisphere can convey meaning by sequences of pictures and the left by sequences of sounds.

It may have struck some readers that we have used the word 'association' in two different ways: with an anatomical meaning and with a psychological meaning. Nerve fibres connecting two parts of the cerebral cortex are called 'association' fibres; and we speak also of the 'association' of ideas. The reason for this is that the first investigators of the anatomy of the cerebral hemispheres introduced the word 'association fibres' for this very reason; they thought that these fibres joined or associated two areas of the cortex, and that this junction formed the basis of the psychological association of ideas and words. Now although this may be so, it was undesirable to use the same word for the two meanings; for it prejudged the whole issue of the neural basis of psychological functioning. Even though the association of ideas certainly needs association nerve fibres, the statement that two areas of cortex are joined by association fibres does not tell us anything about the mechanism of association in the psychological sense. And it may lead us to think that there is no problem here, that psychological association is explained by saying that there are association fibres between two areas of cortex. It must, then, be said that we really do not know what we mean when we use the psychological word 'associate' or when we say that the child learns to associate; we do not know what this means at a neural level, or what are the neural mechanisms involved.

Learning to talk

Deformed babies born without cerebral hemispheres make noises, but they never learn to shape them into the sounds of speech nor to understand that sounds have a symbolic meaning. To grasp that idea needs the cerebral hemispheres.

Human beings are learning language from birth to 90. But the way of learning usually changes around the age of 10. Before that age, one picks it up naturally, that is to say in ways that we are just beginning to learn about; after that time, we learn it in the way we learn at school, learning grammar and spelling with conscious effort.

For the first six months of life both normal and deaf babies babble away, making the same sounds. This shows us that babbling is innate, and that the baby does not need to hear its own voice in order to make these noises. After about nine months of life, a difference between the two begins to appear. The child that hears normally is listening to the sounds he hears. He makes more sounds like those of the people around him, and stops making the sounds that he does not hear. The deaf child does not alter his babbling, and eventually he becomes more and more silent. This ability to hear nuances is remarkable. To hear speech properly, the baby needs to hear all the frequencies used, including overtones; and he must be able to hear differences in timing and duration of sounds. He hears the melody of his mother-tongue, the right intonation.

Therefore, to speak properly, one has to hear normally. The child listens to other people's speech and also to its own sounds. One hears one's own speech by two routes, by air conduction through the external ear, and by bone conduction through the bones of the skull. Other people's speech is heard only by air conduction. A child with much disturbance of hearing cannot hear correctly by either route. Yet studies of the deaf by phoneticians and linguists have revealed that a child deaf over certain frequencies can nevertheless make sounds within this frequency range. We do not fully understand how this can be. It is probably because there may be two or three cues for perceiving a phoneme. A child with normal hearing makes use of all three cues; the deaf child may still perceive the sound by appreciating only one cue; and it may be using cues that are unimportant for normally hearing people.

A child who hears speech incorrectly will model his speech on what he hears, and so he will learn to speak incorrectly. Moreover, hearing his own speech sounding just like their speech, the child cannot grasp why no one understands what he is saying. When his parents correct him, he cannot hear the differences between what they are saying and what he is saying himself. The whole problem is too difficult for him, he probably becomes discouraged, and he may give up trying to speak. He may then be regarded as mentally deficient, or at any rate rather strange and stupid. When the partly deaf child goes to school, he meets a new lot of difficulties as he learns to write. He writes down the phonemes he hears. But as he does not hear what the rest of the world is hearing, he cannot learn to write what the other children are writing. If no one realizes that the child is partially deaf, then the adults again conclude that the child is mentally defective or very dull.

If a parent gets any hint that the child does not hear well, he should get him examined at a clinic specializing in deaf children; and the sooner the better. For children who start learning from specially trained teachers get on better if they start very early.

Not only does the child have to hear properly in order to speak properly, it also has to have the normal sensory input from the mouth, tongue, and lips. When this is absent, the child cannot learn to make the correct movements for shaping the phonemes of its language.

The human baby is born with the right anatomical connections.

To perceive the sound first phonetically, as a total sound or phoneme, and then linguistically, the human uses the left temporal lobe. The baby can make the sounds he hears as there are connections between the speech region of the left temporal lobe and the motor regions of the frontal lobes and the kinaesthetic region of the front part of the parietal lobe.

If a baby or young child has an accident or some malady of the brain that destroys the speech area of the left hemisphere, he loses all the speech he has acquired. The speech area can then be reconstituted in the right hemisphere. Yet this is done only at the cost of functions normally organized by the right hemisphere. This reorganization can take place only during the first years of life. Under the age of 4 it is complete, and the right hemisphere becomes the organizer of speech and thinking based on inner speech. Between the age of 4 and the onset of puberty, the replacement of speech is almost complete. But after puberty, the damage to the left speech area can never be completely compensated for. In adult life, a stroke affecting the left side of the brain causes aphasia, which at its worst is an inability to speak and to understand speech.

All parts of the cerebral hemispheres are not equally replaceable. There are no general rules. Experiments in baby monkeys show that lesions made in some parts of the cortex eventually cause no disability; though when the adult monkey is tired or under stress, the effect of the lesion again becomes manifest. But lesions made in other parts of the cortex cause permanent deficiencies, and there is only a minimal recovery from their effects. Surprisingly enough, the rate of recovery and even the amount is different for the two sexes. This is not the effect of sex hormones; it is genetically determined.

In order to arrive at our present understanding of how parts of the cerebral cortex work together, neurology passed through various phases. At first it was believed that there was no localization of function in the cerebral hemispheres, and that they worked as a totality. The next phase was a belief in very discrete localization of function. In this view, small regions of the cortex were thought of as organizing such complex kinds of behaviour as writing, mathematics, or logical thinking. Our present view is that there is localization of function; but complex behaviour such as reading, writing, adding up figures in columns, turning arithmetic into algebra, or turning algebra into geometry, requires the working together of many different local regions of the cortex of both hemispheres.

Unlearning language

The first neurologist to think that speech might depend on a special, local region of the cerebral hemispheres was F. J. Gall; this idea was a part of phrenology. Before the phrenologists, such a high-level brain function would have been attributed to the activity of the whole brain, in so far as it was thought of as being an activity of the brain and not of a non-entity, the soul. Gall put 'the organ of speech' in the frontal lobes.

A stranger idea than localizing speech in the frontal lobes was that it could be in only one hemisphere. This step was taken by Marc Dax, who was a general practitioner in the southern French town of Sommières. He concluded from the cases he had seen that all patients with a disturbance of the faculty of language had a lesion in the left cerebral hemisphere. By 1836, he had collected over forty cases. He collected others from published records; and he found no exceptions to the rule. He therefore concluded that whenever 'the memory of words is impaired', the lesion will be in the left cerebral hemisphere. This conclusion passed unnoticed until it was rediscovered by an eminent man, Paul Broca. Broca was a professor of surgery, and the founder of the science of physical anthropology. Before Broca published his evidence in 1861, Dax's son, Gustave Dax, had been collecting further evidence in support of his father's views.

Dr Macdonald Critchley has unravelled this history, and I quote the following paragraphs from his paper.

Since he had been a student, the younger Dax had been intensely interested in 'alalia' or speech loss, and applied to submit a thesis upon this subject, but he was not allowed to do so. Patiently he collected case-material and evidence from the literature. He wrote a Mémoire which he presented to his local confrères in 1858 and again in 1860, entitled:

'Observations tendant à prouver la coincidence du dérangement de la parole avec une lésion de l'hemisphère gauche du cerveau'. Later he sent it to the Académie de Médecine, where it was received in 1863. Dax *fils* was bitterly hurt by the fact that subsequent writers continued to pay no heed to his work, and failed to give the credit due to his father .... Lelut commenting upon the younger Dax's report to the Académie, had said that 'that mysterious organ, the brain, would be even more mysterious if its two halves were found to subserve different functions'.

Critchley has added to this history: 'Today the contributions of the two doctors Dax are no longer forgotten in the world of medicine. But even now the quiet little town of Sommières knows little of its two distinguished oppidans. No plaque adorns the wall of their dwelling in the Place du Bourguet, and though a number of eponymous streets are there, visitors will look in vain for a "rue des deux docteurs Dax".' However, that is not the end of the story; for owing to Critchley's investigations, the town has now put up a plaque to honour these two original thinkers who contributed to our knowledge of the brain.

Broca collected the brains of twenty-two patients who had had lesions that had deprived them of speech; in all cases, the lower part of the frontal lobe of the left hemisphere was damaged. He therefore drew the conclusion that this part of the brain was the essential area for speech. He supposed that the lesion in that region had deprived the patients of the memory of the procedure that had to be followed in order to articulate words. For he knew that these patients had normal hearing, and that they had been able to understand speech, both heard and written. He also had one brain in which the lesion was in the same place but in the right frontal lobe. This patient had had no trouble with speech.

The next advance in our understanding of speech was made by Wernicke, who published his conclusion at the age of 24. He had found that there was a region of the left temporal lobe surrounding the primary auditory area that was the essential area for understanding speech.

At present our knowledge of the anatomy of speech is like this. The great majority of people throughout the world are right-handed; propositional speech in them is organized in the left hemi-sphere. This anatomical fixture is finished by the age of 4 or 5. Ambidextrous people have speech essentially in the left hemi-sphere, with a good contribution from the right. Of left-handed people, 70 to 80 per cent have propositional speech organized in the left hemisphere, the rest of them having it on the right or in both hemispheres. People who can do mirror-writing without much effort are left-handed. If the left hemisphere is damaged in early childhood, about a half of the children organize speech in the right hemisphere, while the other half retain it on the left. If the right hemisphere is damaged, there is some disturbance of the organization of speech.

The region of the left hemisphere that organizes speech can be seen in Fig. 20.1: it is covered by the numerals 2,1,3,5, and 4. In order to understand speech, one needs first to realize that the noise coming in is verbal. If it is, then the sounds have to be given meaning. All sounds are heard in the primary auditory areas of both temporal lobes. In the left lobe is the area surrounding the primary auditory area that is needed for understanding the mean-ing of speech. This is often called Wernicke's area; it is marked as (4) in Fig. 20.1. If the area surrounding the primary auditory area is ruined, the patient cannot hear and differentiate the phonemes properly and so he does not get the meaning. In the left frontal lobe is the region that is needed for articulation, the region that, when electrically stimulated, causes movements of the face, lips, tongue, and larynx. It is labelled (1). In front of it, labelled (2), is the region for articulation of words and joining words to make sentences; it has been named Broca's area. In the part of the brain behind and above Wernicke's area is a large region of the brain, the centre of which is an area of cortex called the angular gyrus; this is a region concerned with all aspects of language; it is marked as (5). The pattern of sound of a word is evoked in Wernicke's area. This pattern is sent to the angular gyrus, and then on to Broca's area and other parts of the frontal lobe. Learned visual aspects of the sound are kept in the occipital lobe just behind the angular gyrus. They are the written symbols of the word, written in various alphabets, capitals, small letters, numerals, musical notation, and

the reading and understanding of sentences and other symbols. If
there is some block between the occipital lobe and the speech area,
the patient cannot name the things he sees. He knows what they
are, and he can name them if they are presented to other sensory
channels than the visual. This is a visuo-verbal disconnection.
There is a similar tactile-verbal disconnection, in which the tactile
region of the parietal lobe is disconnected from the speech area.

Man is so visual that one thinks that one needs to see something
in order to give it its name. But this is not so. We know the feel
of velvet better than what it looks like; and we know the smell,
and not the appearance, of eau-de-cologne and we name it when we
smell it.

The band labelled (3) in the figure is a large band of nerve fibres
connecting Wernicke's area to the angular gyrus. Similar fibres
run from the occipital lobe forwards to the angular gyrus. The
band continues forwards from the angular gyrus to Broca's area.
This is a two-way connection so that articulated words and sentences have meaning, and bring up the sound and the visual image
of the thing or relationship given by the word. In Broca's area and
the area behind it, labelled (1), the auditory and visual images of
the word are turned into the muscular patterns needed for saying
the words.

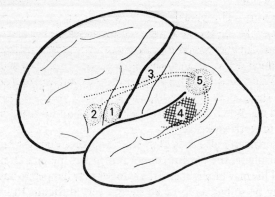

Fig. 20.1 Lateral surface of left hemisphere. (1) Face area of motor cortex; (2) Broca's
area; (3) lesion involving arcuate fasiciulus (dotted lines); (4) Wernicke's area; (5) Angular gyrus.

Speech has two aspects—what is said, and an affective component. For it's not what you say, its how you say it. The propositional aspect of speech is organized by the left hemisphere, by the regions shown in Fig. 20.1. The affective components are organized by the same region on the other side of the brain. When these regions of the right hemisphere are damaged, the subject's speech is devoid of emotional expression. The continuing changes in pitch, loudness, and rhythm that convey emotional meaning are absent. Emotional expression in the face and body is also absent; and a patient who is badly depressed does not appear to be so, for she says she is depressed in a flat and unemotional voice. When the homologous region on the right side to the area on the left essential for understanding speech is damaged, the patient fails to grasp those aspects of speech that are expressing emotion.

When there is any damage to the left cerebral hemisphere affecting the regions marked in Fig. 20.1, there will be some loss of the ability use speech, aphasia. The commonest cause of such damage is a stroke. The various kind of disturbance of speech that occur depend on which blood-vessels are disrupted by the stroke. If the damage is to Wernicke's area, speech is not understood. Written speech is also not understood, and so the patient cannot read. He sees the written words, but what is seen is not interpreted in an auditory form. The patient sees the word written 'Yes', but this does not evoke the sound of yes. If the lesion affects Broca's area, the patient can understand speech and he can read it to himself; but he has much difficulty in speaking and in forming the sounds of speech. When the lesion disconnects areas (5) and (4) from areas (2) and (1), the patient tends to speak a lot, but what he says is all muddled up. When Broca's area is isolated from its visual input it appears to work excessively.

In all or nearly all kinds of speech disorders due to a lesion of the hemisphere, the patient cannot remember the names of many things. This may be slight and the same as may happen to any of us; or it may be so bad as to make speech very difficult. In order to name things that are not there in front of you, you have to have a visual image of the thing. The part of the brain between the temporal and occipital lobes can be damaged by a stroke, and then this ability can be ruined. This results in a kind of aphasia not directly due to a speech deficiency but essentially to a visual defect. This is a two-way pathway. For not only does the image normally bring up the word but the word also brings up the visual image.

We learn our own language by hearing it. We learn dead languages such as Latin and classical Greek by reading and writing. With regard to living languages, how we learn them varies; it is usually a mixture of vision and hearing. These remarks are made as they help us understand what happens to polyglots who have a stroke affecting speech. They do not necessarily retain their mother language, the language they learned first, before they could read and write. When they recover and the ability to use language starts to come back, sometimes a language they learned as a literary language may return before their mother-tongue. In such a case, it is likely that the visual components of speech, served by the connections between the occipital lobe and temporal and frontal lobes, can still work, as these are still intact. Apart from such a result, one sees that often the first language to return after a stroke is the language the patient was usually speaking at the time, and not the language he has known all his life.

We are born with our brains prejudiced in favour of hearing and understanding speech. As Dr B.C.J. Moore puts it: 'no matter how hard we try, it is impossible to hear speech in terms of its acoustical characteristics, i.e. as a series of hisses, whistles, buzzes etc. Rather we perceive a unified stream of speech sounds.'

But when the cortical area for the recognition of speech is cut off from the surrounding areas on both sides of the brain, that is just how speech is heard. Speech is not distinguished from other sounds; it is not known to be speech, it is just a meaningless sound. As one of these rare patients said: 'It is always the same sound.' Another patient with this region cut off from the rest of the brain, said, when tested with a bell, that it was a noise, 'but I don't know what it is'; she thought an alarm clock tone was a whistle. She suggested that five different noises were the sound of a train, although none of them were.

Damage to the speech area of the left hemisphere can cause complete aphasia without a disturbance of musical abilities. There was a Russian composer called Shebalin who, at the age of 57, had aphasia from a stroke. During the remaining six years of his life, he wrote nine works, including a quartet and a symphony. Other similar cases have been described. But this does not mean that all musical faculties depend only on the right hemisphere. Probably the ability to conceive a rhythm, for instance, is organized in the left lobe.

Understanding the sounds of speech is not only auditory; we also may make use of our own articulation. This becomes clear to us when we have difficulty in understanding someone's indistinct speech. We repeat what we have heard, pronouncing it correctly. If we cannot silently articulate to ourselves the sounds of speech that we are hearing, we probably do not understand them. This is one of the ways in which we make corrections for mispronunciations due to speech defects, foreign, or dialect accents. Thus, to some extent the understanding of speech depends on the production of speech. This is so for the sounds recognized as speech sound; but the perception of all other sounds is not done in this repetitive manner. We recognize the sound of thunder without being able to make it; and we comprehend the undeniable statements of music without necessarily being able to produce them.

Severe aphasia is not only an inability to use speech; it is a defect in the use and understanding of non-verbal symbols used in communication. Patients who become aphasic are bewildered because they do not understand the meaning of the gestures used in communicating with others; nor can they make these gestures themselves, as they have lost all meaning for them.

There is another region of the left cerebral cortex that is also closely connected with speech. This part is on the medial side of the frontal lobe just above the corpus callosum (see Plate 12). It is a region concerned with the movements needed for making sounds. People with this part of the brain damaged have to make a great effort to produce any sound, and they may give up communicating.

As speech is organized in the left cerebral hemisphere, the region in the left temporal lobe used for the auditory aspects of speech is larger than that in the right. Changes in the bones of the skull associated with this larger region on the left are found in Neanderthal man, who lived 30,000 to 50,000 years ago, and also in Peking man who lived about 300,000 years ago. However, we do not really know the significance of this asymmetry, for chimpanzees also have it; other monkeys, such as macaques, which we classify as lower in the evolutionary scale, do not show it. Chimpanzees are better at learning the skills we teach them than are the lower monkeys, but they do not possess speech.

Reading and writing

Writing is the most extraordinary thing. It is not only a way of communicating with people who are absent. It is storing information outside the body. Thus, writing enables man to make use of what has been learned. Man has at his disposal not only what he has learned during his own brief life, but also the whole of culture, all that his species has acquired during its progress in and out of various epochs of civilization and savagery. It is thus that each generation, though no more intelligent, can start by standing on the shoulders of the previous generation.

We take writing for granted, except when we are laboriously learning it at school. And yet, as the Lady Sei Shonagon wrote in *The Pillow-book* in Japan at the beginning of the eleventh century (translated by Arthur Waley):

Writing is an ordinary enough thing; yet how precious it is! When someone is in a far corner of the world and one is terribly anxious about him, suddenly there comes a letter, and one feels as though the person were actually in the room. It is really very amazing. And, strangely enough, to put down one's thoughts in a letter, even if one knows that it will probably never reach its destination, is an immense comfort. If writing did not exist, what terrible depressions we should suffer from!

Simple reading and writing can be taught to young chimpanzees. In the United States, Dr David Premack was very successful in teaching one of three chimpanzees to read and write. In the language he made up for his animals, different coloured and shaped plastic labels were used to symbolize objects. One of the animals Sarah, learned to read these symbols, and to put them on a board when it wanted the objects the symbols represented. With time and patience, Premack and his colleagues taught this chimpanzee not only to read and write the names of objects, but also abstract conceptions. It understood prepositions such as 'above' and 'below'. This animal could manipulate the agreed symbols of 'the same as' and 'different from', being able to classify the objects it knew as the same or as different. It understood that objects had common attributes such as shape, colour, and size. It could read, write, and understand the different signs 'red on green' and 'green on red'. The young animal enjoyed the game, and would put out questions for itself which it then answered. It was able to answer such a complicated question as 'apple red, banana yellow, implies that apples and bananas have different colours: true or false?' It even learned the meaning of a conditional 'If . . . then . . .'. After two and a half years, Sarah could construct sentences in plastic signs. Another chimpanzee that had been trained in America to communicate using these plastic signs, on first seeing a duck, spontaneously brought out the two signs 'water' and 'bird', and put them together to name the duck 'water-bird'. Another chimpanzee learned both the English spoken word, an auditory sign for an object, and the visual sign for the object. Thus, this animal knew both the auditory and the visual signs for an object. That is reading.

One cannot conclude that, because a chimpanzee can be taught a kind of reading and writing, these skills are easily acquired. The conclusion is that the chimpanzee is a most intelligent being. There are some children who have great difficulty in learning to read and write, even though they are fully intelligent in other ways. This neurological disorder is called dyslexia or congential alexia. It was first described in 1896 by a general practitioner, Dr Pringle Morgan, of Seaford in England. He wrote of his 14-year-old patient,

His greatest difficulty has been—and is now—his inability to read. . . . He has been at school or under tutors since he was 7 years old, and the greatest efforts have been made to teach him to read . . . he would be the smartest lad in the school if the instruction were entirely oral . . . He did not read a single word correctly, with the exception of 'and', 'the', 'of', 'that', etc.; the other words seemed to be quite unknown to him, and he could not even make an attempt to pronounce them.

This congenital trouble is not often as severe as that. Such a boy probably had some local islands of abnormal development in his brain. Although the condition is not so rare, only one or two brains have been investigated. That is because people with dyslexia don't die from the condition, and when eventually they do come to die, people have forgotten that they had this interesting trouble, and do not get a post-mortem examination carried out. In the brains that have been examined, there is a mixing up of the grey and white matter, and the normal arrangement of the neurons of parts of the cortex has gone wrong. This maldevelopment affects the speech area of the temporal lobe.

Congental alexia runs in families; it is unlikely that it is always due to abnormalities in the speech area of the temporal lobe. Some of these children have associated visuo-spatial troubles, and this is essentially due to the right parietal lobe. Some of them have difficulties in integrating visual and auditory inputs. And some have more obvious troubles with the totality of language and speech. They find it abnormally difficult to understand words or sentences, and to memorize verbal material. In the family, one finds others who were slow starters in talking; and there is also an unduly large proportion of left-handed or ambidextrous people. It is far commoner in boys. This is strange. For although there are sex differences in brains, one would not have imagined that they would affect the speech area. Stammering too is commoner in boys. Some psychologists have obtained evidence that in many of these children there is difficulty in learning to scan from left to right. This also accounts for them often muddling up and reversing letters such as 'p' and 'q', and 'b' and 'd', and also for doing mirror-writing, reversing whole syllables, and writing for instance 'dab' for 'bad'. Most of the children have difficulty in categorizing sounds; and this makes spelling very difficult for them.

Reading entails seeing the written word, and realizing that it is writing, a graphic code having meaning. The grapheme is then turned into a phoneme, a sound. One then has to decide whether the sound is a word or not, whether it has meaning; psychologists call this the lexical address. Writing is doing this in the reverse direction. The child usually makes the sound of speech to himself, then he substitutes the graphemes for the phonemes. A child who speaks a dialect and not the standard language will have similar difficulties to a partially deaf child. For instance, if the aspirate 'h' is dropped in his dialect, the child will write 'come ere' for 'come here'. The partially deaf child cannot hear the phoneme correctly, and so it cannot chose the right grapheme. The Chinese child does not have this obstacle; if he cannot hear normally, he can still appreciate the ideogram. The child is using different parts of its cerebral cortex when he copies letters and when he writes to dictation. When he copies letters, he is really drawing; he does not have to hear the phonemes in his mind's ear, nor does he have to think of the meaning of the phonemes or graphemes. When he writes to dictation, he has to go through the whole process of writing alphabetically, understanding the meaning of the words, hearing the phonemes, and remembering the graphemes that in his language represent these phonemes.

Japanese writing has two different sources; ideograms, taken from China, called *kanji*; and two forms of phonograms, invented by themselves, called *hiragana* and *katakana*. They represent 46 sounds. It is reckoned that for reading Japanese, a minimum of 1800 kanji ideograms must be known. What is interesting and instructive is that when Japanese patients get aphasia, they can get a selective impairment of the *kanji* or the *kana* kinds of writing. Although *kanji* is more difficult to write than *kana*, the brain treats it to some extent like pictures and images, and keeps it, or certain aspects of it, in the right hemisphere. *Kana*, which is more abstract and which is a syllabary, is kept in the left hemisphere.

Even more surprising is the fact that in our Latin script, different typefaces are read by the two hemispheres. Perhaps some part of the hemispheres looks and decides whether what it is seeing is best considered as pictures or as writing symbols; and then sends it off mainly to the appropriate hemisphere.

These examples show us that the ideas of the phrenologists on the localization of our abilities were inspired but naïve. It is only in the last few years that we have begun to understand that functions are localized in the cortex, and it is no simple matter to know what functions underlie our various abilities.

When the child learns to read, it has to repeat the amazing feat of its ancestors: to change an auditory symbol into a visual symbol. It first has to learn that certain seen, heard, and remembered objects have to be associated with a certain sound or group of sounds. Then it has to change these sounds into visual signs. If it is blind, it has to change them into tactile signs. When the child writes, it has to change the visual signs into a set of movements. These very difficult tasks make use of several regions of the cortex. It is not surprising that mentally defective children may not be able to achieve them; it is more impressive to me that ordinary people do learn to read and write.

Nearly all we know about how the brain organizes reading and writing has been learned from patients who have had strokes. What is needed is to study the patient and his disabilities while he is alive, and then to find out the extent and the position of the damaged part of the brain after death. This necessitates, needless to say, removal of the brain in a post-mortem. Often the relatives refuse permission for this. Religion, ignorance, and low intelligence have always been and remain the enemies of scientific investigation and the acquisition of knowledge.

From the brains of patients, it was deduced that the ability to read depends on laying down connections between the visual region of the occipital lobes and the large speech region of the occipital, temporal, and parietal lobes of the left hemisphere. Once the relevant nerve cells are connected, then the seen symbol of a word immediately calls out the word for the object. And so, as we read 'table', we immediately hear 'table' in our mind's ear. There is a favourable time when it is easiest to establish these connections. In some children it is earlier than others, and these children generally show other evidence of high intelligence. It is probable that it is much harder to do it after puberty.

A long time before congenital alexia was recognized, patients were seen who had acquired alexia. Following a stroke, the patient is able to speak and understand speech normally. He understands the meaning of pictures. But he cannot read. Most of such patients can write, but they cannot read what they have just written. Interestingly enough, these patients can usually read the numerals used in Western culture, but cannot read or make sense of Roman numerals; these, of course, are combinations of letters. In such a patient, the part of the brain that has been destroyed is the posterior part of the corpus callosum, the large bridge of nerve fibres connecting the two hemispheres. The nerve impulses can no longer get from the visual region of the right hemisphere across to the speech region of the left. The artery that has been blocked and has caused the stroke had also supplied the visual part of the left hemisphere. The patient thus cannot see the right visual field with the left hemisphere. He is left with the speech area in the left hemisphere intact and the right visual area intact. But what he sees with the right visual area cannot get across the corpus callosum to inform the speech area of what it is seeing. It sees the letters on the page, but they are just dark lines on a white background, strokes and curves without meaning.

This deficiency may not be as complete as has just been described; there are curious cases in which some signs are no longer recognized and others are. For instance, a patient may lose the meaning of arithmetical signs, such as plus and minus. He can do the calculations in his head but cannot do them when they are written down. If you ask him what twice eight is, he tells you it is sixteen; but if you write down $2 \times 8 = ?$ he may write 10 or 6.

Learning braille is learning a sensory tactile skill. One has to learn that palpable spots set out in space can provide a verbal meaning. A blind child learning to read by braille is using its left hemisphere for the symbolic understanding that we call reading, and its right hemisphere for the estimation and remembering of the position of the dots. It has been found that blind children read more efficiently with the left fingers than the right, the left hand being organized by the right cerebral hemisphere.

Making the sounds of speech

For his tongue is exceedingly pure so that it has in purity what it wants in
music.

Our vocal apparatus is a musical instrument, a wind instrument,
like the bagpipes. It is illustrated diagrammatically in Fig. 20.2:

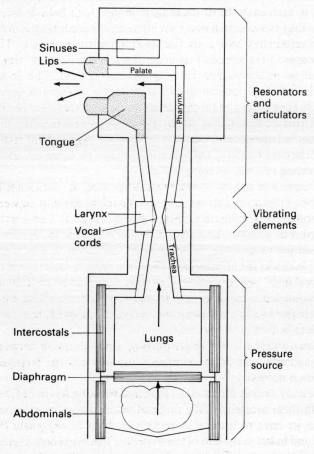

Fig. 20.2 Diagram showing the parts of the body used in making the sounds of
speaking and singing.

The lungs are the bag of air, and they are squeezed by muscles, the abdominal and intercostal muscles and the diaphragm. The windpipe or trachea is the conduit pipe. The vocal folds or cords are the vibrating reed of the bagpipes or oboe. The rest of the apparatus is a variable resonance box, with articulators that alter the sound in amazing ways. Birds make their songs lower down than man. In all vertebrates, the trachea forks into two passages, the bronchi, one going to each lung. Birds make their sounds with both bronchi, and so they can sing two notes simultaneously, producing chords. Other vertebrates have a similar vocal apparatus to man's. The differences in the sounds produced by various mammals largely depend on differences in the resonance boxes used. The South American howler monkey has a resonance chamber developed from its hyoid bones, the two little bones beneath the lower jaw on which part of the tongue is rooted. In this small monkey this chamber is larger than the brain. If one takes this vocal apparatus out of the dead monkey, and blows up the windpipe, one can make the howling noise the monkey makes.

We make the sounds of singing and speaking by breathing in and then blowing the air out through a narrow opening between the vocal folds. The sound is made just as it is when a child lets the air rush out of a toy balloon. As the conduit pipe is narrowed between the vocal folds, the velocity of the expired air is much higher in the larynx. This airstream is continuously interrupted by the vocal folds, and they are worked by small muscles inside them. The sound that comes out of the larynx is incomprehensible, it has to be shaped by the resonance chambers of the pharynx, nose, and mouth to be turned into speech.

Human singing is like feline purring. Careful timing between the diaphragm and other respiratory muscles and the laryngeal muscles is necessary.

The body's needs for air come first, and speaking has to be fitted in with these necessities. We sing and talk while we breathe out, and so we have to breathe in enough air both to oxygenate the blood and to last to the end of the sentence. The messenger in *Alice Through the Looking-Glass* 'was far too much out of breath to say a word, and could only wave his hands about, and make the most fearful faces at the poor King'. The reason was that, after running, he needed all the breathing he could do to get rid of the carbon dioxide from his lungs, and get more oxygen in; and the body considers this to be much more important than speaking to a King. A singer or a wind-instrument player has to train to keep constant both the volume and the force of air coming up the windpipe, so as to keep the note constant throughout its length. In their cases the other requirements of the body have to take second place to the emission of a pure note. When singers take in a deep breath, they must do it quickly so as to go on with the music, and quietly too. When they record or broadcast, and are near the microphone, we may hear them taking their breath in, which is inaudible at a concert.

To make the movements of speech and control the length of syllables, to put stress on them, to emit the proper volume of sound, we have to control our breathing. This comes down essentially to controlling our intercostal muscles. Contrary to what singers believe, we have little conscious control of the movements of the diaphragm. When they think they are working their diaphragms, they are actually working and controlling their abdominal muscles.

The air comes up the larynx with a slight pressure. The stream of air is then interrupted by the vocal folds. When we are not speaking, the pressure is low, between zero and 2 cm of water. The pressure goes up to about 12 cm of water during speaking, and during singing very loudly it goes up to 50 cm. A trained singer can maintain a steady tone for a maximum of 40 seconds.

To convey emotion, we need to control the pitch and the loudness of the sounds we are making. Anger is conveyed by a loud voice and low pitch, joy by loudness and a higher pitch, fear and sorrow by a quiet voice.

The pitch of the note depends on the frequency of vibration, the mass, and the tension of the vocal folds. The resonating chambers of the pharynx, nose, mouth, and facial sinuses make the voice deeper and more resonant.

The fundamental frequency of the male adult voice is between 130 and 145 cycles, and of the female between 230 and 255 cycles a second; thus the female voice is around middle C. The lowest note made by basses of cathedral choirs is about 66 cycles a second, and the highest notes of sopranos are about 1056 cycles a second, some four octaves higher. If one includes the overtones, the male voice makes use of frequencies up to 7500 cycles, and the female voice up to about 10,000 cycles a second. In terms of octaves, most singers have a range of from 2½ to 3 octaves.

The reason why male voices are deeper than female voices is that the vocal folds and the resonance chambers are larger. This increase in size occurs in both sexes at puberty. In boys the lower limit of the voice drops by about an octave, and in girls by about a sixth. If puberty never comes, the voice remains that of a child, but the volume is that of a man. Alessandro Moreschi, the last of the castrati, who died in 1922, fortunately made nine records. The sound is neither like the voice of a woman nor a boy. If castration happens after puberty, the voice is unaffected.

When we play a wind instrument—and that includes singing and even speaking—we have to keep the sound at constant pitch for set lengths of time. To maintain the note constant, both in pitch and intensity, we use our ears; we are monitoring the sound all the time by auditory feedback. It is, of course, well known that good hearing is a fundamental requirement of musicians. To hear oneself emitting a note, and to change it if it is not quite right, takes a certain time, in fact about 140 ms. Thus, the correcting of a note while it is being held can cause a wobble in the voice; 140 ms causes a wobble of about 7 cycles a second. This is the rate of vibrato in singing that sounds pleasant to our ears.

The child learns to make the right sound by listening to the sounds of speech made by those around it. Interestingly enough, the child also looks at lip movements, just as the deaf are taught to do. All the time, the child is imitating the sounds it hears. The delicate movements of the larynx, tongue, and lips that are needed for talking are developed earlier than the movements of the trunk and limbs. This is surprising, and indicates how fundamental speech is for human beings. How the child knows how to turn the sounds it hears into contractions and relaxations of small muscles of the larynx, we do not know.

Eventually, sounds that the child never hears are no longer heard properly. One difficulty in learning to speak a language like a native-born speaker is that the sounds, rhythms, and cadences are not heard. When I asked a Chinese waiter in a restaurant why some prawns were called butterfly prawns, he replied: 'Because they are flied in butter, I suppose.' He could not hear any difference between 'l's and 'r's.

To speak properly, we need to have feedback from the mouth, lips, and palate. One notices that after one has had a local anaesthetic injection for dental treatment, one's pronunciation is not quite perfect. When all the nerves to the mouth and palate have been blocked with local anaesthetic experimentally, speech is slower and pronunciation is less precise.

Saints and other psychotics who hear voices or hear people talking about them are actually saying the words they hear, but enunciating them without forcing any air through the vocal cords. Microphones placed over the larynxes of such people detect the words enunciated, though they detect no sound. These otherwise inaudible sounds have been recorded on tape, amplified, and then played back to the patient. The patients then recognize them as the voices they hear.

21 Learning

For he is docile and can learn certain things.

Each of us possesses two stores of information. One is inherited, the other is acquired. Chomsky has said: 'Learning is primarily a matter of filling in detail within a structure that is innate.' What is innate is far the more important. It is our genes that make us live as human beings and not as wolves or donkeys.

Learning is the process by which experience changes behaviour. We use the word 'learning' only when this change is long-lasting or permanent. In general, we speak of learning and remembering when these activities are performed with consciousness, and when we use these words, we are thinking of psychological activities. In neurology these terms are used more generally. We talk of learning when even a part of the nervous system changes its behaviour permanently owing to experience, though not as a result of fatigue or disease. This way of using the word anchors it in the physiology of the nervous system. For learning is one of the manifestations of neural activity. It occurs in simple single-celled animals. Gelber has shown that paramecia learn to look for food in association with a wire. He put suitable food for them on a platinum wire, and they congregated round the wire. Then he removed the wire and washed it clean. When he put the wire back, the paramecia continued to congregate round it.

Professor Horridge in Aberdeen has done some experiments that show that the lower parts of the nervous system of locusts and cockroaches learn. He cuts the head off the insect, and then suspends the rear end above a dish of saline. When a leg is extended and touches the saline, it gets an electric shock. After about ten minutes, this rear end, consisting of a ventral nerve cord and the trunk and the legs, learns that it must avoid extending the leg to avoid getting a shock. It keeps the limb out of the saline. This lesson is retained. For if the animal without a head is re-tested ten minutes later, it learns to avoid the shock much more quickly; clearly, some of the previous lesson has been retained.

Professor Yerkes showed that earthworms could learn which way to go at a T-junction. When the earthworms went along one limb of the T, they were given an electric shock; they learned to avoid that limb, and always to take the opposite direction. Even when the top twelve segments of the worm had been cut off and thrown away, the rest of the worm still avoided the wrong limb of the T.

This experiment with the earthworm implies something about worms and other animals that is not usually noticed in such experiments: the animal explores. It is interested in its surroundings, and always notices anything new and strange. If a rat explores a similar T-maze every day, it may choose either limb to visit. If you make a change in one limb, say paint it a new colour, the rat immediately notices this, and goes into this limb to explore. But if you first frighten the animal, then it will always go into the familiar limb, and will leave the strange one until a time when it is feeling more confident.

The amount of knowledge that is inborn and the amount that has to be learned varies from species to species. It used to be thought that insects, whose organization is obviously based on inborn knowledge, were incapable of learning. But experiments with ants learning mazes show that these animals can learn, and that some individuals are much better at learning the maze than others.

As the scale of vertebrates is ascended, the proportion of what has to be learned to what is innate becomes greater. Conversely, among the animals lowest in the scale, learning is unimportant. Just how important it is among vertebrates we have only begun to find out during the last twenty years.

We realize now that behaviour is not innate *or* learned; it is innate *and* learned. There is always an interaction between what is inherited and what is acquired from living. What is innate is not necessarily there when the animal is born. Its seeds are present within the central nervous system, and it will come to fruition at some time when the development of the central nervous system and the rest of the body has reached the appropriate state. What is inherited is the potential. This has to be developed. If the circumstances and environment are not right for developing the potential at the correct time, then this potential form of behaviour is wasted and never used.

Further, learning is selective. The young animal is born with the propensity to learn some things and not others, just as we saw in the example of the baby's interest in the human face. The neural process of learning is an active process. It seems that mere repetition can reinforce what has been learned, but something more active has to take place on the first occasion when anything is learned. We have to make efforts to learn, we have to concentrate. This is so whether we are learning a poem by heart, learning to ride a bicycle, or learning Greek.

Learning and changes in neurons

The simplest type of learning is habituation. When a stimulus is regularly and repeatedly applied, the response decreases until finally there is no response. This form of learning occurs within the spinal cord of man. Dr Dimitrijević and I induced it in human beings in whom the spinal cord had been cut through and divided from the brain. It occurs in all spinal reflexes, including the stretch reflex, in which there is only one synapse in the reflex arc.

We have now learned that this fundamental behaviour of habituation occurs in tissue culture. Tissue culture consists of cutting out one or more cells from the tissues of an egg, a foetus, or an adult animal, and growing them in artificial conditions. If one afferent neuron and one motoneuron are grown in tissue culture, a synapse develops between them, the afferent neuron being the pre-synaptic neuron and the motoneuron the post-synaptic, just as in the body. Further, just as in life, the pre-synaptic neuron produces its transmitter substance. If in this culture the afferent neuron is repeatedly stimulated with a suitable electric current, habituation occurs: the afferent neuron gradually stops exciting the motor cell. These two cells have now learned to ignore the stimulus; some lasting change has occurred at the synapse between the two neurons.

The opposite kind of learning is sensitization. As the stimulus is repeated for a short time, the response increases. This also occurs in the human spinal cord and in the monosynaptic stretch reflex.

E. H. Kandel has devoted his life to studying the fundamental changes that occur in nervous systems in a marine snail, *Aplysia*. Examining the behaviour of just a few neurons in this invertebrate, he showed that he could induce sensitization. Lasting sensitization changed the actual structure. Processes grew out of the sensory neurons and reached the motoneurons where they formed synapses. There were also changes in the post-synaptic neurons. This kind of learning affected the structure, increasing the number of contacts between afferent and efferent neurons and also the area of each contact.

In this simplest of examples, we see function changing structure, experience changing the form of the nervous system. One naturally imagined that anatomy came first and that physiology followed, being limited by the rigidity of structure. But we are learning that this is so only with regard to a large and total structure. The actual structure of the minutiae of the nervous system is changed by learning. Changes in the anatomy of cells with learning has also been discovered in bees. To find out the answer to the question how long learning has to go on for, so as to produce changes in the neurons, some investigators in California did the following experiment on the jewel fish. These fish were threatened and made to flee for a period of just nine minutes. This amount of learning, which included fear, caused measurable enlargement of the spines on dendrites of neurons of their brains. The effects were still there twenty-four hours later; in fact, they had become more pronounced.

Rats brought up in a stimulating environment with a lot of things to do have heavier brains than those brought up in boring conditions. The cortex of the cerebral hemispheres is thicker. This is because the neurons have grown more and larger dendrites and the dendrites have more branches and more spines. The rats from the stimulating environment have more protein and more RNA in their brains.

One can now understand how the lack of hormones and of protein in the diet produce unintelligent or even mentally defective children. Normal brains have to grow. If the blocks out of which growth is built, proteins, are not taken in, and if hormones needed for development are absent, then the growth of neurons is less than normal, and their functioning, such as learning and memory, is also deficient. It is also important to note that the changes in the rats' brains with learning by experience were so important that they overcame the adverse effects of removing much of the thyroid gland or of malnutrition.

In the kitten, immediately after birth, most visual cortical neurons can be excited by illuminating either retina. Hubel and Wiesel asked the question if this would be affected by keeping one eye closed. They sewed the eyelids of one eye together in a newborn kitten. After three months they removed the stitches and examined the working of these visual neurons. What they found was that almost none of the neurons connected to the covered eye could be excited into activity. It was the same if, instead of closing the kitten's eye, they covered it with an opaque shield so that diffuse light without any patterning reached the retina. Thus, what had stopped the working of the cortical neurons had been the deprivation of stimulation by contours, edges, moving light, and patterns of dark and shade. In these experiments, almost all the neurons that had been related to the covered eye changed their function, and were now devoted only to the normally seeing eye. The deprivation of excitation causes functional changes in the visual cortical cells within a matter of hours. If the period of covering of an eye is short, recovery occurs, and both eyes again excite the cortical neurons.

Examination of the neurons by microscopy after the animal's death shows that the neural structures connected to the covered eye are not normal. The neurons are small, and dendrites and spines on them are much smaller than in normal kittens. These structural changes due to lack of stimulation do not occur at all times. There is a sensitive period during which the development of neurons laid down before birth is being carried out.

When we ask what these physiological and anatomical findings mean in terms of everyday life, we find that three months' closure of a kitten's eye makes it blind or almost blind in that eye. At best, it can just tell light from dark. Hubel and Wiesel found that if they sewed up the lid of the other eye after opening that of the first covered eye, the previously blind eye recovered within one or two years. But if they did not close the good eye, the previously closed eye never recovered. The cat used the normal eye, continuing to neglect the uncovered blind eye. Here we see the same thing as we saw happening in tissue culture. Repeated stimulation or use affects the synapse between two neurons and lack of use causes the opposite changes in structure.

The same thing can happen with human beings. A young child develops what is called a lazy eye. It may be that the refraction of this eye is abnormal; more commonly we cannot find anything wrong with the eye or its connections. If the child suppresses the visual input from that eye continually up to the age of 5, the eye becomes almost blind.

When rats or mice are raised in the dark, the whole visual system fails to develop normally. The electron microscope shows abnormalities in the rods of the retina, at the synapses between the rods and the neurons connecting to them, in the ganglion cells of the retina, and in the cells of the primary visual area of the cortex. The essential abnormality is that the pathway from the retina to the primary visual area is simplified; only a very few connections are made.

When no impulses pass along a nerve fibre, the number of vesicles in the nerve-ending diminishes. The opposite condition is that the spines on dendrites increase with use; they provide areas for synaptic connections.

Connections that are made when an animal learns should be thought of in terms of large bands of nerve fibres, as well as in terms of synapses. One supposes that when something is learned by the cerebral hemispheres, connections are made between two parts of the brain.

When a blind person learns braille, we presume that connections are made between the secondary tactile area for the index finger and the speech area. When he feels a certain configuration of dots, they automatically bring first the letter, and later the word, to his consciousness.

Much learning of this type also demands connections between the cortex and structures deeper in the cerebral hemispheres, such as the thalamus and the large motor centres in the middle of the hemispheres. Many of these connections could not be made in babyhood or even during early childhood. For when mammals are born, many of the nerve fibres within the brain are rudimentary, and cannot yet carry nerve impulses. The nerve fibres that will become myelinated may not have a myelin sheath at birth, or even for years after birth. If learning depends on these fibres making connections between two regions of the brain, it cannot occur till these fibres have completed their development and are ready to conduct impulses. One reason why certain things can be learned only at certain times is that the neural structures needed for this learning may not yet be adequately matured. For instance, if puppies two weeks old are put on a table, they crawl around and keep falling off, and hurt themselves. At this age, they cannot profit from this experience and learn. The reason is that the parts of the brain needed for acquiring knowledge about edges and ledges is not yet developed, nor is the part of the brain that corrects tendencies to fall when the feet are not placed firmly on a surface. But at this age, when they are placed on their backs, they can turn round and right themselves, for these reflexes have already been developed.

The first step in learning is the sensory input. There must be stimulation from the environment; something has to be experienced, to be seen, smelt, or felt. For learning to take place, the proper stimulation needs to come at the right time. We now know, from much experimental work on young animals deprived of their normal psychological environments and the usual stimuli, that once the right time for acquiring a skill or a certain behaviour has passed, this skill or behaviour can never be properly learned.

The invention of the technique of sensory deprivation has made it clear to us how important the usual enviromental stimulation is for normal development. In this technique, from the time of weaning or earlier, various aspects of the usual environment are removed, and the young animal is brought up bereft of them. Such animals never become normal. The sensory deprivation occurring in infancy and during their early months ruins their ability to learn anything, and they never adapt to many of the features of their environment. Puppies reared in isolation from puppyhood to maturity are always unable to respond intelligently even to danger-ous features of their surroundings. What is very surprising is that they do not respond adequately to painful stimulation, and they cannot localize painful stimuli accurately on their bodies. Such puppies would put their noses into flames and never learned not to do this. They seemed to be indifferent to being pricked with a needle, and they often damaged themselves by bumping into things or falling off heights. When they did fall, or even if someone accidentally trod on one of their paws or on their tails, they never yelped; they did not seem to feel the pain. And when they were obviously hurt they did not learn to avoid the painful stimulus.

It is obvious that if the needed stimulation comes before the nervous system is sufficiently developed to receive it, it can have no effect. But also if the stimulation comes too late, learning does not take place. The sensitive period for learning is particularly short in the case of imprinting in young birds and mammals. It may be as short as hours, according to some investigators, or days, according to others. In birds, this period starts a few hours after hatching, and it never lasts for more than ten days.

Normal social and emotional development probably also needs the correct stimulation at the right time. We can observe evidence of this in those fortunately rare cases of children who have been completely neglected from birth. Sometimes illegitimate children in the country are put away in haylofts or barns to conceal their existence from the neighbours. They are taught nothing, not even to be house-trained or to speak. These children then grow up mentally defective. Even if they are found and rescued by the age of 4 or 5, it is too late; though they can be taught a lot, their speech is always inadequate, and their brains never reach the standards of their siblings. To a lesser degree, the same thing used to happen in orphanages: perhaps it still does in some countries? Rows of beds of illegitimate children fill these institutions. The children never have the love normally given by parents, and they get nothing more than rudimentary care of the body. The usually grow up unintelligent or even mentally defective, and they are equally defective in social and emotional development.

Inadequate food in early childhood causes permanent brain damage; the right amount of the right food must be given at the right time. This environmental influence comes to cause decreased intelligence, and probably also diminished adaptibility.

One now sees that three different influences are necessary for normal development of the nervous system. One has to have protein in the diet, hormones in the bloodstream, and stimulation from the world. We usually classify the last as psychological and the other two as physical or material. As they all cause anatomical events, actual changes in the structure of the nervous system at cellular level, they are, finally, all physical factors.

That we speak our own language perfectly and the languages we learn later imperfectly also depends on learning this skill at the right time. The brain develops in such a way that it is ready to learn to speak between the ages of about ten months and ten years. Languages learned later are not spoken perfectly. The ability to speak a language is a mixed motor and sensory skill, as in fact all skills are. It is necessary to hear all the sounds, the subtle differences between similar but not identical sounds, the rhythm and lilt of the language, where the voice goes up or down, where the accent on a word falls. One has also to work tongue, throat, and lips to control breathing, so that the right amount of force in expelling the air is used. And all this has to be managed at one and the same time. From some time after birth until the age of 6 or 7, normal children can learn all this perfectly; and without much difficulty they can learn two or even three languages at the same time, without finally muddling them up. But later, most of us cannot acquire this skill. We may learn to write and read the new language perfectly; but to acquire the right inflexion and accent, and the ability to speak so that no one can detect that the language is not our mother-tongue, hardly ever occurs. But those of us who still want to learn foreign languages after these early milestones have been passed need not worry; for though we may not learn to speak a new language like the natives, we know from thousands of examples that we can go on learning languages beyond the age of 80. There are so many activities adding up to the simple word 'learning' that, although some of the processes become less efficient with ageing of the brain, our actual experience of learning helps us in learning new material.

The sensitive period during which a language can be learned perfectly is a few years in humans; in most birds, it is a few weeks or months. Thorpe of Cambridge University found, for instance, that the chaffinch has to learn most of its song, and that this learning has to occur during the early weeks of the bird's life, and also during the first spring. If the bird is hand-reared and isolated from other birds from the time of hatching, it sings only very simple songs and it never learns the song of its species correctly. Its song will be elaborated if it hears another chaffinch singing, even though the other chaffinch has also been hand-reared and isolated, and has never heard another bird sing. The singing of these birds is so dependent on learning that chaffinches from different parts of the country sing differently. Just like the human inhabitants of these islands, they have regional accents; though the birds do not base their pecking order on them.

Birds listen to their own singing, and they practise. If a bird is rendered deaf, its song deteriorates. The earlier in its life the bird's hearing is destroyed, the poorer its song will be.

If necessary connections are destroyed, learning cannot occur. When monkeys have had their temporal lobes removed in experimental operations, they can no longer learn what objects are. They pick everything up, smell it and examine it by mouth to see if it is edible, and then put it down. A minute later they pick up the same object without any signs of recognizing it, treating it as though it is something strange and new. They cannot retain anything they may have learned about the object. When certain tracts of nerve fibres are divided in the frontal lobes of dogs or rats, these animals are unable to learn essential social relationships. They treat their fellows as objects, walking on them and taking food even from animals larger and stronger than themselves. Although they get bitten repeatedly, they are unable to learn from this punishment, and keep on doing it.

Learning is made far more effective if strong emotion accompanies it. Indeed, it seems to be that the stronger the emotion, the more firmly fixed the knowledge will be. A child or a chimpanzee will have learned after receiving one prick from a needle on a syringe to fear the needle. When something is learned with strong emotion, it is likely to be retained for years. Something happening only once may be fixed in the memory for ever. Professor Yerkes has recorded that once one of their chimpanzees escaped from its cage, and wandered around the colony making a nuisance of itself, refusing to go back. One of Yerkes's assistants got a revolver, intending to fire a bullet near the animal's legs and frighten it back into its cage. The chimpanzee, who had been born and bred in the colony, had never seen a revolver before. Unfortunately, when the man fired, he hit the animal by mistake in its leg. The terrified chimpanzee immediately rushed back to its cage and stayed there. From that moment the chimpanzee was terrified of the revolver. The staff of the colony could always make the chimpanzee do as they wanted merely by showing it the muzzle of the revolver. As Yerkes points out, the chimpanzee saw the revolver only once and very briefly. Yet the traumatic experience of being shot in the leg fixed the memory of the object for ever. This kind of learning, when something that happened once is retained forever, is usually, perhaps always, associated with fear.

Rats will learn and retain for months an experience that has occurred only once, if it is painful and unpleasant. A rat put in a hammock in a cage, the floor of which is electrified, so that it gets a shock every time its foot touches the floor, will learn after only one shock never to touch the floor of the cage again. In some other experiments, it was shown that when rats learn something to the accompaniment of fear, it will be remembered even after both cerebral hemispheres have been removed. The cortex is needed for learning; but once the task has been learned in association with fear, the knowledge is passed on to deeper levels of the brain. This passing on of acquired knowledge from one set of neurons to another is a feature of neural organization.

Undoubtedly the same thing happens with the young human. An experience fixed with emotion is firmly fixed, and it may remain for life. It can influence the child's behaviour always, forming the basis of certain aspects of its character. Such emotions are terror, disappointment, great interest, or happiness at being rewarded or appreciated.

One of the main theories of Adler's school of psychology is the importance of early childhood memories in the formation of character. Adler considered that the person's first memory was a clue to that person's whole personality. Whatever the person remembers longest has been fixed with a great deal of emotion, and remains a fundamental influence in his character. Looked at from the outside, such an experience may not seem very interesting. But seen with the eyes of the small child, it may have a deep and important meaning.

Emotions such as love, the arousal of interest, and enthusiasm are effective in helping children and adults learn; though few professional teachers are capable apparently of making use of these adjuvants to remembering. The one method they make most use of is boredom; this deters remembering and learning. But rote memory is helped by frequent repetition, even though this is inevitably accompanied by boredom. Physical or psychological pain is effective in fixing things in the memory. For thousands of years teachers and parents have made ample use of physical pain; now that many people disapprove of whipping children, only psychological pain is used.

An animal has to know the results of its behaviour in order to learn. Knowledge of results that alters behaviour can be thought of as a kind of feedback, and it has been called response feedback. Most natural learning is rewarded by pleasure or pain; these emotional accompaniments form a part of response feedback. When an animal learns any skill or the parts of a skill, it gets pleasure; this reinforces what it has learned, and makes it want to do it again. But if the animal makes a wrong response, it is not rewarded or it may even be hurt. The pleasure could be that accompanying satiety from eating or drinking enough, or it could be the feeling of contentment from being in a correctly adjusted environment, correct in terms of humidity, temperature, flow of air, and other physical factors. The punishment could be the mounting hunger felt with the failure to find food, or the mounting frustration and discomfort from failing to find a partner for sexual activity. Punishment may be more forceful than this. If rats are given poison, and they survive, they will always avoid that particular food in the future. In this case there is a long time between the taking of the poisoned food and experiencing its effects; yet these intelligent animals learn straightaway to connect the two.

In the simplest organisms, the reward or punishment must follow the activity quickly for the animal to learn. For such animals do not have memories long enough to connect what they have just done with success or failure, with pleasure or pain, if there is much delay between the act and its reward. For this kind of learning, what psychologists called 'temporal contiguity' is necessary.

For human beings, learning itself can provide the pleasure. We are pleased to have learned something and we may be ashamed not to have done so. But not all learning is rewarded by pleasure. The kinds of learning occurring at the lowest levels of the nervous system occur merely with frequent repetition. Imprinting occurs automatically, provided it comes at the correct time.

For an animal to learn something, it need not make an immediate response. The learning may be all internal; there is no movement, nothing to be seen.

As learning causes changes in our central nervous systems, and as we are learning all the time, we see that every brain must be different from every other one, apart from the fact that each one starts off with a different inherited constitution. Every brain is different according to what its possessor has put into it. One person has learned a new language, another has learned tea-tasting.

Making two brains into one

Weber, who early in the nineteenth century was the first scientific investigator of sensation and perception, observed that children taught to write with one hand could then produce mirror-writing with the other hand, without any further practice. Psychologists later found that this transfer of training occurs for a great many kinds of learning. In all of them, the untrained side of the brain learns more quickly than it would have done had there been no training at all, though it performs less well than the trained side. This kind of learning was investigated in great detail by R.W. Sperry and his colleagues in the United States.

When anything has been learned, some change must have occurred in the brain. In the case of writing, this change has occurred in the left cerebral hemisphere. Without any further training or practice, these changes are transferred to the right hemisphere. When the changes are long-lasting, we speak of memory. Realizing that something physical is conducted from one hemisphere to the other, we can look for the anatomical pathways along which these changes could pass.

The main bridge between the hemispheres is the corpus callosum; this bridge or commissure is shown in Plates 13 and 14. In Plate 14, the middle parts of both hemispheres have been cut away to show the corpus callosum. At both ends it curves round and continues downwards for a short distance, out of sight. On the right side, a part of the frontal lobe has been pulled away so as to show the thickness of the grey matter covering the white matter. The corpus callosum is by far the biggest of all the commissures joining the two halves of the brain. It is the most recent one, having evolved in company with the two cerebral hemispheres, which it links together. The first parts of the hemispheres to evolve were linked by a small structure called the anterior commissure, and by the hippocampal commissure, linking the two hippocampi.

Some functions of the corpus callosum related to vision can now be explained with the help of Fig. 21.1. It will be seen in this figure that each half of the retina receives light from the part of the world opposite it. The right half of both retinae receives from the left visual field, and the left half of both retinae from the right visual field. Each occipital lobe of each hemisphere receives nerve impulses from the half of the retina on its own side; the right occipital lobe receives from the right half of the retina of both eyes, and the left occipital lobe from the left half of both. Thus, what is seen in the right field goes to the left cerebral hemisphere, and what is seen on the left to the right hemisphere. Between these two areas of the hemispheres there are nerve fibres running through the corpus callosum, connecting one point with another of the two occipital lobes.

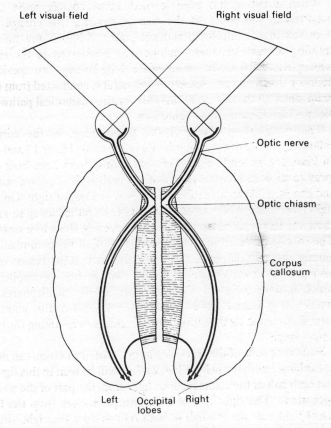

Fig. 21.1 Diagram to illustrate experiments in which the optic chiasm and the corpus callosum are divided.

In order to find out the role of the corpus callosum in visual learning, R.S. Myers cut through the corpus callosum and the optic chiasm in cats. When this is done, all the nerve fibres from the left eye go the left hemisphere and all those from the right eye go to the right hemisphere; for the operation divides those fibres that normally cross. And so, after the operation the left eye and the left cerebral hemisphere form one visual system, and the right eye with its hemisphere form another. These cats were then taught two different solutions of a problem. One solution was taught to the left hemisphere via its eye, and the other solution was taught to the right hemisphere via its eye. For instance, one cerebral hemisphere was taught to make the animal press a lever for a food reward when it saw a white circle, and the other hemisphere to do so when it saw a white square. After the corpus callosum had been cut through, transfer of training did not occur. Each hemisphere then learned independently, and neither knew what the other hemisphere had learned. Each system, consisting of one eye and its hemisphere, functioned well, and behaved as was expected; it acted as if it had no cognizance of the existence of the other hemisphere.

Myers and his colleagues found in further experiments that it was possible to teach each hemisphere an absolutely opposite and contrary solution to one problem. At first, they cut through the corpus callosum in some monkeys. Then they trained one hemisphere to make the animal depress the lever when it saw the outline of a square, and the other hemisphere to make it depress the lever when it saw the outline of a circle. The first hemisphere was also taught that it must not allow the monkey to touch the lever when the circle appears, and the second hemisphere that the lever must not be touched when the square appears. Thus, each hemisphere learns exactly contrary things, the one that the circle is bad and the square is good, and the other that the circle is good and the square is bad. The monkeys with the corpus callosum divided had no difficulty in learning this task. They had no emotional problems and showed no evidence of mental conflict. Intact monkeys would have had severe and intense symptoms of neurosis if they had tried to learn these contrary solutions to problems.

Each hemisphere of an animal with the corpus callosum divided can be taught the contrary solutions to a problem at the same time. In each teaching session, first one hemisphere is taught something via its eye and then the other one is taught the opposite information via its eye; then for the next five minutes the first eye is trained again, and so on throughout the session. A cat or monkey with division of the commissures and the optic chiasm ends up by learning its two different solutions to a problem in the same time it takes the normal animal to learn one solution; and it achieves this without any mental or emotional conflict.

The solution to a food-obtaining problem can also be based on tactile clues instead of visual ones. In this case, the one hemisphere is taught to press a lever when the forepaw examines and feels a certain tactile sensation, and the other hemisphere is taught to press it when exactly the opposite sort of tactile sensation is felt. Again, each sensory cortex learns an opposite solution to the problem, and there is no conflict between the two solutions. What each hemisphere learns via its own sensory input coming from the opposite side of the body is learned better and retained longer than what it learns by transfer across the corpus callosum. What has been learned, for instance, by the left hemisphere coming from the left halves of both retinae (things seen on the right) is well retained, whereas what has been learned in the right hemisphere (things seen on the left) from transfer from the left hemisphere is poorly retained and soon forgotten.

We presume that under normal conditions, what is learned by one hemisphere is automatically transferred to the other via the corpus callosum. It is first learned by one hemisphere, and then a weaker carbon copy, so to speak, is kept in the other hemisphere. We do not yet know how this transfer is done, nor what mechanisms are entailed in the word 'automatically' used in the above statement.

The experimental situation of dividing the corpus callosum has been used in the treatment of certain epileptic patients. The idea has been to stop the severe fits from spreading from one hemisphere to the other, and hence from one side of the body to the other. The effects of the operation were similar to those produced in cats and monkeys. After the operation, each cerebral hemisphere acted independently, as if it were ignorant of the existence of the other.

One great difference between the patients and the animals in which the corpus callosum was cut through is that man possesses language, and the ability to use language depends mainly on the left hemisphere. The right hemisphere had lost its connections with the speech area. There were many consequences of this disconnection. The patient could do some things using only his right hemisphere, but he could not then explain what he was doing, as the right hemisphere had lost its connections with the speech area. He could not write at all with his left hand. Right-handed people, of course, cannot write well with the left hand; but these patients

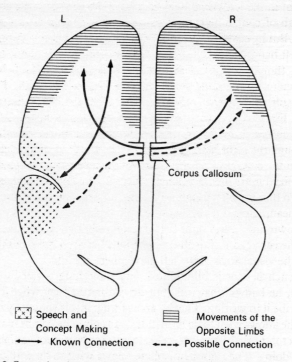

Fig. 21.2 Connections between the speech area of the left cerebral hemisphere and motor regions of both hemisphere.

had not even the slightest idea how to write with their left hands, this hand had no knowledge of the shapes of letters and words.

The anatomical situation is illustrated in Fig. 21.2. This represents a section through the two cerebral hemispheres, made from side to side through the frontal and temporal lobes. The corpus callosum has been divided. This cut separates the right hemisphere from the region of the left hemisphere that organizes speech, reading, writing, and the kind of thinking depending on speech. As the speech region is cut off from the right hemisphere, this hemisphere cannot direct the left hand to do things related to speech, such as writing letters, words, or numbers.

When the pathways through the corpus callosum are cut, there are similar disorders with vision. If we present something to such a patient in the left visual field, he cannot name it or write about it, though of course he can do so when it is presented in the right field. But he can pick the object out of a tray of various things with the left hand. He cannot read anything presented in the left visual field, though he can read it when it is in the right field. His behaviour can be understood with the help of Fig. 21.3. The left hemisphere sees what is in the right visual field and controls the right limbs. The right hemisphere sees what is in the left field and controls the left limbs. When the corpus callosum is divided, although the right hemisphere can still see what is in the left field, it cannot communicate it to the left hemisphere. As reading is organized in the left hemisphere, the patient sees the printed page shown him on the left; but it no longer makes any sense, the letters are meaningless lines of black on a white page. As soon as the page is shown him in the right field, he not only sees it, it makes sense and he can read it. For the connections between the reading areas and the visual areas of the left hemisphere are intact.

If such patient is blindfolded, and something is put in his left hand, he knows what it is, but he can neither say what it is nor describe it in writing. That he knows what it is is shown by the fact that he knows what to do with it. If it is a comb, he combs his hair; if it is a toothbrush, he brushes his teeth. Yet he cannot explain what he is doing. The right hemisphere knows what to do with objects. It is surprising what a patient with the corpus callosum divided

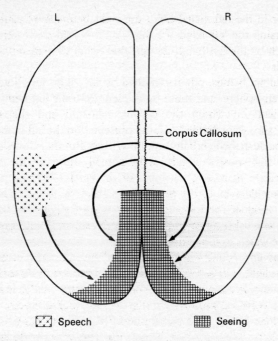

Fig. 21.3 Connections between the two visual areas and the region of the left hemisphere for reading and writing.

can do with the left hand (commanded by the right hemisphere) when material is shown in the left visual field. For instance, a patient shown random pictures of a strip cartoon in his left visual field (going to the right hemisphere) placed them in the correct order using the left hand. But he had no idea what was presented in the left visual field, and no ideas what the left hand was doing. When these patients are shown drawings of landscapes indicating summer or winter in the left field, they can point to the correct name of summer or winter with the left hand. Yet they have no experience of doing anything.

Drawing is affected in all the patients. This shows that it needs the co-operation of both hemispheres. When objects to be drawn were presented to the right hemisphere by being placed in the left hand or in the left visual field, the right hemisphere could draw them using the left hand. In this way it would draw letters that were felt by the left hand, though the letters were meaningless as symbols.

In human beings, odours smelled by the right nostril go to the right hemisphere, and those by the left go to the left hemisphere. In patients in whom the corpus callosum and the anterior commissure were divided, odours presented to the left hemisphere could be described verbally and in writing. But the odours smelled by the right nostril could not be named, although the patients could easily point to the source of the smell. In these patients, nasty smells given to the right nostril and thus to the right hemisphere, produced wincing and withdrawing the nose; but when the patient was asked to say what the smell was, he would say that it must be water, as it had no smell.

Forms and colours are manipulated by the right hemisphere with the left hand; but the left hemisphere can hardly do such tasks. For instance, a patient with the corpus callosum divided is asked to match a coloured geometric design with coloured blocks. This is easily done by the right hemisphere with the left hand. The left hemisphere, using the right hand, does this very slowly and with difficulty. If there are mistakes, and the right hemisphere sees this, it rapidly puts out the left hand and corrects them.

The right hemisphere is better than the left at the recognition of faces, and does it more quickly. The left hemisphere recognizes things by naming them. It has a verbal and conceptual way of apprehending the world. But the right hemisphere is not, as Professor Sperry puts it, 'entirely illiterate'. It reads a word like 'cup', 'fork', or 'cat' in the left visual field, and it also knows some verbs.

For human beings, knowing what something is entails knowing its name and knowing what to do with it. For all other animals, knowing what to do with it is the only knowledge. When the corpus callosum is divided in man, these two sorts of knowledge are split apart. Knowing its name is knowledge of the left hemisphere, knowing what to do with it belongs to the right.

The left hemisphere not only organizes speech; it also provides a detailed conception of time and of ordering events in time. It is good at appreciating detail. It is the main hemisphere for calculation, but probably not for geometry; this is a part of spatial sense, and so it belongs to the right hemisphere.

Visual material may be stored in a visual code, without the use of words, without verbal labelling. This is the same with storing or remembering smells. For seeing and understanding what one sees, both hemispheres are usually used, but probably this visual material is at first coped with by the right hemisphere.

Emotional behaviour and reactions of a vague sort are obtained by showing material with an emotional content to the right hemisphere. A picture of a nude woman presented to the left visual field of a woman with a split corpus callosum induced a feeling of embarrassment with blushing; but the patient could not account for her behaviour. And fear was induced by showing the right hemisphere a terrifying picture. The state of emotion is then totally inexplicable to the left hemisphere. It knows the emotion has occurred but cannot account for it.

These discoveries of hemispheric specialization are so important that ways have been sought of confirming them in normal people. One method has been to present material to each visual field separately. This can be arranged by presenting the material for a very short time to each visual field. In this way there is not enough time to report what we see in one field across the brain to the other hemisphere. Another method is dichotic listening. Different auditory material is presented to the two ears simultaneously. The investigator then notes which the subject attends to. The auditory input goes mainly, but not entirely, to the opposite temporal lobe. These methods have confirmed the findings on cats, monkeys, and patients, and show that lateralization of brain functioning is a reality, and not just a sort of artefact due to surgical lesions of the commissures.

Normally, our knowledge of the world is a product of the organization of the two hemispheres. For all nerve fibres from the left half of both retinae go the left cerebral hemisphere, and all those from the right half of both retinae go the right hemisphere. In order for whole objects to be seen, the two hemisphere inputs have to be joined. This is done instantaneously by fibres crossing in the occipital end of the corpus callosum. Similar fibres in the middle regions of the corpus callosum are used for the integration of sensation acquired through paired limbs. When we feel something with both hands, we make the sensations into a whole; we don't have to think 'On the left hand it feels rough, on the right hand it feels rough too; and so it must be rough all over'. Before we realize what something is, this information from the two sides of the body has been integrated; and the main pathway for this is the corpus callosum.

When we examine patients with lesions cutting off a part of either hemisphere from the speech area, the patient cannot tell us about his defect. Indeed, most of these patients are ignorant of having a defect. This is because 'I'—if we have to use such a philosophical concept—resides somewhere within the speech area on the left. In such a case. 'I' honestly does not know what the right cerebral hemisphere is doing. These patients are difficult to understand, for there is one further problem for the neurologist. In most of these patients, the gap left by the sensory deficiency is filled by confabulation. When a sensory input is suddenly cut off, the result is not usually a state of blankness or nothingness; the patient does not say he feels or knows nothing. Spontaneous input or hallucinations fill the gap. The patient does not say, for example, that his left arm is lacking in all sensibility; he says that that limb is not his, and that it should be thrown away. This has nothing to do with intelligence. The person with the corpus callosum cut through really has a split mind.

From Myers's investigations on cats and monkeys, and from Sperry's work on man, we can draw the following conclusions about the functions of the corpus callosum. It is needed for transferring what one hemisphere learns, and making it a common possession of the brain. It is essential for keeping each hemisphere informed about what is happening in the other one. It is necessary for learning any skill that is bilateral, using both sides of the body. The co-ordination of movements, apart from the reflex part of movements laid down at lower neural levels, depends on the passage of impulses across the corpus callosum between the motor regions of the two hemispheres. It is needed when any motor skill depends on vision. It is also necessary for us to make our visual conceptions of the world, our concept of distance and space.

These experiments on dividing the commissures of the brain have formed the foundation of our knowledge of the different contributions of each hemisphere to our understanding of the world. In right-handed people, the left hemisphere carries out a temporal analysis, the right hemisphere carries out spatial synthesis. The left hemisphere, being the hemisphere of language, is more analytical, for analysis requires thinking in language. It may be that the right hemisphere apprehends the environment in an immediate and total way. The right hemisphere is more important for the recognition and remembering of location, forms and shapes. But internal speech can also be used in remembering those things that are essentially visual. People differ in the degree to which they make use of it. Internal speech is used less when stored visual material has to be recognized than when it has to be reproduced. This use of internal speech of the left hemisphere is made clear when one considers the example of recognizing faces, which is mainly carried out in the right hemisphere. One finds it difficult to put the difference between two faces into words, but one has no difficulty in distinguishing the two. But none of this is invariable. If one needs to distinguish the faces of identical twins, one uses the left cerebral speech region. One starts to say to oneself what minimal differences there are between the two faces. How we do not use speech in remembering is obvious with regard to smell, for putting smells into words does not help at all. It is the same for hearing. Naming a melody may not help one find it in one's musical treasury.

When one is faced with a new occurrence, it seems to be that the left hemisphere becomes dominant if conceptual and verbal understanding of the sensory input is best. The right hemisphere may be dominant when less intellectual examination is more suitable.

It may be said that in these animals and patients with split brains, each hemisphere thinks independently; though this statement depends on how one defines thinking. If thinking requires verbal formulation, then only the left hemisphere thinks. But if one includes in thinking the awareness and memories of colours and shapes, or the scenes of one's dreams, then both sides of the brain are thinking at the same time, unconnected and independently.

22 Remembering

The word 'memory' is used in neurology and psychology to mean a change in behaviour due to the retention of information or an experience. When we speak of memory in everyday life, we either mean recalling an event that we have experienced, or something we have heard of or learned. In neurology this kind of memory is often called highest level memory.

Lower level memory

All essential features of memory occur at the lower levels of the central nervous system. In two examples that follow, the experience has been fixed and retained by neural mechanisms at spinal level.

The first example comes from a patient with cancer. To stop the pain, which was most severe in her case, she had an operation on the spinal cord. This operation makes the whole body below the level of the operation on the spinal cord insensitive to pain. It does not interfere with the tactile forms of sensation, and so the patient can still feel the ground he walks on, and knows where to put his feet. This particular patient had had a car accident six years earlier which had caused a severe and painful fracture of the right knee-cap. The kneecap had been removed, the pain went, and the patient had forgotten all about it. Immediately after the operation on her spinal cord, she found to her amazement that any painful stimulus applied to her right lower limb produced the identical pain she had had in the right knee six years before. The stimulus did not merely produce the pain in her knee; it caused all the sensations which she had had six years previously when her kneecap had been fractured.

The second case shows the same thing. At one time I was studying the problems of pain sometimes experienced by patients after amputations of limbs. One of these patients was a young man who had lost his leg during the Korean War. During the course of a day, I carried out various procedures to the stump of this lower limb, many of which were painful, and all of which had the effect of sending into the spinal cord a barrage of nerve impulses from the limb. On the night after these tests, the patient was suddenly woken from his sleep with severe pain in his absent leg. He immediately knew what this pain was. For five years previously, before he had had his leg amputated, he had been playing ice hockey, had fallen, and had had the outside of his leg cut open by a skate. On the present night he re-experienced the identical sensations in his phantom leg that he had had at that time. It was not that he remembered having had this injury; he felt all the sensations again in his absent leg that he had previously felt.

In these two patients, the pattern of activity of certain neurons within the spinal cord has undergone some permanent change as a result of the pain in the lower limb. What this actual change is, we do not know; but the presence of some change was shown by stimulating the same neurons again on another occasion, several years later.

This is really the same phenomenon as memory, though we do not think of this sort of thing when we use the term. This same sort of memory has also been seen occurring within the neurons of the sensory nerve of the face. During the last war, a dentist and a doctor in the United States became interested in pain in the face that pilots sometimes got during high-altitude flying. This was before planes were pressurized. They found that many of the pilots got pain in the teeth as well as pain located in the facial sinuses, where it might be expected to occur. In going into the dental histories of these pilots, they found out that the pain was felt in those teeth that had sometime before been subjected to some trauma, such as dental treatment. This trauma could have been extraction of the tooth or simply a filling. To reproduce these results once more, and to investigate this phenomenon further, one of the two, the dentist, did some routine fillings. Ten to sixteen days later, the other one, the physician, applied a painful stimulus to the inside of the nose. The pain caused by this stimulus was felt not only at the place where the needle pricked the inside of the nose, but also in the tooth that had been treated a few days before. In a further investigation, they divided the patients into two groups. In one group the dental fillings were carried out under general anaesthesia, so that the patient was unconscious at the time. In the other group the dental fillings were carried out with local anaesthesia so that the nerve carrying impulses from the tooth to the central nervous system was blocked. They found that the phenomenon still occurred in the group of patients in whom the fillings had been done under general anaesthesia: stimulation of the nose still caused pain in the treated tooth. But it no longer occurred in the patients in whom the fillings had been done with a local anaesthetic. This showed that if the nerve impulses were prevented from reaching the brain, the recording and retention of this experience did not occur.

What has happened here is that the painful stimulation has caused some change in the lower level of the brain, in the part to which the nerve from the face goes. It is a permanent or a long-lasting change. This is memory occurring at a low neural level. There is the registration of an experience, its storage, and then its recall. When the material is recalled, it returns with the stamp of the past upon it, and also the sense of familiarity. The experience has become a part of this region of the sensory system, and it alters subsequent behaviour. We presume that the neurons concerned have been altered in some way. When they are stimulated (but not with every sort of stimulation), they work together in the same way as they worked on the previous occasion.

The change in the next case must have taken place among the neurons of the thalamus within the cerebral hemisphere. A builder's labourer had a painful ingrowing toe-nail. He fell off the scaffolding and broke his back, cutting the spinal cord in two. From then on, he was completely paralysed in the lower part of his body, and he could feel no sensation. If he was pricked, pinched, moved, or touched anywhere in the lower part of his body, he could not feel it. If the toe-nail were squeezed or banged, he felt nothing. And yet after this injury to the spinal cord, he still continued to be aware of the painful toe-nail. This means that certain neurons at a higher level than the spinal cord had been changed by the pain. They continued to register pain in the toe-nail, even though all impulses from the foot had been cut off.

Two facts need emphasis here. The first is that these phenomena occur only very rarely. The second is that they exist, whether they are rare or not; and their existence shows that this sort of memory occurs at these lower levels of the nervous system. It is important to realize this, for it appears that many of the functions of the higher levels of the nervous system are elaborations of functions already present at lower levels.

The same sort of retention of change due to experience occurs at higher levels of the nervous system. At this level it involves the thalamus and the neurons of the cerebral cortex. In some patients, when there has been a severe pain going on continually for a long time, the neurons related to this sensation and this part of the body became altered in some way on electrical stimulation of the brain. In normal people, all parts of the cerebral cortex can be stimulated electrically at operation and the patient does not experience pain. When the sensory regions of the cortex are stimulated, the person feels tingling, numbness, or a sensation of the part being moved or about to be moved. But in patients with persistent pain, the electrical stimulation of large regions of the sensory cortex does cause pain, and it causes the identical pain from which the patient suffers. One sees here that the cortex has become altered; areas that normally have nothing to do with pain now subserve the conscious perception of pain. The continuous pain has changed these neurons.

Memory used in skilled movements and perception

A sequence of learned movements is a memory. In dancing, you have to remember the previous gyrations so that the whole series should be made into the required sequence. In drawing, you have to remember how the previous lines were arranged in order to complete the picture. You must also remember the total shape of an object you are drawing from memory. In listening to music, we must remember the first part of a melody for the later part to make sense. One could not appreciate the simplest musical form—a canon, for instance—if one did not remember the phrase that has just been played or sung; and a fugue would be meaningless without a trained memory for musical forms. It is the same with speech. One has to remember the words of the beginning of the sentence for the whole sentence to make sense. Sometimes when we are speaking, we may be distracted in the middle; then the short-term memory may fail, and we have to admit that we have forgotten what we were talking about.

The memories of movement routines are kept in the motor parts of the cerebral cortex. Some disorders of movement, the apraxias, are thought to be due to disconnexions between the cortex, where these memories are stored, and the cortical areas that organize the movements.

Memory is necessary in perception, in the recognition of what one sees and hears. A rose is a rose only when you compare what you are seeing with the memory of previous roses. You know the national anthem because it sounds the same as your stored version of previously played national anthems. If, however, you have no previous version in your memory, then you know that this is an unfamiliar object, something new. This recognition of the familiar based on stored perceptions takes place so quickly that we do not know we are doing anything. We are just seeing a rose. But not all information derived from our sensory apparatus has to be learned and remembered. As we have noted already, some sensory perceptions are innate. The information derived from pheromones is innate, it seems, in all animals; and that must include us. This may be a reason why smells are so difficult to put into words, and also why they are so evocative.

In recent years we have learned a lot about how we recognize objects in the environment, from the work of Professor Mortimer Mishkin in the United States and Professor Rolls at Oxford. Perception depends on memory. What affects the photoreceptors is finally reported to the visual cortex. Each relay into secondary and tertiary regions of visual cortex brings in neurons with larger and more complex visual fields. The first neurons are sensitive to visual elements such as edges and angles. The neurons after the next relay may be fired by the total shape of an object. Finally neurons in the front part of the temporal lobes make perceptions of objects. These neurons are just beside the hippocampus and amygdala (Figs 15.2 and 15.3). They are connected to neurons of these structures; for they are essential parts of the brain that provide recognition based on visual memory. Each temporal lobe is connected to both amygdalae and hippocampi, and so destruction of these masses on one side does not destroy all memory of objects. But if these connections come to be destroyed on both sides, the patient sees things but he does not know what they are; and further, he cannot re-learn it. He is more afflicted than someone who is blind.

It is the same with recognition of how something feels, tastes, or smells. The elements of how an object feels when we take it in our hands and examine it by moving our fingers over and around it are furnished by neurons in the primary tactile, kinaesthetic strip (Fig. 18.1a). Posterior to this strip, other neurons of the parietal lobe add further and more complicated aspects of the object being felt. This region also receives connections from the visual cortex, doubtless providing visual aspects of the object, and also its position in space. These perceptions are reported to the amygdalae and hippocampi for recognition or registration of novelty.

If these pathways are divided experimentally in a monkey, the animal cannot learn. Apparently, it cannot remember the object presented to it; and so each time an object is shown or put in its hand, it treats it as something new. This is applied to all sensory inputs, visual, tactile, smell, and taste—apart from the perceptions that are innate.

There are a few humans in which this memory apparatus has been damaged on both sides of the brain. In them, old memories remain. And so one concludes that there is a store of memories in some other part of the brain as well.

As all the sensory inputs finally connect to the amygdala, it may be that this is the part of the brain that is essential for associating the various aspects of an object so that we know what it is: this red, soft, juicy object with such a smell and such a taste (note how words fail with taste and smell) is a strawberry.

There are also connections between the amygdala and the hippocampi to the hypothalamus. These connections provide the animal with its emotional response. The amygdala and hippo-campi now know what the object is and where it is. They recognize it as something remembered and familiar, or else as something strange. The response has to be arranged accordingly.

Highest level memory

When we speak of having a good memory or of trying to remember something, we are thinking of the highest neural level of remembering. For this kind of remembering, the event has to be registered; then it is retained or stored; and then it is retrieved and reproduced. The memory includes the context of the event: it is localized at a certain time in the past, it is known to have happened to us, and it comes up with the remembrance of the emotions we felt at the time.

We start off with very short-term remembering, what psychologists call memory span. If we are half listening to what someone is saying, and he then accuses us of not paying attention, we find that we can prove him wrong by repeating to him his entire last sentence or more. It has all been recorded for us, just as on tape; but until his accusation we were paying no attention to it. It was being recorded but not thought about, probably not even understood. Then, when we play it back we take in its meaning. This is a remarkable mechanism, and really a most useful one. We can make use of it to take in two conversations at once. We listen to one of them and understand it as we hear it; and we let our short-term memory take the other one down, and then attend to it later.

As we are continually taking in information, the stay of the material in short-term memory has to be very short. This material is either passed on for further processing, or it is forgotten, being replaced by the recording of the next event.

A remembered scene is not the same as the original scene. It is not even a faded photograph of it, it is a reconstruction, based on the original experience. Engineers who work in computers assume that human memory is the same as the memory systems that they build into their computers. When an engineer makes what he conceives as a model of the brain, what he is making is an analogy; he is saying 'The brain might work like this'. And it might not. In the case of human memory, what is remembered is not a run-through of what really happened. What is recollected is a short-ened and compressed version. Much of what really happened has dropped out of the remembered scene, much else has become changed and distorted, and a great deal has been forgotten. How vivid the remembered scene is depends on its importance for the person. If it was important, it will have originally had, or later have acquired, much emotional accompaniment. In the remembered scene the emotion is less.

As the reconstruction is not the same as the experience of the original event, all the neural pathways activated originally are not the same as those activated when the scene is remembered. And further, as there are additions as well as omissions, other neural pathways are involved in producing what has been remembered.

As our memories give us a sort of symbolic representation of the previous event, it was surprising to learn that Penfield evoked such real pictures of the patients' past lives when he stimulated regions of their temporal lobes. For what Penfield obtained was, as he wrote: 'not a memory, as we usually use the word, although it may have some relation to it. No man can recall by voluntary effort such a wealth of detail. . . . Many a patient has told me that the experience brought back by the electrode is much more real than remembering.' Whole scenes from the past were thrust into the patients' consciousness. The patients always recognized the scenes as having happened to them, although till the electrode had been applied to their brains, they had no idea that they had retained these memories.

One might have guessed that memories aroused so unnaturally as by the electrical stimulation of a small part of the brain would have appeared distorted and jumbled up. But this was not so. The scene would appear like a film: in the proper order and at the proper pace. As long as the electrode was kept on the same point of the cortex, the remembered event continued to appear. When stimulation was stopped, the internal film stopped, and the patient no longer remembered the scene from his past; when stimulation was started again, the story went on from where it had been left off, or it began again at the beginning.

The actual reminiscences in most cases were trivial. It seemed most unlikely that they had any special significance for the patient. They were not usually the sort of material that is repressed. Penfield has recounted that one of his patients said to him: 'You forced me to live things again that I'd forgotten. What were you doing? Were you stimulating my subconscious mind?' As Penfield wrote, 'Her question seemed naïve. And then I stopped to consider. Wasn't that exactly what my electrode had done?'

The stimulating electrode breaks into the storehouse of memories, and taps the store. The patient does not have to do the work of recalling. Suddenly, there is a familiar episode out of his past before his eyes. And with the experience there is the emotion felt at the time and the personal associations and reactions to the event. So what is stored is not just the event but the event with its meaning to ourselves. And what is obtained from raiding the patient's store in this way is far more detailed than anything the patient can summon to memory in the normal way.

Had Penfield not shown us this evidence of the existence of these remembered experiences, we would probably not have thought that this sort of record exists. One would have guessed that only a symbolic representation of it is in the brain. For the normal process of recall does not reproduce these realistic scenes, unrolling before one's eyes.

Penfield and some other workers on memory have concluded from their observations when they stimulated the temporal lobes that the record of all that we have experienced remains in the brain. Penfield writes:

Since the electrode may activate a random sample of this strip from the distant past, and since the most unimportant and completely forgotten periods of time may appear in this sampling, it seems reasonable to suppose that the record is complete and that it really does include all periods of each individual's waking conscious life . . . . The stream of consciousness flows inexorably onward, as described in the words of William James. But, unlike a river, it leaves behind it a permanent record that seems to be complete for the waking moments of a man's life, a record that runs, no doubt, like a thread along a pathway of ganglionic and synaptic facilitations in the brain. This pathway is located partly or wholly in the temporal lobes.

Nevertheless, psychologists regard forgetting as a normal and probably necessary process. They think that it is normal to forget the large accumulation of trivialities that are at first committed to short-term memory. We choose to retain some of this material, and not to commit all of it to long-term memory. There is a process of selection and filing going on somewhere along the line. How the content of memory is sorted out so that certain experiences are forgotten and others retained, and how it is divided so that some will be retained for days and others for years, we do not know. One imagines that some sort of review goes on; but this is merely a verbal simile, and brings us no nearer knowing what is happening in the nervous system.

There is evidence from psychology that older memories tend to be retained better than recent ones, and that the longer something has been remembered, the more likely it will be retained in the future. Fixation of what has been retained improves with time, and conversely, the more recent memories are the more vulnerable. This holds throughout the time scale: something registered for a few seconds is more vulnerable than something registered for five minutes, and something retained for a day is more likely to disappear than something retained for a year. If we keep recalling something, it is less likely to be forgotten. Whatever memory is, it improves with repetition.

One naïvely thinks that forgetting is due to the event not being retained. One suppose that it is soon discarded, perhaps leaving no trace, no change in the brain. But the little knowledge we have of this subject indicates that this is not always so. Certainly a great deal of what we have experienced is still there.

Apart from Penfield's striking physiological evidence from stimulating the brains of subjects undergoing operations, there has always been good psychological evidence that far more is retained than might seem possible. Merely carrying out free association shows that one has stored a lot of material one had never realized. We need merely to rest and relax (while remaining vigilant and avoiding falling asleep, which is easier said than done) and all sorts of things come to mind that we did not know we knew, or thought we had forgotten. We suddenly see a face, and we realize we saw that face yesterday in front of the British Museum. It is the same with dreams. A strange episode appears to be the product of fantasy. But if we let ourselves associate to that episode, we recognize it as a distortion of an insignificant event which happened the previous day. It was so unimportant that we would not have imagined that it could have been recorded, stored, and recollected.

One or two curious cases have been reported of patients with Parkinsonism who become mentally excited with the drug L-dopa. During the excitement, memories of their earlier lives crowd into their minds. As they relive their previous experiences, these patients use the slang and fashionable expressions of the time. Until that moment they had no idea they still retained the memories of forty or fifty years ago. When the amount of the drug is reduced, the recollections pass away with the excitement, and the patient once again is no longer aware that the memories are hidden in his mind.

During psychotherapy, similar memories from the past roll up, though they had not been recalled before. Often they return with full emotion; and the adult will be raging at the way one of his parents was treating him at the age of 4. This again surprises us, for we did not know we had retained the memory of these experiences.

The ability to recall is not the only criterion there is of an experience having been retained. This can be deduced also from the ease of re-learning. If one knew a language at the age of 5, had never spoken it since that time, and had apparently forgotten it completely, one will learn this language far more quickly at the age of 20 than someone who had never known it at all. Something, then, must have remained.

The ability to recognize also shows us that something has been retained. When we fail to remember something, and somebody else reminds us of it, we then recognize that what he has remembered for us is correct. This shows us that we had registered and stored it; the failure was only in recall. Recognition is sometimes used as a test of memory. Objects are shown to the patient, and then removed. A few minutes later some of these objects are shown to him again, this time together with new objects he had not seen before. If some memory traces remain, the patient will be able to divide the material into two groups, the part that is familiar and the part that is new.

An example of failure to recognize a retained experience as a memory was recorded by Claparède, the founder of the Geneva school of psychologists. He had a patient who had the typical disturbances of memory due to years of alcoholism. To test her memory, he concealed a pin in his hand and stuck it into her fingers while shaking hands. Some minutes later, as he was leaving her, he proffered his hand to shake hands with her again. She pulled her hand away, but she apparently had no idea why she did so. When he asked her why, she said 'But hasn't one the right to withdraw one's hand?' And when she was questioned further, she said that he might have a pin hidden in his hand. When Claparède asked 'What makes you think I want to prick you?' she replied that it was an idea that came into her head. Then, when she was asked to explain this surprising idea, she said 'Sometimes people do have pins hidden in their hands'. But she never remembered that she had been pricked a few minutes before, and she did not recognize these ideas as being based on memory.

Recognition has many degrees; one can recognize something completely, or one may merely recognize it as being vaguely known. There are also degrees in the amount of forgetting. If the material is almost completely forgotten, its buried presence is shown only by the saving of time in re-learning. If it is more easily available, this is indicated by recognition. When it is least buried, it can be mustered by the usual processes of recall.

When something is remembered, it comes back correctly ordered in time. This ordering in time may be a separate function. For where there are defects in remembering, this function alone may be disturbed. The person remembers that he was on the way to Scotland, but he does not remember if the event occurred on his 1985 or 1987 visit. He may remember an event, but cannot relate it in time to other events.

When something is recognized, it evokes a feeling or emotion of familiarity. In fact, familiarity is a necessary part of recognition. Whether this emotion of familiarity is the same as the strong sense of familiarity discussed in Chapter 18, is not known. Certainly, the sense of familiarity occurring before an epileptic fit or that occurring during stimulation of the temporal lobe at operation feels different to the patient from merely recognizing a familiar object or event. But under these abnormal conditions, the emotion is pure and isolated, and so one might well expect it to feel different.

Familiarity is a part of all behaviour. Animals behave differently to something familiar than to something new. What is familiar evokes the previous pattern of behaviour. Something new brings out exploratory behaviour; it may cause a startle reaction; it evokes vigilance. Familiar and not dangerous brings out one kind of behaviour; familiar and dangerous brings out another. But unfamiliar brings out quite different behaviour: careful, vigilant, exploratory, a mixture of curiosity and fear. Recognition being a part of remembering, and familiarity being an essential part of recognition, we see that familiarity is an essential part of remembering.

In certain disturbances of the brain, such as may occur with chronic and prolonged alcoholism or after severe head injuries, material may be registered and retained, yet when it is reproduced, the sense of familiarity is lacking and the subject does not recognize it.

The failure to recognize one's own thoughts as coming from something one has read leads to literary plagiarism. The sense of familiarity and localization in the past does not accompany the thought as it arrives in consciousness. That is why, if one wants to write one's own thoughts, it is essential not to read what other people have written on the subject; one cannot trust one's memory. The mechanisms of recognition may be dormant; and what has been taken in from reading or hearing may appear to be one's own marvellous contribution.

A blow to the head temporarily stops the higher levels of brain function; this is well known and is the condition of concussion. During this time the patient does not always lie pallid on the ground. As many footballers know, he may go on with what he was doing at the time. This state was first described in 1501, by the first great Mogul Emperor, Babur. He wrote in his *Memoirs*:

As I turned round on my seat to see how far I had left them behind, my saddle-girth being slack, the saddle turned round, and I came to the ground right on my head. Although I immediately sprang up and mounted, yet I did not recover the full possession of my faculties till the evening and the world, and all that occurred at the time, passed before my eyes and apprehension like a dream, or a fantasy, and disappeared.

During this time, mental functioning is apparently normal; it is only the continual registration and storage of experience that is not working. Mental testing during this time may reveal that the person is not working at his most efficient intellectual level, or it may not show anything abnormal. The case of one patient has been recorded in which the patient's mental functioning was so good that he learned touch-typing; yet this period was included in the patient's period of absence of memory. Although he always remembered how to type, he never remembered learning the skill. Cases such as this show us that memory for recent events can be normal while complete memory during that period is deranged.

The reproduction of retained material without knowledge that it belongs to oneself may cause some strange abnormalities of memory in patients after head injuries. One patient I saw during the Second World War had a vision of a horse in a cloud as he recovered consciousness. He had a clear view of the horse. He said it was a brown cob, galloping with its head up, coming from right to left. This vision soon passed, and he then became conscious that he was in bed and that two nurses were making his bed. He asked them what had happened. They told him he had had an accident. He then asked whether it was anything to do with a horse, and they replied that they did not know but that he had already told them that it was due to a horse. He himself had no recollection of having spoken to them before, no knowledge that he had had an accident, and no memory of the horse. Later it was confirmed by the police that a runaway horse was the cause of his accident, and that it must have passed by the patient from right to left. Even when the story of the accident was pieced together and told to the patient, he could not remember anything about it; nor could he remember the horse as he saw it in the vision.

Sometimes a vision of what had actually happened occurs suddenly, and the patient does not know why he is seeing this vision. Something, perhaps an episode in a film or the sight of a car, brings the whole event back to his mind, even though he did not know that he had retained any recollection of the event. Professor Ritchie Russell, who studied thousands of cases of head injury over the past forty years, has reported the case of a patient who was injured while standing on a tramway island. He recovered consciousness twelve hours after the head injury. On several occasions in the ensuing weeks he would suddenly have a vision of the huge tyre of a motor lorry bearing down on him, while he threw up his arms unable to escape. In fact this was exactly what had occurred. But the patient could never remember these details of the accident. The vision that spontaneously came into his mind might just as well have happened to someone else.

In cases such as these material has been retained. It is unaccompanied by the usual sense of familiarity or by the feeling of myness, and the patient cannot recall it by voluntary effort.

A patient who has had a severe head injury may come to the doctor two weeks later and say that for the past two weeks he does not know what has happened, that he has no memory of anything that happened since a minute before his accident. During most of this time he may have been normally reading, writing letters, playing cards, as patient do. Although he has been behaving normally, in the true sense of the word he has been unconscious; he recovered consciousness only when he started to have continuous memory. During the period between his head injury and the day when he came to, he remembers either nothing or a few scattered isolated events.

From cases of head injury, we have learned that the first part of memory, the fixation of the experience in memory, takes time. This time varies from a split second to about a minute. On recovering consciousness after a head injury, the patient never remembers this short period. The events that the patient was living through during that time must have been registered in the usual way, for the head injury had not yet occurred. But it is impossible to bring back the memories during this split second or seconds. If the head injury is more severe, the period of permanent absence of memories is longer. The more severe the damage to the brain, the longer this period will be. There may be obliteration of all memories for months or even years: what had been registered and stored has disappeared. The most recent memories disappear with less severe head injuries, the older memories go when there is more severe damage to the brain. Although we usually consider memory as short-term and long-term, these divisions are really matters of degree, the one merging into the other. The longer a memory has been established, the more firmly it is fixed. As time fixes memories, it is those things that have been retained for a short time that may disappear for ever. The result of this for young children is that a severe head injury can sometimes obliterate the child's memories of its entire life before the injury. The child's mental state is then reduced to that for babyhood. Everything he ever learned, he has to learn all over again.

We understand very little of the neural processes underlying the retroactive effects of damage to the brain; we understand still less about the recovery of some of the forgotten material. For sometimes, months after the head injury, when the patient's cerebral processes are again normal, the period of absence of recollections before the head injury shrinks, so that in the end the patient recalls a large period of the time that he had previously forgotten, and he ends up with just a short period of amnesia just before the injury.

When we recall something from the past, we may have to make some mental effort. We search for what we hope we have retained. Exactly what parts of the brain are used for this activity, and what we are doing in terms of the physiology of neurons and synapses, we do not yet know.

Whatever the physiology of this recalling ability is, a conscious effort to look for the past experience is not always the best way of finding it. The retained experience may come to mind spontaneously. After we have suspended control, suddenly what we were trying to remember is there before our eyes. This may also happen when we are asleep; on waking up, we find we have remembered it. Whether the process of searching goes on when we are asleep, we do not know. Certainly, memories may return during dreams, under hypnosis, and during various states of dimmed consciousness. More automatic and less controlled thinking can be more effective for recall than conscious control. And so one should have confidence in unconscious processes of thought to fulfil one's needs. They mostly do so, though they sometimes arrive too late. Only after one has written a paper or given a lecture does one suddenly know how one should have done it.

Memories can be brought to mind by the psychological process of free association. When we do this, we relax, and let one memory bring up another. Sometimes an event reminds us of a similar event that occurred before, or a sensation brings to mind another occasion when the same sensation was experienced. The sense of smell, as is well known to us all, is particularly evocative of memories.

Memory is an important ingredient of creative thinking. Strange as it may seem, creation comes from pouring a great mass of ill-assorted things into the mind, leaving them to ferment, and then getting something new out of it. The mechanism of getting something out is an ability that depends on character as well as on intelligence. It is done with effort, with searching concentration, with merely sitting and waiting, or with sleeping, lying around, or doing other things. A lot has to be put in, and all of it has to be stored. For memory consists of experiencing, retaining the shadow of the experience, and recalling; these are also the essentials of creation.

As the biological purpose of memory would seem to be the organization of present behaviour in the light of previous experience, it is obvious that some sort of classification is necessary. It seems likely that the contents of the mind are classified and cross-indexed in many different ways. When we try to remember something, we can seek it via many different routes. If, for instance, I try to remember the name of a particularly beautiful East African starling, I first remember that the name was that of a German, then that it probably ended in 'dt'. I also know that it is in J. G. Williams's book on *Birds of East and Central Africa*, and that in this book, the colour plate of the starling and the description of the bird are on different pages. And I also remember that this starling has an orange eye. Thus I find that in my mind Hildebrandt's starling is classified under the heading of foreign names of birds, sub-heading German, birds in Williams's book, sub-heading starlings, and most important of all, I have in my filing system a visual picture of the bird, so that I can match a proffered picture of it against my visual memory of it, and then recognize the bird.

It is probable that the more cross-indexing there is, the better. Material is probably classified according to its effect, pleasant or unpleasant, as usual or unusual, as what happens on holidays, as games to be played at silly parties, as nursery rhymes, as jokes to amuse 10-year-old children, and so on.

But this is all armchair psychology, and tells us nothing about how the brain organizes these psychological mechanisms. Penfield has reported the case of an epileptic patient who shows us other aspects of this mechanism of classification. The patient was a young man who would get fits when he saw someone grab something from someone else. On one occasion he saw someone snatching a rifle away from a cadet on parade, on another a man snatching his hat away from the cloakroom attendant; on both occasions he had a fit. Seeing someone grab or snatch something, would immediately produce a vivid recollection of an occasion when he was 13 years old. At this time he was playing with a dog, grabbing a stick from its mouth and throwing it. The patient would associate the two events, become confused, and have a seizure. As Penfield was operating on the left temporal lobe, he stimulated one point, and the patient suddenly cried out: 'There he is!' When Penfield questioned him, he said: 'It was like a spell, he was doing that thing: grabbing something from somebody.' As any sort of grabbing of something from somebody precipitated his fits, this brain must have classified experience to include a category of grabbing something from somebody.

The anatomy of highest-level memory

When we think about the highest-level memory, we have to separate the different kinds of memory that are covered by this one word. There is memory for the events that occurred to one in the distant past, memory for what happened yesterday, and memory for what you read in the sentence before this one.

We have already related how Penfield found that when he stimulated certain parts of the temporal lobes, he brought back memories that the patients did not know they still had. Penfield made many other important contributions to this subject by studying the effects of cutting out parts of the temporal lobes in the treatment of brain tumours and of epilepsy. When large parts of the hippocampus are cut out, the record of a life is cut out with them. It is as if one's memory is a filing cabinet, and someone has taken it away. In principle, just like a tape-recorder, what is stored in a person's memory could be consulted by anyone. We have two ways of doing this. We have the psychological way of asking its owner to tell us what is there; and we have the physiological way of electrically stimulating certain parts of the brain. This aspect of one's memory should perhaps be emphasized, as we regard our memories as so personal, so much a part of ourselves, almost as ourselves. Yet in fact, once the registered experience is stored, it is there to be tapped, almost regardless of us.

Each neuron or each circuit of neurons within the hippocampus is not the repository of something experienced; it is not a kind of pigeon-hole in which a memory is stored. Penfield has emphasized that when he stimulates a little spot of the cortex and this stimulation produces a flashback, cutting out that little spot does not remove the flashback. After it has been cut out, the patient can still remember the whole episode by using his memory in the ordinary way; the remembered event has not gone. It is only when a very large area of the temporal lobes of both hemispheres is destroyed that the entire memory is ruined.

In Chapter 23, certain aspects of a case will be related in which this operation was done. The disastrous result was that the patient could not recognize anybody. He treated his own mother, to whom he had been very attached before the operation, in the same manner as he treated the nurses in hospital, calling her 'Madam', and he no longer showed any emotional attachment for her. Here we see that his sensory input is normal, and that he makes perception from what he receives. He can recognize the moving object as a woman. But the significance of that particular woman depends on previous experience of her; that is to say, it depends on memory. With no remembrance of her, there is no accompanying emotion, such as one is used to having in relation to one's mother. He perceives a woman, and behaves to her as he would to any unknown woman. He 'not only could not remember anything that had happened recently, he could not remember anything of his past'. When the doctors tried to get him to talk about the town he lived in, his own house, his family, he could not answer the questions, and did not seem to understand them, 'as if their object was entirely unknown to him'. The patient lived without a past and without a future.

Scoville, a neurosurgeon working in the United States, tried to help patients with most severe epilepsy and mental disorders by removing or disconnecting the deeper parts of the temporal lobe; the important parts were the uncus and amygdala, and the anterior part of the hippocampus and the hippocampal gyrus. One of his patients was extensively studied by Professor Milner over a period of years. This patient had the most severe loss of recent memory. After the operation, he had completely forgotten everyone in the hospital and could not recognize any of them. He could not find his way about. He did not remember that he had been in hospital before the operation, and had no memory of the previous two years. But he remembered his life before that.

Ten months ago the family moved from their old house to a new one a few blocks away on the same street; the patient still has not learned the new address, though remembering the old one perfectly, nor can he be trusted to find his way home alone Moreover he does not know where objects in continual use are kept; for example, his mother still has to tell him where to find the lawn mower, even though he may have been using it only the day before. She also states that he will do the same jigsaw puzzles day after day without showing any practice effect and that he will read the same magazines over and over again, without finding their contents familiar. This patient has even eaten lunches in front of us without being able to name, a mere half-hour later, a single item of food he had eaten; in fact, he could not remember having eaten luncheon at all.

Yet to a casual observer this man seem like a relatively normal individual, since his understanding and reasoning are undiminished.

The two essential structures for memory are the amygdala and the hippocampus. If either is damaged memory is impaired, but if both are badly damaged on both sides of the brain, the effect is disastrous. It is probable that things are put into the hippocampus for transient storage, pending a decision whether the information is to be passed to other regions for permanent memory.

It has been found in a few patients in whom a large part of the hippocampus has been cut out on one side when the other side is already damaged, that information cannot be stored. They can remember something for a minute or two, but any new event immediately obliterates what has just been experienced. And so, finally, nothing is remembered, and learning is impossible. Professor Milner wrote that she gave one of these patients a number to remember and then went and had lunch. When she came back and asked the patient for the number, he gave it correctly. She then diverted his attention from the number by talking to him about other matters. At the end of that, she asked him for the number again. He said, 'What number?' The conversation in between had washed away all trace of a number to be retained.

In acute and severe alcoholism, a sudden delirium, called delirium tremens, or dt.'s for short, can occur. The person is suddenly very ill and confused; and a few of these patients have frightening hallucinations, such as the traditional pink elephants. The patients are unsteady and have paralyses of the eye muscles, so that they squint and see double. The parts of the brain most severely damaged in this state are regions surrounding the ventricles of the centre of the brain, parts of the hypothalamus and thalamus. When this state is cured or alleviated by the injection of vitamin B, the patients are usually left with confusion, apathy, and indifference to everything, and outstandingly, a severe defect of memory. Chronic alcoholism damages the same parts of the brain; the resulting mental state of these patients is called Korsakoff's psychosis. Although their lack of memory is outstanding, these patients have other intellectual defects as well. They have lost recent memory, although they still retain what happened up to few years before the final damage to the brain. They can hardly learn anything new, as they cannot remember what they have just taken in for more than a few minutes. And of course, if you cannot learn, you cannot remember, for there is nothing in the store to retrieve. But one of the patients described by Korsakoff in 1889 could still play a good game of chess. He could not remember all the moves that had brought about the position of the pieces on the board, but he could still work out the probability of moves yet to be made. These patients fill out the gaps in their memories by confabulating, and the likely stories they make up are often quite convincing.

Cases such as these show us that severe disruption of memory can be due to damage of a small region of the hypothalamus near the ventricle, and to parts of the thalamus. The surgical cases show that memory is also ruined by removal of a large part of the hippocampal regions of both sides of the brain. The hippocampus is directly connected to the relevant part of the hypothalamus. Although the hypothalamus and the thalamus are essential for memory, we do not yet know the relation between these parts and the temporal lobes in the total functioning of remembering.

Total remembering, the storage of what has been experienced, is one kind of memory. The memory necessary for recognition (re-cognition—knowing it again) depends partly on the regions of cortex around each sensory area. Recognizing what we see depends on the visual areas of the occipital lobe, knowledge of things smelt depends on areas around the olfactory area, and so on for other sensations.

There is verbal memory, that is memory for what you heard spoken; a variation of this is memory for what you saw written. These compartments of memory depend on different parts of the cerebral hemispheres. Verbal memory needs the front part of the left temporal lobe. The cortex of this region stores the sounds of words, regardless of their meaning; the sound and the meaning rely on deeper structures of this lobe. Complex visual patterns, such as the human face, are stored in the right temporal lobe. The location of objects in space is automatically coded, and does not need to be learned; this depends on the right temporal lobe. Retaining an internal map so that one knows how to get around one's house, one's town, one's country, depends mainly on the region on the right between the occipital and the parietal lobes. But also patients with damage to the temporal lobes have difficulty in remembering the places they know and how to get about.

For knowing where one is and getting around, one does not have to have such a large and complicated brain as man has. Insects with far simpler brains are good at it. Bees have maps just as people have, with their hives as home. And hunting wasps and ants can be seen climbing to the tops of plants to see where they are.

There is the sort of memory needed in playing cards; you have to remember the cards played by yourself and other people, or the cards that are now lying face downwards on the table. Some people's ability to remember is amazing. Blindfolded chess champions can play twenty games of chess simultaneously. They are told the various moves, announce their own moves, and remember the strategy of twenty games at the same time so well that they win them all. Stanley Spencer said that he never made sketches when he was out walking. For those detailed and realistic paintings of his, such as the *Magnolias* or the *Path Through a Field*, he had remembered everything he had seen when he was out. He remembered the exact appearance of every ear of wheat, of the curls of the petals of the magnolias, of the way the light and shade was laid on every leaf.

People remember in different ways, just as they learn in different ways. Learning a list of words, using rote memory, is quite different from learning the meaning and the contexts of the words; and learning shapes and forms is different from learning words. Each difference means using a different part of the brain. Some people remember more verbally, using the temporal speech area; others remember more visually, using the visual occipital regions. The verbal person says it silently to himself, then repeats this when he recalls it. The visual person sees the situation in his mind's eye, and has a picture of it in his memory.

Perhaps the anatomy of remembering is something like this. When something happens to us, this affects the neurons of all sensory parts of the brain. Something has been seen and experienced. Messages are also sent to the association areas of the cortex, to the speech area, to areas providing us with emotion and feelings. Messages are sent to the hippocampus of both temporal lobes. From there they are sent to lower parts of the brain, to the septal region, the hypothalmus, and the midbrain. When we remember the event, the same parts of the brain that were active when the event was being experienced are reactivated. But these are not exactly the same neurons, for the event is not re-experienced exactly as it was. When we remember, we activate the hippocampus, for the event is either stored there or else the hippocampus contributes essential mechanisms for the storage of memories.

23 Personality and the brain

For he is a mixture of gravity and waggery.

It is only during the last thirty years that research workers in the many branches of neurology have come to investigate the physiology and anatomy of personality. Before then, the subject of character and personality had been left to psychologists and psychiatrists. It may have been reckoned that ultimately this subject would have to be related to the physiology and anatomy of the brain, but it appeared as if everyone had agreed that the time when this correlation would be made would always lie in the future. Freud, who was a neurologist before he invented psychoanalysis, always thought of psychoanalysis as being based on the physiology and anatomy of the nervous system. Yet, as it turned out, psychoanalysis, and especially Jung's contributions, increased the distance between a scientific study of the neural aspects of personality and psychology and psychiatry. Those influenced by Freud, Groddeck, Jung, and their successors, seem to have known nothing of the scientific method. Such psychotherapists established schools, behaving more like priests than scientists.

That the frontal lobes are somehow related to personality could have been deduced during the past eighty years or so. But this did not happen. Most neurological textbooks merely stated that the frontal lobes have to do with man's intellectual attainments. There was no evidence for this belief. It seems to have arisen merely because the frontal lobes are large and well-developed in man, and man is an intellectual animal.

Scattered throughout the pages of medical literature are the names of certain famous patients. We have already mentioned two of these, Dr Beaumont's Alexis St Martin, and Wolf and Wolff's Tom. More incredible is the case of Phineas Gage, reported in the Boston Medical and Surgical Journal of 1848 by Dr J. M. Harlow.

Phineas Gage was a capable and efficient foreman who, in 1848, suffered an extraordinary accident. During some rock-blasting operations, an iron bar 4 feet long was blown through his left cheek and out of the top of his head. The bar entered the left side of his face below his eye, and passed out through the top of his skull. Gage was taken in an ox-cart a distance of three-quarters of a mile, and then about one hour after the injury got out of the cart by himself, and walked from the cart to the surgery. While the doctor examined the hole in his head, Gage 'related the manner in which he was injured to the bystanders'. From the position of the bar it may be deduced that the greater part of the left frontal lobe and the front part of the corpus callosum were destroyed.

This damage to the brain brought about a great change in Gage's personality. Dr Harlow reported that

The equilibrium or balance, so to speak, between his intellectual faculties and animal propensities, seems to have been destroyed. He is fitful, irreverent, indulging in the grossest profanity (which was not previously his custom), manifesting but little deference for his fellows, impatient of restraint or advice when it conflicts with his desires, at times pertinaciously obstinate, yet capricious and vacillating, devising many plans for future operation, which are no sooner arranged than they are abandoned in turn for others appearing more feasible. . . . His mind has radically changed, so decidedly that his friends and acquaintances say he is 'no longer Gage'.

He died, in the words of Dr Harlow 'twelve years, six months and eight days after the date of his injury'. The skull of Phineas Gage is now in the museum of the Medical School of Harvard University.

Until that time, it was generally held that the entire cerebral hemispheres worked as a totality to produce thinking and intellectual activities. But here was a case in which a large amount of the hemispheres had been destroyed, and yet purely intellectual activities had not suffered. Also till that time, it had not been appreciated that the brain had anything to do with personality and character. It was true that this was indeed claimed by the phrenologists, but they had been relegated to the realms of quackery. Here was a case in which the personality and character had been disastrously altered by a lesion of the frontal lobes.

Although the case of Phineas Gage became famous in medical literature, all the implications were not fully grasped. Doctors were amazed that such a large amount of the brain could be damaged and that the patient could walk and talk immediately after the injury, and go on living for years. They were also amazed that so much of the frontal lobes could be damaged without causing a great defect in speech, calculation, and thinking ability. That character and personality could be changed so disastrously came as a striking fact to all who knew about the case; but still no one seems to have drawn conclusions about the frontal lobes being related to personality and social relationships.

For a hundred years or so, no more cases like this were reported, but now there are others. In the Second World War, two officers were playing Russian roulette, a game in which a revolver with one bullet in it is put to the temple and fired. The idea is that the single bullet in one of six chambers will fall to the bottom, this chamber being the heaviest, and that the chamber fired will contain no bullet. An officer put the revolver to his temple and fired, and was surprised to see the face of his friend turn ashen grey. He then put his hand to his temples on both sides, and found they were wet and sticky, and the cause was blood. Realizing that he had shot himself, he fell to the ground. But then he thought that there was no need to fall, that he had done so only because it seemed the correct thing to do, so he got up again, and walked off to see a doctor.

A similar case was reported in March 1977 at Troyes in France. A workman had a quarrel with his wife, told her he was going to put an end to his life, left the room, and returned in a few minutes saying: 'Ça y est, je me suis suicidé.' His wife took no notice of this histrionic remark. She did notice a few drops of blood on his pillow in the morning, but did not think anything of it. But her husband seemed a little odd all day, and could not remember that it was Friday, although he was repeatedly told what day it was. The wife and son thought they had better go and see the doctor, owing to his defective memory and odd behaviour. They all walked to the doctor next day. An X-ray examination of his head showed two bullets from a rifle in the front of his brain. The man had never said anything about it, apart from his first announcement, as he could not remember what he had done.

So we see that the front part of the brain is not necessary for living; one can pass in a crowd without it. Not only the frontal lobes are important for character and general behaviour; parts of the temporal lobes are also of fundamental importance. In Chapter 13, the role of these structures was recounted, both as it appears in strange forms in epilepsy and as it can be seen on the electrical stimulation of the brain. The main mass of the temporal lobes have been removed bilaterally in the monkey by Klüver and Bucy. As these monkeys could not recognize any object by vision, the connecting nerve fibres between visual areas and the amygdala and hippocampus having been divided, they brought all objects to their mouths, smelling, tasting and chewing them. But in addition to this, the hypothalamic areas for eating and for sexuality had become disinhibited. The monkeys would chew sticks and ate meat, which these monkeys never do. They had the same voracious appetite for sexual activities. They masturbated the whole time, and regarded both female and male monkeys, and even cats and cushions, as legitimate sexual objects. Later experiments in which only limited regions of the temporal lobes were removed showed that one area was responsible for limiting the excessive sexual activity and another area for limiting the voracious appetite.

The animals with the temporal lobes removed showed an abnormal passivity and lack of aggression. The operations in which the commissures connecting the two hemispheres were divided have now been combined with removal of the amygdala on one side of the brain. At first the optic chiasm, the corpus callosum, the anterior commissure, and the hippocampal commissure are divided in a ferocious macaque monkey. This produces a monkey in which things seen with the right eye go only to the right side of the brain and things seen with the left eye go only to the left side. The situation is illustrated in Fig. 23.2. There is no connection between the two sides of the brain; but unless one makes special tests on such abilities as the transfer of training, one will not recognize that this monkey's brain is abnormal. Now the tip of the right temporal lobe including the amygdala is cut out. Normally cutting out one amygdala has no effect; one has to remove both to get the results described by Klüver and Bucy. An amazing thing is now found. If the right eye of the monkey is covered with an eye-shield, it sees people with its left eye, and this eye is connected to the amygdala in a normal manner. The monkey reacts to people in its usual way, emotionally and aggressively. Now the left eye is covered, and the monkey sees people with its right eye; but this eye has no connections with the amygdala, for it has been removed. The animal is now quite indifferent and docile when he sees human beings. As Downer, who did these remarkable experiments, wrote: 'One can in effect "remove" and "replace" the amygdala, and thereby change the animal's emotional state, merely by opening and closing the appropriate eye.' We are seeing two totally different personalities in one monkey. One half of the brain makes the monkey behave in its usual aggressive way towards people. The other half makes it behave in a docile manner to the very same people.

Similar operations have been carried out on patients in North America before it was understood what disastrous effects would occur. Those patients who have effectively had the amygdaloid nuclei removed on both sides of the brain show a similar increase in sexual behaviour, combined with a lack of the conventional social inhibitions. They also have a voracious appetite for food. One of these patients ate as much as four normal people. They tend to eat anything, with no preferences for any particular food. One patient was observed 'to look for a secluded corner far from anyone, eat everything voraciously, lick the dish incessantly, and after fifteen minutes asked for more'. Another patient, whose case has been well documented by Terzian and Dalle Ore, had this operation performed on account of extremely severe epilepsy originating in these parts of the brain, and uncontrollable outbreaks of aggression and rage, making him dangerous to everyone, including himself. He also had terrifying hallucinations and automatic behaviour during which he often tried to strangle people or to commit suicide; at times he would fly at people, including the doctors. After two operations, one on each temporal lobe, the

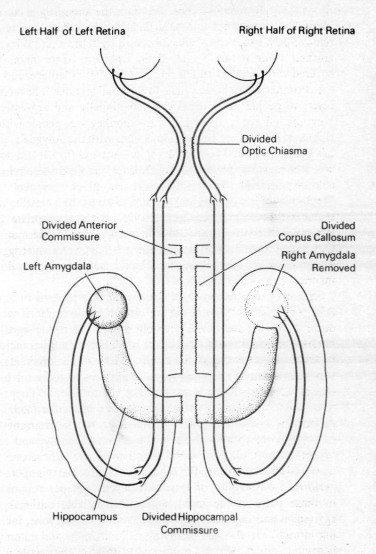

Left Half of Left Retina

Right Half of Right Retina

Divided
Optic Chiasma

Divided Anterior
Commissure

Divided
Corpus Callosum

Right Amygdala
Removed

Left Amygdala

Hippocampus

Divided Hippocampal
Commissure

Fig. 23.1 Diagram to illustrate experiment in which the corpus callosum, other commissures, and the optic chiasm are cut through; in addition the right amygdala has been cut out.

patient's personality was completely changed. He showed no aggression and no emotion of any sort. Terzian and Dalle Ore reported:

The patient no longer manifested the slightest rage reactions towards the nurses and doctors upon whom before the second operation he used to rush as soon as they came into sight. The patient on the contrary now assumed an extremely childish and meek behaviour with everyone and was absolutely resistant to any attempt to arouse aggressiveness and violent reactions in him. He was completely indifferent towards everyone, including his parents.

He not only expressed no emotion, it was clear that he felt none. He was unable to display emotion to such an extent that even his voice became monotonous. His face usually wore 'a conventional and unmotivated smile. An emotional expression was noticed in the patient's face only once when he saw his image in a mirror, betraying a childish satisfaction because he had found human features in a lifeless object.'

When neurologists and psychiatrists learned of the importance of the temporal lobes for controlling and organizing drives, such as sex, hunger, and aggression, they began to examine some psychotics and aggressive psychopaths to see if they had abnormalities in their temporal lobes. In fact, brain tissue damage is a rare cause of such abnormalities of personality.

At the same time as we were learning about the effects of removing the anterior deep parts of the temporal lobes upon personality, similar observations were being made on the effects of removing the anterior parts of the frontal lobes in chimpanzees. After this operation, the animals became lethargic and apathetic; they no longer took any interest in life. And, what turned out to be more important, the animals no longer became worked up or upset about things. If, before the operation, a chimpanzee had been upset by failure to do a psychological test, after the operation it no longer cared.

Damage of the same sort as that caused by this operation to both frontal lobes may occur in man. It often results from people trying to shoot themselves without knowing how to do it properly. They usually put the barrel of the revolver against the right temple, and fire. If this does not kill them, and it may well not do so, it usually causes what is called a through-and-through gunshot wound; the bullet goes through one side of the head and comes out of the other. It commonly damages one or both optic nerves, making the person blind in one or both eyes. What may also happen in such patients is that, after this damage to the frontal lobes, the depression has gone. Their personalities are now more like those of the chimpanzees with front parts of the frontal lobes removed. They are indifferent to everything.

In the wars and the everyday violence that characterize the present century, damage to the frontal lobes occurs. The strange kind of indifference that is a feature of damage to the front parts of the frontal lobes is made clear if I quote from the notes I made on a patient I saw in Italy during the war in 1944. The patient was a lieutenant in the New Zealand army. He was picked up soon after being wounded, and it was noted that his brain was oozing out of the wound in front of his head. When he was operated upon twenty-four hours later, the roofs of both his orbits were found to be shattered, and the front of the brain on both sides was reduced to pulp. Twenty-one days after the injury, his state was as follows:

His condition is best described as one of apathy. He lies in bed doing nothing and responds to nothing, except that sometimes he follows with his eyes anything that is happening. He leaves his lit cigarette on the bed; he holds up the paper in front of him as if he is reading it, when it is put in his hand. Recently I observed him lying on his back with the paper held up in front of him; on his chest was the feeding cup where someone had put it, and the spout was between his lips; but he was making no attempt to drink from it, nor did he put it down, he just lay there with the feeding cup full of tea touching his lips, his paper in his hand; and he did nothing. The greater part of the day he spends sleeping or lying on his bed with a paper held in front of him, pretending to read it, but never turning over the pages; however when I handed it to him upside down, he did turn it the right way up.

But this is not the whole picture, for he does sometimes get up and put on some of his clothes, go to the table to eat or look out of the window. Such activities are done with an intense preoccupation with what he is doing at the moment and an equal indifference to any circumstances relating to other people. What he does, he carries out perfectly, as he puts on his shoes and laces them, eats his food with the other officers with correct manners; he spreads jam on his bread and cuts it and makes a sandwich of it all neatly. While I was talking to him and trying to take a medical history from him, he got up, put on the top of his pyjamas and went and looked out of the window, all while I was asking him questions and attempting to examine him; he went through these activities just as if I were not there. As I talked to him and examined him, he repeatedly stretched out to get a cigarette and light it, although I kept moving them away from him. I had the impression that each time he began again, he did not realize that he was not to do it. Once as he walked about the ward, he defecated while walking, showing no interest in this act whatsoever.

His speech is entirely normal and he seems to understand everything or at least everything simple. It seems to need much effort for him to speak, and he does not make this effort.

This picture of apathy and total indifference to social relations does not last, though the amount of recovery varies from case to case. Actually, that young man's father wrote to me from New Zealand eight years later, and told me that his son had eventually made a good recovery and satisfactory adjustment. However, after such lesions the patients are usually left with some degree of apathy or restlessness, tactlessness, and lack of self-control, difficulty in maintaining attention, and thus difficulty in learning and in planning, easy fatigability, and a lack of interest in things and other people.

Patients with damage to this part of the frontal lobes also lose spontaneity of speech. Even if they do answer questions, this seems to be an effort for them, and their answers are very brief. They often merely repeat the question they have just heard, but making the question into a negative or affirmative, without any elaboration, and they give up when they are asked to discuss the question further.

In 1935, Moniz, a neurologist working in Portugal, came to the conclusion that if the operation of dividing the frontal lobes from the rest of the brain reduces the anxiety and frustration of the chimpanzees, it would probably do the same in patients. He therefore invented the operation of prefrontal leucotomy for the treatment of certain psychiatric patients.

The first results obtained with prefrontal leucotomy were the same as those obtained in the chimpanzee. When much of the frontal lobe was divided from the rest of the brain, the patients had no energy, and they showed little spontaneous activity arising from internal motivation. In most severely afflicted patients, the lack of initiative was such that the patient would stay in bed until he was got out of it. If food was put in his mouth, he may have done nothing about it, merely leaving it there without chewing or swallowing it. When the effects of the operation were less damaging, the patients were just placid: whatever they did, they did slowly and without much interest. They lacked emotion, or rather they lacked any persistence in emotion. They often had sufficient insight to explain that since the operation they had no feelings. As one previously hypomanic and intelligent patient put it: 'I am dull, a bore, and I know it.' These patients did not have enough initiative to start doing anything, and they could not concentrate for long. The patients who were less damaged could carry on a routine, doing the things that they knew well how to do. But they undertook no new projects, made no plans and lived without enthusiasm. Intelligence was unimpaired.

A further feature of these disastrous operations was that the patients were distractable. They would show a momentary interest in anything that came along, and would let this interfere in the plan of what they were carrying out. Nothing was irrelevant; everything might be attended to and allowed to interrupt the current activity. Thus, the patient's behaviour was fragmentary and inconsistent. What was worse, they were uninhibited. Some were sexually disinhibited; some ate excessively. Although they were not aggressive, they could easily lose their tempers, particularly when their distracted activities were interrupted. They were unable to resist the first impulse that occurred to them, and these impulses were not curbed by the reactions of other people, as they had lost much of their feeling for others and also the ordinary social inhibition. A patient who had had a leucotomy would start undressing and going to bed in front of his guests because he felt sleepy.

A much smaller operation, consisting of cutting the white matter of the lower part of the front end of the frontal lobe, is still done.

This operation helps more than half the patients with severe chronic depression and the same proportion of patients with very severe obsessional neurosis; it is best for the patients with agitated depression, those who cannot settle or rest, who are actively tormented by worry and anxiety as well as by depression.

From observations on neurotic or psychotic patients it is hazardous to draw conclusions concerning how these various parts of the brain contribute to our personalities. But recent investigations of patients with destruction of the front parts of the brain that occurred in Americans in their war against Vietnam have confirmed these findings on patients with leucotomies.

It may be concluded that the amount of energy one has depends on the frontal lobes. Damage to one frontal lobe causes different defects in personality from damage to the other lobe. To consider the frontal lobe as one entity is inadequate. For damage to the upper part of the front of the lobe causes different defects from damage to the orbital region, that is the part that lies above the orbits and behind the eyebrows. The ability to sustain attention depends on the right lobe and on its upper or dorsal part. Patients with this part of the right frontal lobe damaged are more psychologically upset than those with damage to the left lobe.

The frontal lobes are not particularly the region of the brain concerned with the intellectual attainments. The popular concept of a highbrow with a tall forehead fits better with someone with hydrocephalus, associated often with defective intellectual ability.

Clearly, the frontal lobes are necessary for many aspect of living. They are important for establishing the social feelings and reactions that we learn in childhood. The control of instinctual endowments needed for living in a community partly depends on the frontal lobes. They have been affected by the experience of living, by years of upbringing, and by our knowledge of how to relate ourselves to other human beings.

Not the whole of the frontal lobes are devoted to these general activities. The parts in front of the primary motor region are also concerned with movements, with turning, with speaking and swallowing, with all the skills we have learned. The parts nearest the mid-line are also related to the hypothalamus. These are the parts of the brain used for the control of the bowels and the bladder, and they are also concerned with sexual activity. When this part of the brain is removed, none of these activities are controlled; they are no longer fitted into the rest of the patient's living, and tend to lead an independent existence, the bowel and bladder emptying when they are full, and sexual urges demanding immediate gratification.

When the changes and deteriorations of old age affect the brain, the results vary according to what parts are chiefly affected. It is common for the memory to go, as we all know. When the memory becomes severely impaired, learning is no longer possible. Commonly, when intellectual capacities are much diminished, the senile person confabulates. Perhaps the ability to recollect if an event is a part of one's own past or is something one has heard about becomes disturbed; and this may contribute to apparent confabulation.

Similar changes are seen in the realms of personality, of emotion, of social relationships. The senile person is less able to control his emotion, or rather the manifestations of emotion; yet most of such people will say that the emotions they are showing are not deep. They may cry if they see anything sentimental or are reminded of an emotional occasion. Patients relate that they cry when they hear 'God Save the Queen' played in a crowd.

When the oldest parts of the temporal lobes degenerate, the effects are similar to those produced by removal of these parts at operation. One such patient would stuff everything into her mouth, which included her flowers and handkerchiefs, and would chew and try to swallow them. When the front parts of the frontal lobes become atrophic, the patient loses finer sensibilities, and may become indifferent to the feelings of others. As the lobes become more atrophic behaviour becomes more ruled by the needs of the moment and less cognizant of social requirements. One patient I saw threw a chamber pot out of the window of a top floor of the house; she explained that, as she had finished with it, she threw it away. These old people become indifferent to personal appearance; the preening instinct ceases to be important. Certain basic features of their personalities come out. The obsessional personality becomes more marked; rituals and compulsions dominate their lives, the patient worries about the few things he has to do, and cannot think of anything else. The choleric person loses his temper even more readily. The jovial person becomes fatuous. The ability to make use of symbols deteriorates. The patient still understands the concrete, but no longer understands abstractions.

When intelligence decreases, the patient can no longer read a book, but can still read the newspaper. For he cannot remember enough of the book to keep the general scheme in mind or to remember the plot of a novel; but he may still have enough memory to remember the theme of an article or an essay. He has difficulty in composing letters, in thinking what to write, though he still retains the mechanical part of writing. When the right parieto-occipital region of the cortex atrophies. the old person has great difficulty in finding his way about. This may not be noticed as long as he remains at home; but it becomes clear if he is taken away. When these patients come to hospital, they cannot find their way to the bathroom, and on returning to the ward they do not remember which is their bed. This difficulty in getting their bearings is always worse at night, in the dark. In the daytime, there are numbers of sensory clues, everything is clearly seen. At night, they may have to feel their way about, the light being inadequate to show up the total environment.

Eventually their exhibition of facile emotions goes off, and they become indifferent to everything. This indifference of senility may perhaps be a further stage in the contentment of later middle age that comes when desires have become less urgent and demanding. Between the indifference of age and the urgency of youth, there may be a period of serenity—or is that saying too much?

What we are seeing when the cortex becomes atrophic is the decay of the functions organized by this part of the cerebral hemispheres. According to the principle deduced by Hughlings Jackson, the most recently acquired functions disintegrate first, leaving the oldest established to the end. He also pointed out that when the higher level of function goes, the lower level one is released and manifested in an exaggerated form. The higher functions are often related to lower functions by exerting an inhibition on them, and this inhibition is removed when the higher functions go off.

One cannot sum up in a few well-chosen words the relation

between the cerebral hemispheres and the hypothalamus and the thalamus—mainly because we do not really know what it is. It is not simply, as the early psychoanalysts conjectured, that there are lower parts which are a pool of instinctual urges, controlled by the educated and trained cerebral hemispheres above. The relationship between the two levels of the brain is a reciprocal one. Each part can bring the other part into activity, and then the two parts of the brain work together.

It is on account of the reciprocal and intimate relation between the cerebral hemispheres and the hypothalamus and thalamus that psychotherapy is possible. The whole of our nervous systems, and secondarily of our bodies, can be influenced by all we experience, all we hear. Frequently repeated persuasion and explanation, the awakening of emotion, the reliving of experience, and re-awakening of memories; all of this can have effects on our personalities and behaviour because the cerebral hemispheres influence the rest of the brain. The hypothalamus controls the autonomic nervous system and the endocrine system of the body, and in turn they affect many parts of the brain. Patients find it very difficult to understand how 'just talk' can help them or even cure their ills. But everything we have ever experienced and which made us what we are has entered our brains through some sensory channel, through the skin, the nose, the eyes, or the ears. For us humans, a good deal of it has entered via the ears, in the form of speech. And so there is no reason why further talking should not continue to affect us and influence our personalities.

The discoveries obtained from using the scientific method of investigating the universe and everything in it proceed at a great rate, possibly at a frightening rate. Lest we have some illusions about what science can do, we should be clear about one thing. Science brings knowledge, and this knowledge allows us to make new things, to change the world, and to have new ideas. But science does not bring happiness, except perhaps to those whose lives are dedicated to its service.

Glossary

Weights and measures are now expressed in SI units (Système International d'Unités)

Å = Ångstrom unit = 0.1 nanometre = 10^{-10} metre.

acetylcholine: the transmitter used by vertebrate motoneurons, parasympathetic neurons, and by some sympathetic neurons.

adrenal glands: a pair of endocrine glands resting on the kidneys. They consist of two parts, the adrenal cortex and the adrenal medulla. The cortex forms hormones playing a part in metabolism of carbohydrates, fats, and minerals, in sex, growth, and response to all sorts of stress. The medulla supplies the body with adrenalin and noradrenalin, which are needed for activity.

adrenalin: one of the two hormones secreted by the adrenal gland, and also emitted by neurons as a transmitter.

adrenocorticotrophin (ACTH): a hormone secreted by the pituitary gland that stimulates the adrenal cortex to release its hormones.

afferent nerves: nerves taking impulses to the central nervous system.

amino acids: chemical substances containing an amino group (NH_2), a carboxyl group (COOH), a hydrogen atom, and another group, attached to a central carbon atom. Amino acids are the components of proteins; there are about 300 amino acids in a protein.

amygdala or amygdaloid nuclei: large groups of neurons in the front part of the temporal lobe.

anion: a negative ion.

anterior horn: the anterior part of the grey matter of the spinal cord, in which the motoneurons lie.

anthropoids: a sub-order of the primates. Living forms of anthropoids are the chimpanzee, gibbon, gorilla, man, and orang-utan.

aphasia: a difficulty in organizing language, there being no paralysis of the muscles needed for making the sounds of speech.

arthropod: a member of the largest division of the animal kingdom, which includes insects, spiders, and crustaceans, animals characterized by having an exoskeleton and externally jointed limbs.

axon: the central part of the nerve fibre. It is an elongated process of a neuron, usually single, sometimes double or triple, which conducts nerve impulses over long distances in the central and peripheral nervous systems.

brain stem: the parts of the brain between the cerebral hemispheres and the spinal cord, including the medulla oblongata, pons, and midbrain.

calcite: calcium carbonate

cation: a positive ion.

cerebellum: part of the brain superficially resembling the cerebrum, hence its name of little cerebrum. It is usually considered to be part of the brain, but W. S. Gilbert (1882) established another convention, thus:

> When in that House M P.'s divide,
> If they've a brain and cerebellum, too,
> They've got to leave that brain outside,
> And vote just as their leaders tell 'em to.

cerebral cortex: grey matter of the cerebral hemispheres, forming the outermost part of the hemispheres.

cerebral hemispheres: the largest and most recently evolved part of the brain.

cerebrospinal fluid: liquid circulating throughout the ventricles of the brain, and surrounding the whole of the central nervous system. When a patient has a lumbar puncture, some of this fluid is taken by means of a needle introduced between two vertebrae in the lower back.

cerebrum: the two cerebral hemispheres.

cholinergic: nerve fibres emitting acetylcholine as transmitter substance.

cholinesterase: enzyme that breaks down acetylcholine into inert choline and acetic acid.

cilia: fine motile hairs that are outgrowths of cells. Their arrangement is the same in all organisms, there being a ring of nine with two in the centre.

code: a system of signals used to convey information.

commissure: a transversely running band of nerve fibres connecting homologous parts of the central nervous system across the mid-line.

confabulate: to recount made-up experiences glibly, mostly about oneself; it is done to fill in gaps in the memory, or to try and put sense into a state of confusion.

convergence: the principle according to which many neurons send their axons to a few neurons, thus bringing much information to a few channels.

corpus callosum: large commissure joining the two cerebral hemispheres together.

cortex: Latin for the bark of a tree; used in anatomy to mean the outer layers of any structure.

cutaneous: adjective pertaining to the skin.

cytoplasm: the living components of plant or animal cells, apart from the nucleus. Together with the nucleus, it forms the protoplasm.

DNA: deoxyribonucleic acid. A long thread-like molecule which is the hereditary material of the cell; it reproduces itself, and provides the cell with instructions for making proteins.

dendrite: a branching process of a neuron, specialized for receiving nerve impulses from other neurons.

divergence: the principle according to which one or a few neurons send branching axons far and wide to many neurons, thus sending information to many parts of the nervous system.

dopamine: a monoaminergic transmitter substance.

echo-location: echo-ranging: a method for finding objects and measuring distances utilizing the time taken for sound waves to travel.

efferent nerves: nerves taking impulses away from the central nervous system.

electroencephalogram: the waves of change of electrical potential of the cerebral hemispheres recorded by means of electrodes fixed to the scalp.

electrolyte: a chemical substance that can form ions.

encephalopathy: disease of the brain. Wernicke's encephalopathy is a disorder affecting particularly the hypothalamus due to lack of vitamin B and chronic alcoholism.

endocrine gland: a gland which passes its secretion into the bloodstream directly and not through a duct or pipe.

enzyme: a protein which speeds up metabolic activities.

epilepsy: a disease characterized by the spontaneous or induced discharge of groups of neurons of the forebrain.

ethology: the scientific study of the behaviour of animals in their normal environment.

excitability: a characteristic of cells that allows them to respond to irritation; very marked in neurons and receptors.

excitation: the process of arousing a cell or a group of cells or an organism into activity.

extensor muscles: the muscles that straighten out the back and the limbs.

feedback: a term borrowed from radio technicians to mean the diversion of a small part of the output to control the input. It occurs both in natural and in man-made systems.

firing: the neuron is said to fire when it sends off a nerve impulse.

flexor muscles: the muscles that bend the trunk and limbs.

forebrain: the part of the brain in front of the midbrain.

fovea: a small area of the retina composed of cones; light rays are automatically focused here for greatest visual resolution.

fusimotor: the name for motoneurons or nerves going to the small muscle fibres within the muscle spindle.

GABA: inhibitory transmitter.

ganglion or ganglion cells: a group of nerve cells collected together having a common function.

grey matter: the parts of the central nervous system made up mainly of neurons.

gyrus: smooth folds of the cerebral hemispheres and cerebellum.

hair-follicle: a little sac in the skin from which a hair grows. It is supplied by several nerve fibres.

hallucination: perception of a non-existent object.

hippocampus: a part of the temporal lobe of the cerebral hemisphere, of great importance for memory.

homeostasis: the capacity of animals to preserve a constant composition in the face of a changing environment.

hormone: chemical substance secreted by endocrine glands or neurons.

horseshoe crab: an ancient and primitive arthropod.

hypothalamus: the central and basal parts of the brain.

Hz: 1 Hz = 1 cycle per second.

inertia: a fundamental property of matter, making it resist change in its motion.

inhibition: the opposite of excitation.

ion: an electrically charged particle of an electrolyte, carrying either a positive or a negative charge.

kinaesthesis or kinaesthesia: the sense of the movements and / or position of parts of the body.

lsd: lysergic acid diethylamide. It causes hallucinations and abnormal behaviour.

lesion: damage to tissues by trauma or disease: may be made surgically as treatment or for experiments on animals kept in laboratories.

limbic lobe or limbic system: a group of nuclei within the brain that are essential for feeling and expressing emotion and instinctual drives, such as sex, aggression, fear, eating, drinking.

mammals: vertebrates with mammary glands and hair.

medulla: the marrow or inner part of any structure.

medulla oblongata: the lowest part of the brain, situated immediately above the spinal cord.

membrane: a boundary layer forming the walls of cells or tissues.

membrane, basilar: a layer within the inner ear which is thrown into folds when sound waves are transmitted to the inner ear.

membrane, tectorial: a layer within the inner ear covering the receptor cells.

metabolism: the life process of cells and organisms, comprising the building of tissues, anabolism, and the breaking down of tissues, catabolism.

midbrain: the part of the brain above the pons and below the hypothalamus and thalamus.

migraine: a particular sort of headache, characteristically restricted to one side of the head; hence the name, which is a contraction of hemicrania.

millisecond: ms: 10^{-3} second.

molecule: smallest particle of a substance that retains all the properties of a larger mass of the same material.

monoamines: the chemical substances used for monoaminergic transmission in the central and the peripheral sympathetic nervous systems.

motor end-plate: the special end-organ where the nerve fibre terminates in the muscle.

muscle: a tissue of animal bodies consisting of protein fibres which contract when they are stimulated. Organs such as the heart and the bladder are made almost entirely of muscle. Limbs consist essentially of muscles attached to bones which are hinged at joints.

muscle spindle: receptors of the muscles.

myelin sheath: a fatty sheath surrounding axons of myelinated nerve fibres.

myelinated nerve fibres: nerve fibres surrounded by myelin sheaths.

myo-neural junction: another word for neuro-muscular junction.

μ**m:** micrometre: 10^{-6} m.

nerve fibre: the long process of a neuron consisting of the axon surrounded by supporting cells.

nerve impulse: the brief activity passing along nerve fibres that constitutes the message. It is usually detected in experimental investigations by the electrical phenomena; but there are other aspects of it, such as visual and thermal phenomena and chemical events.

neuroglia: cells needed for the nutrition and support of neurons in the central nervous system.

neuron: nerve cell: the essential conducting unit of the nervous system. It consists of cell-body, dendrites, and one or more axons.

neuro-muscular junction: the modified synapse where nerve impulses are transmitted to the muscle.

noradrenalin: the main transmitter of the sympathetic nervous system; also used in the central nervous system.

nucleus: a collection of neurons grouped together, all having the same function.

oestrogen: any compound which acts as a female sex hormone.

olive: a structure in the medulla oblongata consisting of neurons and making an eminence on the surface, which recalled an olive to earlier anatomists.

ommatidium: the unit of the compound eye of arthropods.

optic chiasm: the point of crossing of the optic nerves behind the two orbits.

optical isomers: chemical substances having the same composition and the same molecular weight, but different properties with regard to the transmission of light.

oval window: small membrane covered opening between middle and inner ear.

ovary: egg-producing organ in the female animal and plant.

parasympathetic nerves: a system of motor nerves going to viscera; their main neurotransmitter is acetylcholine. In general, the action of these nerves is the opposite of the sympathetic nerves.

peptides: a class of chemical compounds formed of two or more amino acids; they are linked together as follows—NH = CO. Depending on the number of amino acids in the molecule, they are called di-, tri-, tetra-peptides, and so on. Proteins are made up of many peptides.

perception: the interpretation of sensation.

piezoelectric effect: when certain crystals are subjected to mechanical stress they produce an electric charge. Conversely when a charge is applied to such a crystal, the crystal shows a slight change in dimensions. This principle is used in making high-frequency loud speakers, microphones, and gramophone pick-ups.

polarity: a field or circuit in which ions and electrons are flowing between positive and negative poles.

pons: the part of the brain situated immediately above the medulla oblongata.

posterior horn: the posterior part of the grey matter of the spinal cord in which afferent neurons lie.

potential, electric: the work done on or by a unit positive charge as it moves from infinity to some point in an electric field, or as it moves from one point to another in an electric field.

primates: order of mammals characterized by having nails on some of the digits. Living forms of primates are the tree-shrews, lemurs, tarsiers, monkeys, and anthropoids, including man.

progesterone: hormone concerned with pregnancy, produced by the ovary.

proteins: a class of compounds made up of 100 to 1,000,000 molecules of 20 amino acids, joined together as peptides. Many biological proteins are active, and perform all the functions of living cells.

RNA: ribonucleic acid; it has a long thread-like molecule consisting of a single polynucleotide chain. Messenger RNA carries the information encoded in DNA to the sites of protein synthesis outside the nucleus of the cell.

receptor: a neuron or a non-nervous cell specialized to respond to stimuli from the external or internal environment. If the receptor is not itself a neuron, it converts forms of energy into nerve impulses.

reciprocal innervation: organization making a muscle relax when the muscle with an opposing action contracts.

reflex: an innate, stereotyped, immediate response of muscle or gland to a particular stimulus, involving the central nervous system. 'Reflex' is both an adjective and a noun.

round window: small membrane-covered opening between middle and inner ear.

Schwann cells: cells surrounding and nourishing nerve fibres of the peripheral nervous system. They form the myelin sheaths of peripheral myelinated nerve fibres.

sensitive period: the time during which the nervous system is best prepared to develop a program depending on its inherited proclivity.

serotonin: a monoaminergic neurotransmitter.

servo-mechanism: automatic mechanism in which the output is partly controlled by feeding back a part of the output to the controlling elements.

sex hormones: masculinizing or feminizing hormones produced in the testes and ovaries. These steroid chemicals cause the secondary sexual characteristics. Their production and release into the bloodstream is controlled by the pituitary.

sign or signal: the element in a communication system that carries the information.

somatic: having to do with the skeletal part of the body, being opposed to 'visceral', having to do with the internal organs. Often used as the adjective for body, as in somatotrophic, making the body grow.

species: a basic unit of classification of all living organisms. All members of a species have the same set of genes.

steroids: chemical substances with the characteristics of lipids. They have a particular chemical configuration, with at least 17 carbon atoms and four rings.

swim-bladder: a thin-walled sac lying in the body cavity in front of the vertebral column in fish, filled with gas, and used in helping the fish live at various depths with their different pressures.

sympathetic nerves: a system of motor nerves going to blood-vessels, sweat glands, and viscera; their main neurotransmitter in mammals is noradrenalin. In general, the action of these nerves is the opposite of the parasympathetic nerves.

synapse: the region where two or more neurons meet, and where impulses are passed from one to the others (divergence) or from others to one (convergence).

testosterone: a steroid hormone produced by the interstitial cells of the testis, causing masculinization.

thalamus: a large ovoid mass of nuclei in the centre of the cerebral hemisphere, consisting chiefly of relays between the cerebral cortex and lower level structures of the central nervous system.

tissue: a group of cells with the same structure and with the same or similar function. The body of a plant or animal is considered to be made up of many kinds of tissues.

vertebrate: an animal having a backbone.

vertigo: sensation of rotation in which either the surroundings seem to rotate around the subject or the subject seems to rotate.

white matter: the parts of the central nervous system made up mainly of nerve fibres.

Index

abacus, 273
acceleration, 71, 72, 75–6
acetylcholine, 97, 98, 99, 100, 101, 105–6, 363
acromegaly, 199
action potential, 84–5, 87, 130
acupuncture analgesia, 161–3
adenosine triphosphate, 99
Adler, Alfred, 310
adrenal glands, 143–4, 363
adrenalin, 97, 99, 100, 102, 103, 183, 199, 203, 363
adrenocorticotrophin, 203–4, 363
advertising industry, 246
aggression, 147, 150, 170, 171, 172, 182–3, 188, 203, 206–7, 254, 352
alarm calls, 244
alarm reaction, 187
alcoholism, 335, 336, 344–5
Aldini, H., 222
Alexander the Great, 248
alexia, acquired, 292–3
algae, 68
alimentary canal, 183, 184
ambidextrous people, 283, 290
amnesia, 337–9, 342–3
amphibia, early, 34
amputation, and painful phatom limbs, 153, 156–7, 158, 265–6, 324–5
amygdala, 185, 186, 196, 230, 252, 262, 329, 343, 344
analgesia: acupuncture, 161–3; chemical, 156, 159–60; conditioned, 160–1; electrically induced, 159; local anaesthetics, 88, 326
androgens see testosterone
anencephalics, 113, 167, 278
anger, 183, 187, 231, 234
angina, 101
angular gyrus, 283, 284
antelopes, 134, 135, 182
ants, 7, 56, 300

anxiety, 133, 150–1, 183, 229–30
aphasia, 280, 285–7, 291
Aplysia (marine snail), 179, 302
Aristotle, 152, 195, 204, 208
arithmetic, 219, 263
Aschoff, J., 178
aspirin, 156
association: areas, 216; fibres, 277–8; of ideas, 277–8
astronauts, 76
Aubrey, J., 151
auditory cortex, 261–2
aura of epilepsy, 221–2, 231
automatic behaviour, 239–40
autonomic nervous system, 179–84
aversive centres, 168–9
axon, 3, 84, 87, 103, 363
axonal transport, 103

babbling, 278
babies: and sucking, 177; hearing of, 278–9; play of, 122; reflexes of 109–10, 113–14; sense of smell of, 47; sounds of, 278; vision of, 255, 256
Babur, Mogul Emperor, 337
bacteria, 68
Baker, Robin, 69
balance, 70–5, 77, 116–19
ballet dancers, 131, 276
Bancaud, J., 227
Bartholow, Roberts, 222
basal ganglia, 71, 118–19
basic functions of living, 132–3
basilar membrane, 28–9, 30, 31, 35
bats, 32, 37–43, 148
bears, 55, 134
Beaumont, Dr., 149
bees, 7, 20, 36, 48, 52–3, 55, 68–9, 267, 302
Beethoven, Ludwig van, 272
birds, 20, 21, 22, 33–4, 43–4, 69, 104,

birds (cont.):
137, 142, 145, 188, 192, 195, 211, 243,
247, 248, 267, 271, 308; see also under
individual birds
bitter taste, 58
bladder, 64, 70
Blakemore, C., 259
blindness, 39, 250, 251–5, 293, 304–5
blindsight, 260
blood pressure, 101, 102, 151
blushing, 88
body awareness, 264–6
bombykol, 53
bone, damage to, 154
boredom, 147, 310
Bouillaud, J., 220
Bourne, Geoffrey, 272
boxing, 187
braille, 293, 304–5
brain, 3–4, 7–8, 140, 155; bullets
through, 350–1; electrical stimulation
of, 159, 165–6, 167–8, 171, 173–4,
222–39, 331–3; gender of, 193; motor
areas of, 216–17, 226–7, 305; plan of,
208–17; sensory areas of, 215–16,
228–9; see also auditory cortex; visual
cortex; size of, 210; speech areas see
speech centres; see also under individual
headings, e.g. cerebral hemispheres;
hypothalamus
breathing, 81, 166, 295–6
Broca, Paul, 220, 281, 282
Broca's area, 283, 284, 285
Browning, Robert, xiii
Bucy, P., 351–2
bullets through brain, 350–1
Burdenko, N.N., 136
butterflies, 6

Cajal, Ramon, Y., 90
cameras, 10, 11, 12
cancer, 154, 169, 233, 324
Cannon, Walter B., 180
carbon dioxide, in blood, 81–2
carnivores, 15, 18; see also under individual animals
castrati, 202, 297
castration, 196, 207, 297
cataplexy, 125–6
catatonia, 146

catfish, 69
cats, 20, 58, 62, 107, 124–5, 129–30, 137,
147, 174, 184, 196, 204–5, 258–9
cattle, 134
cell membrane, 84–5, 88, 105
central nervous system, 2, 3–4, 180; see
also brain; spinal cord
centre-surround antagonism, 15
cerebellum, 119–20, 209, 213, 215;
damage to, 120–1
cerebral cortex see cortex, cerebral
cerebral hemispheres, 3–4, 119, 120, 135,
184–8, 209; and movement, 121–6;
electrical stimulation of see brain, electrical stimulation of; evolution of,
210–12; left/right, 123–4, 262, 263–4,
280, 281, 282–3, 286–8, 291, 311–23;
reorganization of, 280, 283; short-
circuiting of, 187; see also communication, language; learning; memory;
personality; sensation, meaning of
chaffinches, 308
chameleons, 181
Chaucer, Geoffrey, 243
chemoreceptors, 8, 46, 57, 81–2, 211
chess, 346
chickens, 111, 165–6, 206
chimpanzees, 122, 123, 146, 149, 182–3,
207, 242–3, 271, 272, 288–9
Chinese, 161, 162, 291
Ching, James, 105
cholecystokinin, 102
cholinesterase, 364
Chomsky, Naum, 299
Christianity, 208
chromatophores, 181
cicadas, 34
cilia, 25, 29, 50, 72–3, 364
circadian rhythms, 177–9
Claparède, E., 335
clock, internal, 178–9
cochlea, 34, 35, 39
cochlear nucleus, 261
cockroaches, 299–300
colliculi, 113
colour, 11, 20–1, 252, 253–4
colour-blindness, 20–1
commissures, 214
communication: and learning speech,
278–81; and losing speech, 281–8; and

making sounds of speech, 293–8; and reading/writing, 288–93; by gesture, 267–8, 270–1; by sound, 268; by symbols, 270–2, 273–4, 275; emotions as, 147–8

Conan Doyle, Arthur, xiii

concussion, 336–9

condor, 21

conduction of messages along nerve fibres, 83–9

cones, opitcal, 12

confabulation, 321, 359

congenital non-progressive sensory neuropathy, 157

connection between senses, 262–4, 274–5

consciousness, 142–3, 212

control circuits, 16–17

copulation, 124, 134, 142, 172–3, 174, 181, 196, 205, 206, 246

coronary thrombosis, 154

corpus callosum, 312–19

cortex, cerebral, 131–2, 210, 214, 215–16, 217, 257

Cowles, John T., 272

cranes, 118

creative thinking, 340

crickets, 6

Critchley, Macdonald, 254, 281–2

Cushing, Harvey, 223

cybernetics, 17

Dalle Ore, G., 352

Dax, Gustave, 281–2

Dax, Marc, 281, 282

daydreams see imagination

deaf children, 278–9, 291

deaf-mutes, 271

decibels (dB), 24

deer, 123, 134

defence reaction, 170–2, 180, 181

déjà vu, 235–6

delirium tremens, 344

Dement, W.C., 136

dendrites, 92, 95–6, 302, 304

dental treatment, 325

depression, 102, 150, 231, 232–3

deprived children, 306–7

Descartes, Réné, 213

diabetes insipidus, 203

diabetes mellitus, 203

diaphragm, 296

Dickens, Charles, 235

Diderot, Denis, 251

diet, choosing, 143–5, 177

Dijkgraaf, D., 38

Dimitrijevic, M.R., 301

dogfish, 47

dogs, 32, 112, 125, 138, 167

dolphins, 44–5, 123

dopamine, 100, 102

Doppler effect, 40, 261

Dorset, Earl of, 151

Dostoevsky, F.M., 222, 230–1, 232

douroucouli (South American night ape), 13

drangon-flies, 18

drawing, 318–19

dreaming, 137, 138, 229

drinking, 176–7

drug addiction, 162–3

ducks, 243, 244

dynorphin, 160

dyslexia, 289–90

ears, 9, 24–45; evolution of, 34–5; structure of, 25–7, 28–9, 39; see also hearing

earthworms, 23, 300

eating, 169, 174–7, 187, 351

echo-location, 37–45

eels, 111

efference copy, 119

electric eel, 68

electrical stimulation of brain see brain, electrical stimulation of

electroreceptors, 68

elephants, 35–6, 135, 148–9

Eliot, George, 219

embryo see foetus

emotions: and cataplexy, 125–6; and electrical stimulation of brain, 229–34; and learning, 309–10; and left/right cerebral hemispheres, 263, 320; and speech, 285; as communications, 147–8; physical effects of, 148–51, 181; reactions to, 148; recognition of, 148; reproductive, 146–7; see also

emotions (*cont.*):
  reproductive behaviour; social, 146; *see also under individual emotions*
encephalitis lethargica, 135
endocrine gland, 190
endorphins, 157, 160, 162–3
enkephalins, 160
epilepsy, 35, 173, 221–2, 223, 224, 230–1, 232, 234, 239–40, 315–16, 341
Euler, U.S. von, 99
eunuchs, 201–2, 207; *see also* castrati
excitatory *v.* inhibitory impulses, 93–6, 98, 128
extensor thrust reflex, 117
external ear, 32, 33
exteroceptive receptors, 7
eyelids, 128
eyes, 9, 10–23; and reciprocal innervation, 110; compared to camera, 11–12; lazy, 304; structure of, 10–11, 12, 17; *see also* vision

Fabre, J.H.C., 52
faces, recognition of, 256
fakirs, 116
familiarity *see* recognition, 336
Fantz, R.L., 256
Fawkes, Guy, 161
fear, 147, 151, 170, 171–2, 183, 230, 309
Fechner, G., 60
feedback, 16, 106–7, 119–20, 212, 310–11
field of vision, 17–18, 19, 258
fish, 6, 13, 18, 35, 36–7, 46–7, 52, 68, 69, 73, 111, 211, 302; *see also under individual fish*
fistula, gastric, 149–50
fleeing, 182, 183, 187
flexion reflexes, 114–15, 128–9
flies, 6, 36
flight of birds, 104
flowers, 20, 47–8
focus, 15, 16–17
Foerster, O., 223
foetus, 31, 113–14, 193–4
follicle-stimulating hormone, 190
follitrophin, 200
forebrain *see* frontal lobes
foreign language, 307–8

forgetting, 333; *see also* memory
fovea, 12, 15, 16–17, 21
frequency: of sound, 24–5, 30; of voice, 296–7
Freud, Sigmund, 140, 250, 348
Frisch, K. von, 20, 36, 48, 55, 267
Fritsch, G.T., 222–3
frogs, 35, 97, 111
frontal lobes, 209; damage to, 348–51, 354–9
function of nervous system, 1, 83

Gaddum, J.H., 99
gag reflex, 115
Gage, Phineas, 348–50
Galambos, R., 38
Galen, 179–80
Gall, Franc Josef, 218, 219, 223, 281
gamma-aminobutyric acid (GABA), 98
ganglia, 180
gastric function, 149–51
Gelber, B., 299
gender differences, 193, 195–6, 290
geniculate nucleus, 257
geographical knowledge, 262, 360
geometry, 273, 319, 320
Geschwind, Norman, 274
gesture, language of, 267–8, 270–1, 287
gibbons, 122
gigantism, 199
giraffes, 114
glucose, in blood, 82
gnu, 123
goats, 123
Golgi, Camillo, 90, 91
gonadotrophin-releasing hormone, 190
gonadotrophins, 200
gorillas, 122, 123, 146, 149
graphemes, 290, 291
grasshopper, 196
gravity, 70, 73, 108, 116, 117
Green, Hon. Philip, xiii
Gregory, R.L., 253
Griffin, D.R., 38, 41, 44
Grinnell, A.D., 41
growth/growth hormone, 199–200
guacharo (Peruvian nocturnal bird), 43–4
guilt, 230–1

habituation, 301–2
hairs, and vibration, 25; see also cilia
Hall, Marshall, 107
hallucinations, 142, 166, 225, 229, 230, 238, 321
hamsters, 62, 198
Harlow, J.M., 348–50
Hartline, H.K., 14
Hartridge, H., 38, 105
head injuries, 337–9
hearing 255; and echo-location, 37–45; conduction of sound in, 27–8; damage to, 31; foetal, 31; localization of sound in, 32–3; mechanism of, 26–7, 28–30, 32–3, 34–5, 36–7, 39, 40; of bats, 37–43; stereophonic, 32–3; see also deaf children; deaf-mutes
heart, 106, 154
Heath, R.G., 169, 232–3, 234
Hediger, H., 134–5, 146, 170–1
hemiplegia, 125
herbivores, 18, 134–5; see also under individual animals
Hess, H.R., 164–5, 166, 170, 172, 174
hibernation, 145, 167, 198
hierarchical organization of brain, 167, 359–61
hindbrain, 209
hippocampus, 185, 186, 196, 216, 262, 329, 342, 344, 345
Hippocrates, 208
hippopotami, 128
Hitzig, E., 222–3
hoarding, 177
Hodgkin, A.L., 84
Hogarth, William, 18
Holst, E. von, 110–11, 165–6
homosexuality, 196
Homskaya, E.D., 256
hormones, 82, 141, 173, 189–207; and eating, 145; and meaning of objects, 247; and movement, 124–5; digestive, 184; sex, 174, 179, 190, 193–6, 198, 200–2, 204–7
Horridge, G.A., 299–300
horses, 135, 248
horseshoe crab, 14–15
howler monkey, 295
Hubel, D.H., 303–4

Humboldt, Baron von, 43
humming-birds, 20, 104, 142
humpbacked whale, 45
hunger, 145, 175–6, 187
Huxley, A.F., 84
hypergraphism, 232
hypogonadism, 207
hypothalamus, 82, 135, 164–88, 209, 213, 345, 359, 361

ideograms, 291
imagination, 147, 229; and hormones, 192; see also hallucinations
impotence, 101, 173
imprinting, 200, 244
Infant Hercules syndrome, 198
inflammation, 155–6, 157
inhibitory impulses see exitatory v. inhibitory impulses; social inhibition
innate abilities, 11–12, 121–2, 124–5, 242–8, 249, 268, 300–1
inner ear, 25–6, 35, 70
insects, 47–8; see also under individual insects
instinctive energy, 140–2
intelligence, 250, 277, 302–3, 306–7; and nutrition, 303, 307
intensity of stimulation, 8–9, 64
internal environment, control of, 80–2
internal speech, 124, 256, 269, 322
interoceptive receptors, 7; see also receptors, for inner world
intestines, 70, 155
intra-uterine events, 31

Jackson, Hughlings, 220, 221–2, 230, 234, 235, 239, 274, 360–1
Japanese writing, 291
Joan of Arc, 161
Joints, 79
Jung, Carl, 348
Jurine, Charles, 37

Kandel, E.H., 302
kangaroo rat, 43
Kellogg, W.N., 45
Kerwin, Joseph, 76
kidney stones, 155
Kleitman, N., 136

Klüver, Heinrich, 351–2
knee-jerk, 79–80, 108, 109, 115
knowledge: acquired, 249–61; see also learning; inborn, 242–8; see also innate abilities
Koehler, Otto, 248
Korsakoff's psychosis, 344–5
Kozak, W., 116
Kreidl, A., 73

labyrinths, 18–19
Lack, David, 246
language, 219; learning, 278–81, 297–8, 307–8; loss of, 281–8; making sounds of, 293–8; reading/writing, 288–93
laughter, 125, 126
lazy eye, 304
L-dopa, 102, 344
learning, 299–323; and cerebral hemispheres, 212; and changes in neurons, 301–11; and corpus callosum, 314–19; and emotions, 309–10; and innate abilities, 300–1; and left/right cerebral hemispheres, 311–23; and movement, 122–3; 124; and punishment/reward, 309–11; and stimulation, 302–7; and vision, 11, 250, 251–6, 303–4; at cellular level, 301–3; correct time for, 123, 249–50, 252–4, 255, 303–4, 305–8; language, 278–81, 297–8, 307–8
left/right cerebral hemispheres, 123–4, 262, 263–4, 280, 281, 282–3, 286–8, 291, 311–23
left-handedness, 283, 290
Lennox, W.W., 240
lens of eye, 10–11
leucotomy see mutilation of human brain
Lewes, G.H., 219
lexical address, 291
light see eyes; vision
light, effects on behaviour, 22–3, 197–8
limbic lobe, 185
limbic system, 231
lions, 182
Lissman, H.W., 68
lobes of brain, 214–15
location of stimulation, 8–9, 64–6
Locke, John, 251
Loewi, Otto, 97

Lorenz, Konrad, 140–1, 142, 243, 267
LSD, 232, 367
Luria, A.R., 256
luteinizing hormone, 190
lutrophin, 200

macaque monkey, 206, 288, 351
magnetic field detection, 68–9, 178
marijuana, 232
marsupials, 128
marten, American, 205
maternal behaviour see reproductive behaviour
mathematics, 271, 273; see also arithmetic; geometry
mechanoreceptors, 8, 61–2, 63, 64–6, 152–3
medulla oblongata, 3, 159, 183, 209, 213, 215
melatonin, 197, 198–9
memory, 324–47; and brain mutilation, 342–4; and concussion, 336–9; and electrical stimulation of brain, 238–9, 331–3; and pain, 324–7; and perception/skilled movements, 327–30; and recognition, 334–6, 345; classification in, 340–1; highest level, 330–41; highest level, anatomy of, 341–7; inaccuracy of, 274, 330–1; lower level, 324–7; short-term, 328, 330, 343–4
Menière's disease, 76
mice, 47, 53, 55, 200
midbrain, 209, 367
middle ear, 26–7
migraine, 101, 367
migration, 145, 201
Milner, Brenda, 343–344
Milner, Peter, 167–8
Mishkin, Mortimer, 328
Molyneux, 251
money, 272
Moniz, Edgar, 356–7
monkeys, 53, 130, 148, 149, 175, 242, 258, 271, 288; see also under individual monkeys/apes
Moore, B.C.J., 286
Moreschi, Alessandro, 297
Morgan, Pringle, 289–90

morphine, 159–60, 162–3
mosquitoes, 6, 54
moths, 36, 41–2, 52, 53
motion, detection of, 71, 72, 73, 75–6
motion-sickness, 75, 76
motivation, 140–2
motor areas of brain, 216–17, 226–7, 305
movement, 104–26; and cerebellum, 119–20; and cerebral hemispheres, 121–6; and hormones, 124–5; and learning, 122–3, 124; and nerve messages, 105–6, 242; innate, 121–2, 123; perception of, 15, 21–2; see also motion, detection of; reflex, 106–19; speed of, 104–5
multiple sclerosis, 89, 120
muscle sense, 79
muscle spindles, 77–9, 108
muscles: and pain, 154; and stretch reflexes, 108–9; contraction speed of, 104–5; nerve messages to, 105–6; skeletal, 106
music, 262, 287, 327–8
musical abilities, 287–8
musical notation, 272
mutilation of human brain: and left/right cerebral hemispheres, 315–20; and memory, 342–4; and motor skills, 217; and pain, 153–4, 263; and personality, 325, 354, 357–8; and social inhibition, 357–8; dehumanizing effects of, 342–3, 254, 357; present-day, 358
myelin sheath, 86–8, 89
Myers, R.S., 314

narcolepsy, 138
Neanderthal man, 288
needs, 140–6
Nernst, W., 84
nerve fibres, 2; conduction of messages along, 83–9; transporting substances inside, 103
neural tube, 1–2
neuralgia, post-herpetic, 156
neuroglia, 92
neuromodulators, 100–1
neurons, 2–3, 90–2, 210, 217, 241, 257–9, 302–4; and pain, 157–8, 325–7;

damage to, 101–2; passing messages between, 93–6
neuropeptides, 101
neurotransmitters, 97
nociceptors, 8, 61, 62–4, 153, 156; see also pain
nocturnal animals, 13–14, 32, 43–4; see also under individual animals
noradrenalin, 97, 99, 100, 102, 103, 183, 203, 368
nose, structure of, 48–50
nystagmus, 74–5

oestradiol, 197, 200, 206
oestrogens, 54, 194, 196, 204–5
Olds, J., 167–9
ommatidia, 14–15
opossum, 13
orang-utan, 122, 123
orientation see position detectors; spatial sense
Orlovsky, G.N., 121
otosclerosis, 28
ovaries, 204–5, 207
owl, 32
oxytocin, 202, 203

pain, 7–8, 62–4, 152–63, 263, 306; and analgesia, 158–62; and memory, 324–7; and reflexes, 128–9; central, 155; chronic, 157–8, 160, 326–7; function of, 153, 157; indifference to, 154, 157, 161; referred, 63–4; theories of, 152–3; types of, 63, 154–6; see also nociceptors; torture
painting, 275–6
pallor, facial, 182
paralysis, 112, 125
paramecia, 299
paraplegia, 112
parasympathetic system, 97, 106, 166–7, 180, 181, 183–4
Parkinsonism, 334
Patterson, Margaret, 162
Peking man, 288
Penfield, Wilder, 223, 225, 228, 234, 235–6, 239, 288–9, 331, 341, 342
penguins, 34
Peon, Hernandez, 129–30

peripheral nerves, 2, 83, 180; and pain, 154–5; effects of cutting, 66–7, 80, 156–7; see also receptors
peritonitis, 155
personality, 348–61
perspective, 18
pH of blood, control of, 81
phantom limbs, 153, 265–6, 324–5
pheromones, 51–6; alarm, 52, 56; human, 47, 54; in mother/offspring communication, 47, 54–6; sex, 52–4, 246; territorial, 55
philosophers, 208, 251
phonemes, 290, 291
photoreceptors, 10, 11, 12–13, 14, 15, 23; see also eyes; vision
phrenology, 218–20, 281, 291
Piaget, Jean, 269–70
piano-playing, 105
pigeons, 69
pigs, 54, 227
pineal gland, 22, 197, 198
'pins and needles', 66
pitch of notes, 296–7
pituitary gland, 22, 190, 197, 198, 199, 201, 203–4
plagiarism, 336
play, 122, 123
pleasure centres, 167–8, 169, 184, 232–4
Ploog, O., 268
polyglots, 286
pons, 209, 213
porpoises, 133–4
position detectors, 73
posterior horns, 63, 65
posture, 107, 108, 116–19
prawns, 73
Premack, David, 288–9
progesterone, 194, 195
prolactin, 124, 201, 205
proprioceptors, 7, 77–80
prostaglandin, 99, 156
proteins, 103, 197, 303
psychoanalysis, 348
psychotherapy, 334, 361
puberty, 54, 196, 198, 199, 200–2, 297
pupil, 17
Purkinye cell, 91–2

quantitative theory of pain, 152, 153

r.e.m. sleep, 136, 137–8
rabbits, 173–4, 248
rage see aggression; anger
Rank, Otto, 31
rats, 53–4, 59, 143–4, 145, 167–8, 190–1, 195, 201, 206, 207, 248, 300, 302–3, 311
Rauwolfia, 102
reading/writing, 288–93, 316–17, 319
receptors, 5–9, 61; cutaneous, 60–9; for inner world, 70–82; gustatory, 6, 57–9; light, 10–23; olfactory, 46–56; sound, 24–45; see also sense organs
reciprocal innervation, 110
recognition, 256, 334–6, 345
reflexes, 79–80, 106–19; above spinal chord, 113–15; and posture, 107, 108, 116–19; changes in, 115–16; flexion reflexes, 114–15, 128–9; for standing, 116–19; in babies, 109–10, 113–14; of spinal chord, 111–12, 116; stretch reflexes, 108–9, 117; see also under individual reflexes
re-learning, 334
releasing mechanisms, 141
religiosity, 232
reproductive behaviour, 146, 190–2, 195, 197–8, 201, 243–4, 247
reptiles, 23, 211; see also under individual reptiles
reserpine, 102
reticular formation, 132–3, 210
retina, 10, 11, 12, 14–15, 21–2
Reynolds, D.V., 158–9
Richter, C.P., 143, 144
robins, 246–7
rods, optical, 12, 13, 21
Roeder, K.D., 41–2
Rolls, E.T., 258, 328
Romans, 186
Russell, Ritchie, 338

saccule, 34, 71, 72, 73
salivary glands, 181, 184
salt, craving for, 144
saltiness, 58–9
scent-marking, 55, 112

schizophrenics, 102, 169, 234
Schwann cells, 92
Scoville, W.B., 343
scratch reflex, 115
sea-lions, 44
Sei Shonagon, Lady, 288
selection of sensory input, 127-31
self: concept of, 264, 321; perception of, 264-6, 321
semicircular canals, 71, 72, 74, 76
Senden, M. von, 252
senility, brain deterioration in, 359-60
sensation, meaning of, 241-66
sense organs, 2, 5-9, 210-12; see also under individual organs
sensitive periods see learning, correct time for
sensitization, 302
sensory deprivation, 305-6
septal region, 168, 169, 232-4
serotonin, 100, 103
servo-mechanism, 16-17, 106-7, 370
Severin, F.V., 121
sex hormones see hormones, sex
sexual behaviour, 52-4, 172-4, 179, 195, 196, 204-5, 233, 351; see also copulation
Shakespeare, William, 207
sharks, 47
sheep, 134
Sherrington, Sir Charles, 110
Shik, M.L., 121
shingles, 156
shivering, 166
short-term memory, 328, 330, 343-4
shrews, 14, 205
sign-stimuli, 242-8
silkworms, 53
singing, 295, 296-7
single-celled organisms, 10
skin, 60-9, 154-5
skunk, 51
sleep, 132, 133-9; and dreaming, 137, 138; disorders of, 135-6, 138; length of, 134, 135; phases of, 136-8; waking from 135, 138-9
sleep paralysis, 138
sleep-walkers, 137
smell, sense of, 6-7, 41, 46-56, 319; and

brain, 210-11; and pheromones, 51-6; mechanism of, 50-1
snakes, 35, 47, 67, 111
social inhibition, 349, 357-8, 359-61
social needs, 146, 306-7
social rank, 206
somatostatin, 102
soul, 208, 213
sound, 24-5, 30; conduction of, 27-8
sour taste, 58
Spallanzani, Lazzaro, 37, 38
spatial sense, 262-3, 265, 273, 319
speech, 267-98; see also communication; internal speech; language
speech centres, 264, 283-4; damage to, 275-6, 280, 281, 282, 283, 285-7, 291
speed of nerve impulses, 86-8
spelling, 290
Spencer, Herbert, 220
Spencer, Stanley, 346
Sperry, R.W., 312, 319, 321
spiders, 6, 141, 245
spinal cord, 1-2, 3, 63, 79-80, 83, 111, 324; effects of severing, 111-12, 116
squint, 9
squirrel monkey, 268
squirrels, 122
St Martin, Alexis, 149
stammering, 290
standing, 116-19
statocyst, 72-3
stereophonic hearing, 32-3
stereoscopic vision, 18-20
steroids, 197, 203
stimulation, need for, 147, 302-3, 306-7
stimulus-specific theory of pain, 152-3
stomach, 155, 176
strange experiences, 234-9
stress, 176, 199, 203-4, 206; see also pain
stretch reflexes, 108-9, 117
strokes, 275-6, 280, 285-6, 287, 292-3
structure of nervous system, 1-4; see also brain; nerve fibres; receptors
submission, 244
sucking, 177
sunbirds, 20
supplementary motor area, 216-17
suprachiasmatic nucleus, 179
surround inhibition, 66

sweat glands, 83
sweet taste, 58
swift, 135
swimming, 122
symbolic reasoning, 274
symbols, 269–75; as shorthand, 270–2, 274–5
symmetry bilateral, 213–14
sympathetic system, 106, 166, 179–84
synapses, 93–6, 180; chemical transmitters at, 96–102
synaptic gap, 93–4, 95, 98
syphilis, 80

tactile placing reaction, 110
Tailarach, J., 227
talopoin monkeys, 206
target cells, 196–7
taste, sense of, 57–9
tectorial membrane, 29
teeth, 65, 154, 325–6
television, 277
temper, losing, 187
temperature control, 80–1, 166
temporal lobes, 216, 225, 231–2, 258, 261, 263, 346, 351, 359
tension, physical/pschological, 79, 133
termites, 68–9
territorial behaviour, 170, 188
Terzian, H., 352
testes, 204, 205
testosterone, 54, 125, 200–1, 205, 206, 207, 371
thalamus, 257, 361, 371
thermoreceptors, 8, 62, 67–8, 80–1, 105
thinking, 275–8; and left/right cerebral hemispheres, 322–3; auditory, 276; creative, 340; influences on, 277; olfactory, 276; symbolic, 274; see also symbols; visual, 275–6
third eye, 23
thirst, 176–7
Thorpe, W.H., 22, 308
thyroid gland, 190, 204
thyroid-releasing hormone, 190
tick, 5
tickling, 153
tics, 158
Tinbergen, N., 243, 248

tissue culture, 301–2
toads, 52, 58, 111
Tolstoy, Count Leo, 263
torture, 138
touch, sense of, 60–9; and left/right cerebral hemisphere, 317–18; electroreceptors, 68; magnetic field detection, 68–9; mechanoreceptors, 61–2, 63, 64–6, 152–3; nociceptors, 61, 62–4, 153, 156; thermoreceptors, 62, 67–8, 80–1;
tracking, 106–7, 120
Treat, A.E., 41–2
Trevor-Roper, P.D., 254–5
trophic activity, 103
tuatara, 23
tumours, 198, 201; see also cancer
Turner, Joseph M.W., 11
tympanic membrane, 26, 28
tyrosin, 101

Uexküll, J. von, 243
ulcers, 149
uncus, 343
urination, 55, 112, 125, 148, 149, 167
utricle, 71, 72, 73–4

vacuum activities, 141–2
Van Gogh, Vincent, 32
varicosities, 100, 180
vasoactive intestinal peptide (VIP), 101
vasopressin, 202–3
verbal memory, 345–6
vertebrates, early, 1, 34
vertigo, 75, 221, 293
vestibule, 70–6
vibration, perception of, 8, 25, 34
vipers, 67
viscera, sensations from, 64, 70, 153, 155
vision, 7; and learning, 11, 250, 251–6, 303–4; and left/right cerebral hemispheres, 312–15; and orientation in space, 71, 75; colour 20–1; field of 17–18, 19, 258; mechanism of 14–17, 257–9; movement, 21–2; nocturnal, 13–14; stereoscopic, 18–20;
visual cortex, 257–61
visual memory, 346

vocal apparatus, 294–7
voices, hearing, 298

walking, 117–18
Wallace, J.G., 253
wasps, 6, 246
Weber, E.H., 60, 311
Weber-Fechner law, 60
Webster, Douglas, 43
Wernicke, C., 282
Wernicke's area, 283, 284, 285
Westerman, R., 116
Wever, R., 178
whales, 45, 210
Wiener, Norbert, 17
Wiesel, T.N., 303–4

Williams, J.G., 340–1
Wilson, E.O., 56
Wolfe, John B., 272
Wolff, H.G., 149
Wolff, S., 149
wolves, 170
writing *see* reading/writing

Yerkes, R.M., 146, 182, 272, 300, 309
yoga, 116

Zen Buddhist monks, 161
zoos, 146, 147

Index compiled by Peva Keane